Diversity and Visual Impairment

The Influence of Race, Gender, Religion, and Ethnicity on the Individual

**Madeline Milian
and Jane N. Erin, Editors**

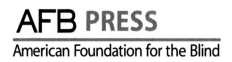

AFB PRESS

American Foundation for the Blind

Printed in the United States of America
2008 printing

Library of Congress Cataloging-in-Publication Data
The American Foundation for the Blind (AFB)—the organization to which
Diversity and visual impairment : the influence of race, gender, religion,
and ethnicity on the individual / Madeline Milian and Jane N. Erin, editors.
     p. cm.
     Includes bibliographical references and index.
     ISBN 978-0-89128-383-6 (alk. paper)
     1. Visually handicapped—United States—Social
conditions. 2. Blind—United States—Social conditions. 3. Minority
handicapped—United States—Social conditions. 4. Blind women—
United States—Social conditions. I. Milian, Madeline. II. Erin, Jane N.

HV1795 .D58 2001
305.9´08161—dc21   2001022263

AFB—the organization to which Helen Keller devoted her life—is a national nonprofit devoted to expanding the possibilities of the 10 million Americans who are blind or visually impaired.

Cover: *Eagle Man* by Michael A. Naranjo, 1994, Bronze, 14 × 7 × 15 inches. Photo by Mary C. Fredenburgh.

To the memory of my immigrant parents.

M. M.

To my parents,
John and Elizabeth Newton,
who taught me to value diversity
and to honor humanity.

J. N. E.

Contents

Acknowledgments

There are many people who made this project a reality and deserve our recognition and gratitude. The authors of individual chapters were approached with the difficult task of writing about a topic that has hardly been explored in the field of blindness. They enthusiastically accepted the challenge and developed chapters that will become the first ever written on the topic. We are grateful that they joined us in writing this book.

Many individuals with visual impairments and their family members shared their experiences and opinions with the authors of the chapters to make this work a true representation of diverse voices. Without their stories, many of the chapters would have depended solely on published scholarly material and would have lacked the important connection to people's lives. We are grateful that they perceived this project to be a vehicle in which their experiences and opinions could be shared with a general audience.

Bill Morrison and Eva Kenny, doctoral students at the University of Northern Colorado, spent many hours in the library locating resources to facilitate our work. We sincerely thank them for their efforts and support.

Stan Luger patiently read many of the chapters and provided an outsider's perspective on the content and writing style. His suggestions assisted in keeping many of the chapters free of the type of professional jargon that often interferes with understanding. We appreciate his encouragement and willingness to help.

Three anonymous readers provided lengthy and thoughtful suggestions that improved the quality and clarity of our work. Their recommendations were immensely helpful to all the authors and to the editors. We thank them for their insightful contributions to our work.

Natalie Hilzen, editor-in-chief of AFB Press, was always patient, wise, and enthusiastic. The challenge of integrating multiple perspectives into a coherent book often seemed insurmountable. Without Natalie's belief in the importance of our project, we could not have made our concept a reality.

—M. M. and J. N. E.

Foreword

Education in the United States today is characterized by national, state, and local reforms aimed at improving outcomes for *all* students. Recently, these efforts have been expanded to include a specific focus on ensuring that individuals with disabilities have access to the same quality of education that is provided to their nondisabled peers so they are ultimately prepared to live independently, pursue postsecondary education, make a successful transition into the labor force, and be fully integrated into our communities. Despite standards-based reforms, there continues to be a significant gap between outcomes for individuals with special needs (such as students with disabilities, those from low-income backgrounds, students of color, and students for whom English is not their first language) and their middle-class, majority-group peers. A contributing factor is that educators and policymakers have essentially ignored the country's changing demography and the increasing diversity of American society. In too many instances, programs and services address disability-related needs but are inconsistent with the individual's racial, linguistic, cultural, socioeconomic, and other background characteristics. As a result, the very programs designed to improve outcomes for individuals with disabilities become part of the problem, not the solution.

As we grapple with the complex issue of how to best serve multicultural populations with special needs, we typically turn to the literature to find answers, or at least direction. However, the preponderance of available books and articles on diversity focus on individuals without disabilities or on individuals with mild disabilities. Very little is written about diversity among low-incidence populations. The literature is virtually silent on the topic of diversity and visual impairment. Madeline Milian and Jane N. Erin take us a giant step forward by addressing this void. They go beyond the traditional focus on the interaction among disabilities and language and culture to address such other important topics as race, gender, religion, and sexual orientation. The contributors offer excellent discussions of how all of these factors influence the life experiences of individuals with visual impairments. They also offer superb recommendations for serving individuals who experience "multiple jeopardies" as a result of the combination of their disability and their race, gender, religion, and/or ethnicity.

Perhaps the most important message in *Diversity and Visual Impairment: The Influence of Race, Gender, Religion, and Ethnicity on the Individual* is also the simplest one: A visual impairment does not define the individual. People with visual impairments will be in a better position to contribute to their communities when members of the society at large view their abilities and interests as more important than their disability. To that end, increasing the participation of individuals with visual impairments in education, labor, and community activities is key to engendering positive viewpoints of people with disabilities. However, given the changing demography, the goal of increased participation can be best met only if programs and services that serve individuals with disabilities reflect multicultural perspectives.

In programs that incorporate multiculturalism, individuals with visual impairments see themselves, their contemporary life experiences, language, culture, norms, and values, reflected in the programs and services in which they are involved and in the texts and related materials that support their education and training. Programs with pluralistic views guard against stereotyping by continuously reinforcing that there is as much diversity within as across groups.

Meeting the needs of individuals with visual impairments requires high-quality, intensive professional development to ensure that all personnel have the skills and knowledge to work with diverse groups. The goal of such training should be to ensure that service providers understand that diversity is a reality, that multiple world views are a reflection of that diversity, and that differences do not equate with deviance or incompetence. The diversity of students and clients requires that professionals demonstrate cultural competence. Culturally competent professionals understand and value their own identities, are able to interact successfully cross-culturally, and can assist in developing programs and services that are responsive to the particular needs of their clients. Moreover, professionals who themselves accept, respect, and value diversity contribute in important ways to reducing prejudices that serve to limit the potential and status of individuals with disabilities.

The readers of *Diversity and Visual Impairment* will be enriched not only by the discussions of the multiple factors that shape our identities, but also by the voices of diverse individuals with visual impairments that are heard throughout the book. The text provides valuable insights and practical suggestions about how to create a culturally responsive service delivery system for individuals with disabilities. It is an excellent reference for all educators and other service providers who work with special populations.

Alba A. Ortiz
President's Chair for Education Academic Excellence
Professor, Department of Special Education
Director, Office of Bilingual Education
University of Texas, Austin

About the Contributors

Madeline Milian, Ed.D., is Associate Professor at the University of Northern Colorado, College of Education, School for the Study of Teaching and Teacher Education, in Greeley. She is the author of numerous articles, chapters, monographs, and reports focusing especially on bilingual education and the education of students with limited English proficiency who are visually impaired. Dr. Milian is the recipient of the 1996–97 College of Education Service Award and the 1995 Outstanding Dissertation of the Year Award from the International Council for Exceptional Children, Division on Visual Handicaps, among others.

Jane N. Erin, Ph.D., is Associate Professor and Director of Programs in Visual Impairment in the Department of Special Education, Rehabilitation, and School Psychology at the University of Arizona at Tucson. She served as editor-in-chief of the *Journal of Visual Impairment & Blindness* from 1998–2001 and is a former executive editor of *RE:view*. Her writing and research interests are in the education of students with visual and multiple disabilities, braille reading, and parent and family issues related to visual impairment. She co-authored *Visual Handicaps and Learning*, and has written numerous articles, chapters, and presentations. Dr. Erin previously held presidencies of state or local chapters of the Association for Education and Rehabilitation of the Blind and Visually Impaired (AER) and the Council for Exceptional Children in Arizona and Texas, and she is the recipient of the 2000 Margaret Bluhm Award and the 1996 Mary K. Bauman Award for contributions to education in visual impairment, both from AER.

Eugene Bender, M.A., is a vocational rehabilitation counselor for the Office of Vocational and Educational Services for Individuals with Disabilities, New York State Education Department, White Plains.

Virginia Bishop, Ph.D., is Adjunct Professor at the University of Texas at Austin, at Texas Tech University in Lubbock, and at Stephen F. Austin University in Nacogdoches. Her previous publications include *Teaching Visually Impaired Children,* as well as many articles and book chapters. She is the recipient of the 1996 Berthold Lowenfeld Award from the Association for Education and Rehabilitation of the Blind and Visually Impaired.

Lila Cabbil, M.S., is Supervisior of Occupational Information and Children's Services at Upshaw Institute for the Blind in Detroit, Michigan.

Paula Conroy, Ed.D., is a teacher of students with visual impairments and orientation and mobility specialist at the Boulder Valley Public Schools in Boulder, Colorado, and has published in the *Journal of Visual Impairment & Blindness.*

Vivian I. Correa, Ph.D., is Professor in the Department of Special Education, College of Education, University of Florida at Gainesville, and holds the 2000–2001 Matthew J. Guglielmo Endowed Chair in Mental Retardation at California State University, Los Angeles. Dr. Correra is the co-author of *Interactive Teaming: Enhancing Programs for Students with Special Needs,* has published numerous book chapters and articles, and was co-editor of *Teacher Education and Special Education.* She has been involved in many research projects in the areas of early childhood and special education.

Kay A. Ferrell, Ph.D., is Assistant Dean of the College of Education, University of Northern Colorado in Greeley. She is the author of *Reach Out and Teach: Meeting the Training Needs of Parents of Visually and Multiply Handicapped Young Children* and has published extensively on the development and education of infants and young children who are visually impaired. Dr. Ferrell is the recipient of the Distinguished Service Award from the Council for Exceptional Children, Division on Visual Impairment and the Alumni Award for Research in Special Education from Teachers College, Columbia University.

Moniqueka E. Gold, Ed.D., is Assistant Professor of Education at Austin Peay State University in Clarksville, Tennessee.

Patrika Griego, M.A., is a teacher of a first-grade inclusion class at Valencia Elementary School in Los Lunas, New Mexico, and a doctoral candidate at the University of Northern Colorado.

Carol Yumiko Love, Ph.D., is a teacher of students with visual impairments and an orientation and mobility specialist at the St. Vrain Valley School District in Greeley, Colorado. She has published in the *Journal of Visual Impairment & Blindness (JVIB)*, has presented papers at a variety of conferences, and is a peer reviewer for *JVIB* and *RE:view.*

L. Penny Rosenblum, Ph.D., is Adjunct Assistant Professor in the Department of Special Education, Rehabilitation, and School Psychology at the University of Arizona in Tucson. She is co-author of *Finding Wheels: A Curriculum for Nondrivers with Visual Impairments for Gaining Control of Transportation Needs.* Dr. Rosenblum has published various articles in the *Journal of Visual Impairment & Blindness* and has presented papers at a variety of conferences.

Sandra Ruconich, Ed.D., is a teacher at Utah Schools for the Deaf and Blind in Ogden; Assistant Professor in the Department of

Special Education of the University of Northern Colorado in Greeley; and Adjunct Faculty Member in the Department of Special Education at the University of Utah, in Salt Lake City. She is president of the Utah chapter and past president of the Kentucky chapter of the Association for Education and Rehabilitation of the Blind and Visually Impaired.

Katherine Standish Schneider, Ph.D., is Senior Psychologist and Coordinator of Training at the University of Wisconsin at Eau Claire Counseling Services.

Irene Topor, Ph.D., is Adjunct Associate Professor at the University of Arizona in Tucson, and an allied health professional at the Children's Rehabilitative Services of the Arizona State Health System for Children. She has written a number of chapters, including several on vision assessment and intervention with infants and children.

James Warnke, M.A., M.S.W., is a psychotherapist in private practice, a consultant in blindness and visual impairment, Priest Associate at St. Paul's Church in Englewood, New Jersey, and Retreat Leader and Spiritual Director in the Upper Room ministry. Mr. Warnke is former chairperson of the Psycho-Social Division of the International Association for the Education and Rehabilitation of the Blind and past-president of the New York Milton H. Erickson Society for Psychotherapy.

Introduction

Many professionals in special education and rehabilitation can remember taking a university course that introduced them to experiences related to visual impairments. These courses often require students to read autobiographies, do volunteer work, and listen to presentations by people who are blind or visually impaired. Typically, an introductory course in visual impairments urges students to consider how everyday experiences, such as eating in a restaurant, negotiating familiar and unfamiliar settings, establishing and maintaining social interactions, and applying for a job, are different when a person has a visual impairment. In essence, the focus is on how low vision or blindness shape the human experience.

However, there is a risk in presenting blindness or visual impairment as the major influence on personal experiences. Too much emphasis on visual impairment may result in the disregard of the other variables that shape human behavior. This book is intended to remind readers that human behavior is a product of a multitude of factors and that a visual impairment may not necessarily be the dominant one. Other personal characteristics, such as gender, race, culture, religious beliefs about disability, or an individual's social status within a given society, are also powerful forces that articulate the human experience. These variations are interwoven with a visual impairment to produce unique experiences and to influence social perceptions about low vision and blindness. A central theme of this book is that a visual impairment affects a person's lifestyle, but does not create it.

It is our hope that this book, which introduces an area of study that is in its infancy in our field, will encourage readers to consider the multiple dimensions of their own identities and hence to appreciate the forces that have shaped their clients, students, and colleagues. The book is directed to those who have professional contacts with people who are blind or have low vision, whether new or experienced; however, it may also be useful to people with visual impairments, their family members, and others who want to understand the complex patterns of human diversity. We hope that it will add a new understanding to the ways in which readers view the individual differences that form personality and interpret disability.

We selected authors who can speak from experience as well as from a scholarly perspective. Thus, readers will not only learn about research and resources related to each topic, but will hear the voices of personal experience. The authors of many of the chapters on race and ethnicity have written from their own experience as members of minority cultures in the United States, and each author has included the voices of individuals with visual impairments who are members of the ethnic and racial minorities, religions, or gender groups under discussion and who were interviewed for this book. Some chapters were written by authors who are visually impaired, who used their own experiences, in addition to those of others, to describe the interaction of visual impairment and the other characteristics that define their personalities and perceptions of disability.

DIVERSITY AND VISUAL IMPAIRMENT

In Part I, the editors expand on the overall themes of the book. In Chapter 1, Erin addresses society's perceptions of disability and visual impairment and ways of altering negative stereotypes. Milian continues the exploration of diversity in Chapter 2, considering the multiple dimensions that contribute to an individual's self-identity and how these characteristics affect the work of professionals with individuals who are blind or visually impaired. The subsequent sections examine three major factors in creating individual identity: race and ethnicity, religion, and gender.

ETHNIC AND RACIAL DIVERSITY

In explorations of human variations that can influence perceptions of disabilities and adaptation to a disability, ethnicity and race play a central role in understanding students and clients who are blind or visually impaired. No person exists as one thing at a time; instead, each individual's reality is intricately created by all the attributes that define the person. Of these factors, ethnicity and race are probably the most influential in an individual's development of a cultural understanding and a group's development of a group identity. Therefore, teachers and rehabilitation professionals need to understand the values and traditions of an ethnic or racial group to be able to help interpret the behaviors, perceptions, and reactions of individual students and clients to the educational and rehabilitation process.

The United States is a highly diverse country. Consequently, the selection of which groups to examine as part of a discussion on ethnicity and race is always difficult. The groups that were selected for discussion in Part II—African Americans (Chapter 3), Asian Americans and Pacific Islanders (Chapter 4), Latinos (Chapter 5), and Native Americans (Chapter 6)—are four of the largest demographic groups in the country and ones that vision professionals are most likely to encounter in their work. Although there is great diversity among Americans of European background, the cultures of the various European American ethnic groups are more likely to be similar to the mainstream American culture—if there can be said to be such a thing—and thus familiar to most professionals.

In struggling to determine which groups to include, the editors decided that the aim of a discussion of ethnicity and race is to provide a framework for acquiring sensitivity to the beliefs, values, and mores of another culture that teachers and rehabili-

tation professionals can follow when they encounter other diverse groups, and we believe that the authors of these chapters
have done so. The chapters included in this section emphasize
the demographics, history, health, perceptions of disabilities,
and cultural values of the selected groups. Ultimately, teachers
and rehabilitation professionals face the challenge of discover-
ing how three sets of values—their own, those of the system in
which they work, and those of their students or clients—can interact in a positive and empowering coalition.

RELIGIOUS VARIATIONS
AND VISUAL IMPAIRMENT

Planning the section on religion and visual impairments presented unique challenges to us. In contrast to most other variations described in this book, religious beliefs may be chosen by
an individual. Religious preferences are highly personal and are
not visible to others. In addition, religious considerations are not
included in the job roles of most professionals in the field of visual impairment. Furthermore, because federal law requires the
separation of religion and the state, public schools and agencies
do not directly address this issue.

Ultimately, the decision to include this section on religion was
driven by these factors. Although knowledge of religions may
not be necessary to the professional role, personal belief systems
clearly influence the lives of visually impaired people just as they
do the lives of others. Many blind people describe the importance of religious beliefs and values during their adjustment to
blindness. Families of some visually impaired children pray for
their children's vision to be restored, and others interpret their
parenting role as being a part of a divine choice or plan. Regardless of their beliefs, it is vital that professionals understand and
respect the importance of religion for many of their students and
clients. In some cases, religious beliefs and ethnic backgrounds
are parallel, and awareness of an individual's religion can enhance understanding of that person's community and culture.

The two chapters in this section represent two different aspects of the religious experience. Chapter 7 describes the religious communities and value systems of people with visual impairments. In this chapter, readers will hear voices from a wide variety of religious backgrounds describing the meaning of religion for them, especially as it supports their experiences with visual impairment.

Chapter 8 focuses on various religious communities, providing suggestions for professionals and others who want to facilitate the participation of blind and visually impaired individuals in them. It reminds professionals that many of the practical adaptations that can be made in the school or work setting can easily be accomplished within a religious community. A lack of knowledge about how best to meet the needs of a visually impaired member of a congregation may be the primary barrier to religious inclusion.

This section is offered to encourage readers to consider the importance of a personal belief system and how it connects with the experience of visual impairment. For many people, religious beliefs are instrumental in forming their personal identities. Professionals who acknowledge this influence can be more effective in supporting people to reach their chosen goals.

GENDER, SEXUAL ORIENTATION, AND VISUAL IMPAIRMENT

In any discussion of human behavior, the topic of gender is certain to unearth strong opinions about the influences of biology and environment. Although people have different views about the nature-nurture conflict, few disagree that gender is a powerful force in forming human experiences. It shapes people's behavior, communication, socialization, and long-term partnerships.

Views about the influence of gender have changed from generation to generation. In the late 1940s and the 1950s, following World War II, the United States saw a return to traditional gender roles, with more women becoming homemakers and men returning from the armed forces to enter the workforce. By the 1970s more women began to work outside the home, and the social view of gender reflected strong environmental influences on women's roles, with the result that many people believed that gender roles were completely a result of learning and environment. The 1990s saw a new acknowledgment of innate differences between the sexes, with an emphasis on the equal importance of different characteristics.

The understanding of gender roles is now broadening to include the experiences of gay men and lesbians, who were rarely considered a social force in the past. Religious communities, businesses, and political decision makers must consider the existence of same-sex unions and the fact that primary relationships can be homosexual as well as heterosexual. The nature-nurture debate is active with respect to the experiences of gay and lesbian people, and biological influences on homosexuality have recently been acknowledged.

For all people—with and without visual impairments—the achievement of the best quality of life must include the opportunity to be secure with their gender identities. When a person is visually impaired, that opportunity can be curtailed by social expectations related to gender roles and behavior. In many communities, gender roles are defined by appearance; clothing and hairstyles, short-term fads, and subtle variations in accessories can affect gender identity as others perceive it. Information about appearance is less available to the blind or visually impaired person who cannot observe others or monitor her or his own appearance. In addition, the assumption that the individual is dependent can neutralize the perception of gender identity by others.

In Part IV, readers will hear the voices of many people with visual impairments—women (Chapter 9); men (Chapter 10); and gays, lesbians, and bisexuals (Chapter 11)—as they describe how they worked to develop identities related to gender and sexual preference. They are not always easy stories to read: girls who saw themselves as socially separate and boys who were denied access to the sports culture because of their blindness had to work harder to become secure with their roles. Visually impaired people who are gay or lesbian face the additional stress of dealing with the implications of homosexuality in the general society, as well as of interpreting their visual impairments to gay or lesbians friends and partners.

Few people will read this section without reflecting on their own gender identities and how they became comfortable with the persons they are. That is our intent. In understanding the complex forces that shape one's own identity as male and female, one is more open to consider the experiences of others. We are confident that readers will connect the stories from the men and women that follow with their own experiences, reinforcing the idea that gender identity is a complex and important influence on the quality of one's life.

PROFESSIONAL PRACTICES AND DIVERSITY

Part V focuses on two areas that will provide practical information to both practitioners and university personnel. Chapter 12 discusses language diversity, which then leads to the topic of providing services to individuals who speak languages other than English. Although the topic is complex and probably deserves an entire book, this chapter introduces readers to some of the main areas of concern when working with this population. The chapter ends with two case studies that illustrate how two teachers managed to incorporate students who were learning English into their caseloads.

Chapter 13 should be useful to teacher educators and rehabilitation professionals at the university level and to others who provide training in professional development for two reasons. First, it provides a rationale for supporting and encouraging cross-cultural competence in the field of blindness and visual impairment so that professional practices become more culturally responsive to the students and clients who receive services.

Clearly, many university programs, school districts, and agencies have already achieved this goal. However, since the needs of communities vary according to changes in population, this chapter may be a starting point to those who are beginning to develop programs that will meet the communities' needs. Second, the chapter presents a list of competencies that will assist university programs and staff development personnel in designing new courses or including multicultural competencies within existing courses or in-service training programs. It is our hope that these two chapters will serve as a foundation for professionals who want to include the topic of diversity in their teaching.

Perhaps the most important messages of this book are the recommendations for professionals. Although no person can walk in another's shoes, a professional can take steps to travel in harmony with a student or client who knows a different lifestyle. The first and most important step is to show respect for the route that others have already traveled. The experiences presented in this book are an important reminder that people are resilient; they use what they have learned in past journeys as they move into the future. People of all backgrounds and beliefs can incorporate visual impairments into their life experiences, and they can use their own experiences to become competent as visually impaired individuals. Professionals who can reshape their skills to meet individual situations will be effective in supporting this change.

PART I

Diversity and Visual Impairment

Individual and Societal Responses to Diversity and Visual Impairment

Jane N. Erin

Marian is going to a party with several friends who are faculty members at the university where she teaches. Because she has been blind all her life, she knows that there will be some awkward moments when she is introduced to new people at the party. It will be up to her to put out her hand so that others will know that it is appropriate to shake the hand of a blind person, and she may have to enter some conversations without being sure whether she is welcome. As a young African American woman who teaches at a college where most faculty and students are Anglo, she occasionally wonders whether new acquaintances seem uncomfortable interacting with her because of her blindness, race, or faculty status or because she is new to the university.

When Marian was younger, she used to try to separate people's responses to her different characteristics. Now these characteristics do not seem to matter as much to her: She has learned that she has some visible differences from many others in social situations, but she has also learned that she can break down communication barriers by taking the initiative in communicating with others and putting them at ease. Although she knows that some people will have stereotyped ideas about blind people or African Americans, she tries to dissolve these stereotypes by presenting herself as a person with interests, abilities, and opinions. Furthermore, she has learned that being different has some advantages: People notice her, and she has the opportunity to make a memorable first impression. Occasionally, she feels frustrated that she must exert extra effort every time she is in a new situation, and she wonders how much her experience is different from that of other newcomers in social situations.

Marian's story is fictitious, but it reflects the experiences of many people who have several characteristics that are different from most others with whom they associate. Marian has become comfortable with the responses of others even though she may not know the reason why they behave as they do toward her. She understands that the immediate responses of others to a new acquaintance are often subconscious and are based on a variety of factors, including appearance, speech patterns, and movement. When two people have continuing contact, however, their responses to one another become more complex. Qualities, such as communication styles, introversion and extroversion, and shared experiences, influence their reactions toward each other.

This chapter examines variations in how human beings respond to differences in others. The nature of human differences and the origin of stereotypical thinking are described as the bases for a discussion of social responses that invites readers to consider their own ways of responding to human differences. These patterns are applied to visual impairment, which has some distinctive characteristics when compared to other disabilities. The chapter concludes with a discussion of attitudinal changes, with the hope that professionals can demonstrate positive attitudes toward individuals with all differences, including visual impairment. As the anchor chapter of the book, this chapter is intended to stimulate readers to consider how they shape attitudes toward human differences.

STEREOTYPE, STIGMA, AND HUMAN DIFFERENCES

Stereotypical thinking evolves with the mind's innocent attempts to cope with differences. All people are creatures of routine, and they learn from childhood through repeated experiences that help to form mental constructions of concepts and ideas. Human beings categorize their experiences because doing so helps them make sense of an otherwise random and complex world. In organizing ideas into categories, however, people magnify the importance of characteristics that are common to all members of a group (Schmelkin, 1988). A stereotype is the assumption that people have characteristics because they belong to a specific group, regardless of whether the characteristics are desirable or undesirable. Stereotyped responses can be positive or negative, overt or unconscious.

When new information is encountered, an individual can interpret it only in the context of what he or she already knows. A sighted woman imagines that blindness must impose helplessness and frustration because these are what she experiences when she searches for a candle in the dark during a power outage. A Caucasian man assumes that Hispanic people are not intelligent because his grandmother had a Mexican housekeeper who could not read. The generalization of a single characteristic to an entire group of people represents stereotypical thinking. If an individual has limited contact with a group of people, the stereotype is strengthened even if the person knows of only one or two members of the group with a specific characteristic.

Overgeneralizations about groups of people usually describe undesirable characteristics, which are known as stigmas. Stigmas allow people to feel in control, to resolve the threat of the unfamiliar, and to strengthen their own identities and status. Negative stereotypes about racial or ethnic groups, gays or lesbians, or women reinforce beliefs about ability or status by representing the stigmatized individual as less important or less powerful than others.

Stigma associated with disability is more complex, however, because it may not appear to be negative and is often demonstrated through socially acceptable or altruistic responses. Responses by nondisabled people, such as more assistance than the person wants or needs or being too solicitous, may appear to be altruistic when they actually mediate the nondisabled person's efforts to deal with discomfort and anxiety. Makas's (1988) study of disabled and nondisabled individuals' perceptions of "positive attitudes" toward disability found that the nondisabled respondents thought their positive attitudes reflect "a desire to be nice, helpful, and ultimately place the disabled person in a needy situation" (p. 58), whereas the disabled respondents thought that positive attitudes promoted the rights of people with disabilities.

People who are involved in charitable or altruistic efforts may have motivations in addition to helping others. They may want to draw attention to themselves or to present an image of themselves as kind and considerate. In discussing the motivation of individuals who undertake altruistic efforts for self-serving reasons, Longmore (1997, p. 135) said this about the cultural dilemma of public fund-raising activities such as telethons: "Telethon donation is a collective rite designed to enable Americans to demonstrate to themselves that they still belong to a moral community, that they have not succumbed to materialism, that they are givers who fulfill their obligations to their neighbors." Although such practices as telethons benefit both givers and receivers, they reinforce simplistic and stereotypical views of people whose only common characteristic may be a similar disabling condition.

Like people with disabilities, women may experience stereotyped generalizations that appear to be positive but actually have an elusive, negative impact. The assumptions that women are kind, gentle, dependent, and nurturing may appear to be complimentary in a social context, but they can be the root of women's limited opportunities for leadership and economic independence.

In contrast, the responses to other stigmatized groups in American society are clearly negative. Members of cultural and religious minorities and people who are gay or lesbian may encounter overt or hidden negative assumptions by others about their abilities, personalities, and lifestyles. Inappropriate assumptions about people with disabilities may not be noticed because they reflect socially acceptable behaviors such as giving assistance, speaking of a disabled person with excessive affection, or protecting disabled people from the responsibility of work. Negative and positive stereotypes are different in form and function, but they both erode opportunities for people to be viewed as individuals.

SOCIAL RESPONSES TO DIFFERENCES

Although stigma, or negative stereotype, is an undesirable generalization, it originates from a normal psychological struggle to resolve the unexpected and unfamiliar. To improve stereotypical attitudes toward differences such as visual impairment, it is important to understand what causes these attitudes. Stereotypical thinking is tangled in early experience and assumptions about others that can be modified only by altering later experiences. Thus, true attitudinal changes take place not from a single contact or the acquisition of new information, but only after people are given the opportunity to test and rethink their original assumptions.

Research has identified variations in the way nondisabled people react to specific disabilities, although these findings have not been consistent across studies. Stovall and Sedlacek (1981) found that undergraduate college students in one eastern college reacted more positively to the idea of social interaction with students who were blind than with those who had physical disabilities; however, they were more negative about engaging in academic interactions, such as study groups, with students who were blind. Yuker (1988) reported similar findings, indicating that nondisabled persons had stronger positive attitudes toward blind people in social situations, more moderate attitudes in "service" situations like interactions between professionals and clients, and more negative attitudes in employment situations than they did toward people with other types of disabilities. Teachers who worked with students with disabilities viewed students with physical disabilities as the most desirable to teach, followed by those with sensory disabilities (including blindness), those with mental retardation, and those with behavioral and social disorders (Hannah, 1988). This finding reflects the tendency to be more favorable about disabilities that are beyond the control of the person who experiences them.

Several factors—familiarity, perceptions of competence, socioeconomic status, and physical status and appearance—influence the degree and nature of stereotypical thinking. Each factor is described here in the context of attitudes toward disabilities, especially visual impairment.

Familiarity

When nondisabled people encounter others with disabilities, they generally feel uncomfortable—a finding that has been widely reported in the literature on social responses to disability. Their discomfort is manifest in such physiological changes as variations in voice stress, physiological arousal, and decreased eye contact (Makas, 1993). This discomfort generally decreases as people have greater contact with individuals with the same disabilities.

However, most nondisabled people rarely encounter people with specific disabilities, and hence their levels of discomfort do not naturally decrease. A few meet people who are blind in their schools or workplaces, but the majority encounter them only briefly, perhaps while passing on the street, waiting at a bus stop, or attending a religious service. Because of this limited contact, they tend to overgeneralize the characteristics of the blind individuals they do encounter. For example, if they meet a blind person who talks excessively, is below average in intelligence, or is highly dependent, they may assume that this characteristic is directly connected with blindness because they do not know any other blind person. In contrast, they would not draw such casual conclusions if they met a nondisabled person who was talkative, had low intelligence, or was dependent. The rarity of blindness alone leads them to the conclusion that all other characteristics of a blind person must be connected to blindness.

The discomfort caused by lack of familiarity may be one reason why many people choose to affiliate with people whose characteristics are similar to their own, that is, to form homogenous groups. When they do so, they may perpetuate the stereotypical thinking of others about people who are different from themselves. Preston (1994, p. 203) stated that many deaf parents want to have children who are deaf, because deafness is normal in a household in which both parents are deaf, and "there is tension around any variation from the norm." Fichten, Robillard, and Judd (1989) found that students with physical and visual disabilities had the same stereotyped beliefs about individuals with a disability other than their own as did nondisabled individuals.

Perceptions of Competence

A second factor that influences people's responses to differences is their perception of competence, according to the established standards of the majority culture. In the United States, value is placed on intelligence, and individuals who do not meet the standard of expected intelligence are often viewed negatively. Although the term *mental retardation* is perceived as undesirable, to the point that some professionals no longer use it, the term *giftedness* has undergone no such censure because it represents competence in a society that values intelligence and achievement. In addition, competence in the United States is strongly associated with health and physical intactness, independence, and proficiency in communication.

Attitudes toward the competence of people with disabilities are frequently subjected to the same overgeneralization that is evident in other forms of stereotypical thinking. When a disability affects competence in one area, the individual may be assumed to be incompetent in all ways. The common tendency to treat those with disabilities as childlike or to assume that they cannot make their own decisions is one example; other examples include the assumptions that someone who cannot walk needs assistance preparing food or that a person who is blind cannot make financial decisions, even though there may be no functional relationship between the disability and the task. This type of overgeneralization distances individuals from comfortable social interaction with others. Although some people with severe disabilities cannot reason well enough to make their own life decisions, most people who have disabilities can make their own life choices, even though their means of communicating or gaining information may vary. A disability may affect competence in one area but not *general* competence.

When an individual has an exceptional competence in one area, it may serve to offset stigma related to his or her other characteristics. This concept, known as "competency/deviancy" theory (Gold, 1975), states that special abilities or talents increase tolerance of other differences that are typically perceived negatively. Albert Einstein's wild hairstyle or eccentric social behaviors were tolerated because of his genius as a scientist, and the manneristic rocking of some people with mental retardation and blindness is accepted when these people have special musical or mathematical abilities. Competencies, as defined by the majority culture, have a strong influence on how persons with disabilities are perceived. Through overgeneralizations related to function, an individual's abilities can be greatly exaggerated or diminished.

Socioeconomic Status

Socioeconomic status both influences and is influenced by the presence of a difference. A stigmatized individual is often automatically assigned a lower social status. Longmore (1997) pointed out the similarities between race and disability, stating that both function as the "bottom marker" of social status for those who are searching for some measurement of their own relative status to others. He drew from the writings of James Baldwin to support the idea that stigmas associated with being both disabled and African American allow others to feel socially elevated. As he noted, "disability has implicitly been offered as a replacement for race. People with disabilities are ritually presented as the new mudsill, the bottom of the social ladder below whom 'we' must never allow ourselves to fall" (p. 154). Longmore presented as primary evidence the telethons and fundraising activities that emphasize the dependence and neediness of people with disabilities.

Murphy (1995), a university professor who began to use a wheelchair as an adult, described a variety of status changes that he experienced after the onset of his physical disability. He noted that "lower-status" people in his world showed a new connection with him. For instance, his students tended to reinforce their sense of closeness, and an African American campus policeman, who had ignored him when he was able bodied, began to greet him regularly. In contrast, some "higher-status" people unconsciously distanced themselves from him. For example, a dentist patted Murphy on the head, and physicians expressed surprise when they were told that he had a full-time job. Murphy stated that a notable feature of responses to people with disabilities is the "withdrawal of deference" that is usually accorded to those who are perceived to have higher social status in this society. Because the symbols of this deference are subtle and often nonverbal, they are almost imperceptible until they are withdrawn.

The result of membership in a stigmatized group is frequently reduced economic status. Both people with disabilities and those from other stigmatized groups experience discrimination in the employment market, but there are differences in how stigma affects economic status. People who are members of cultural minorities may experience ongoing economic difficulties because of the lack of opportunity and social discrimination to which their groups have been subjected for generations. In contrast, people with disabilities may experience the combined effects of discrimination, functional limitations, and lack of appropriate training. These factors may result in lower earning power than other family members and a decrease in their families' economic status for the next generation.

Physical Status and Appearance

Social expectations of physical normalcy and physical attractiveness are important influences on how others respond to persons with disabilities. Although cultures vary in their emphasis on physical normalcy, most have ranges of values that define typical appearance and features that are exceptionally attractive or unattractive. In relation to appearance, people with disabilities may experience different degrees of stigma in different cultural groups. Furthermore, expectations and resultant stigmas may be different for women than for men.

With respect to visual impairment, the role of physical attractiveness and social acceptance has not been thoroughly explored. The social separation experienced by some adolescents with visual impairments may be closely connected to their inability to monitor their physical appearance or to adhere to relatively narrow standards of physical attractiveness valued by the adolescent culture, and physical appearance is a critical variable in determining everyone's first impressions, whether by teachers, prospective employers, or social acquaintances.

Deviation from conventional physical appearance can create a negative impression, especially when the observer believes that the other individual should be able to improve his or her physical appearance. Thus, although nondisabled people may think a person who is blind has little or no control over differences in the appearance of eyes, facial expressions, or posture, they may view wearing unkempt clothing, being overweight, or being poorly groomed as controllable and therefore more negative.

The visibility of a disabling condition may also play a part in the reactions of others. A number of studies have noted that individuals with more severe and obvious disabilities may experience less rejection than those who have milder or less-visible disabilities (French, 1994a). Individuals whose disabilities are not apparent may be more greatly misunderstood by the general public, may need to explain their own abilities to others more carefully, or may be faced with choosing whether to explain their functional differences to every new person they meet. For example, people with low vision may be perceived as seeing well in some instances and as functionally limited in others, and must decide when and whether to describe their conditions or to request adaptations.

In some ways, the experiences of people with less severe, less-obvious disabilities are similar to the experiences of people whose cultural backgrounds, religious affiliations, or gender preferences do not fit into easily defined categories. A multiracial person in a racially segregated environment, a person from a mixed religious background, or a transvestite who is heterosexual may have difficulty forming an identity as part of a subgroup when his or her membership in that subgroup is based on a characteristic that only partially defines the individual's experience.

MANAGING STEREOTYPING RESPONSES

Stereotypical thinking represents a simplistic attempt to explain variations among human beings. People who have uncommon characteristics can deal with such unidimensional thinking more successfully if they understand the function it serves and the factors that influence it. There are several possible types of responses to stereotyped social expectations:

Reinforcement. A person who is the target of stereotyped expectations may reinforce the stereotype by becoming what the public expects him or her to be. If people around the person believe the stereotype, they may unconsciously reinforce behaviors that reflect their thinking, thereby encouraging the individual to behave according to the stereotype. The passive blind child who behaves helplessly, the Hispanic student who makes no effort to achieve academically, or the gay man who behaves effeminately may respond in these ways because they have been influenced by the expectations of others.

Opposition. The individual may rebel against the stereotype by making an extraordinary effort to contradict it. A blind person who refuses to use a cane, a woman who is excessively assertive and uncompromising, and a Japanese American student who refuses to apply herself in school may be taking control of their identities by actively refuting stereotypical social expectations.

Integration. An individual may manage the stereotype on the basis of its origin and function. For instance, a man who is blind may realize that the stereotype of helplessness originates from an exaggerated perception of the amount of assistance needed by people who are blind. He is aware that people who are blind do need assistance with some tasks that could be done more independently by sighted people, and he is skilled in requesting the specific type of assistance he needs, in monitoring the type of assistance provided, and in reciprocating in socially appropriate ways. He manages the stereotype by understanding its roots and by developing abilities that do not magnify it inappropriately.

People who are affected by stereotypical attitudes can benefit from the opportunity to discuss and implement strategies for managing inappropriate responses related to stereotypical thinking. Professionals who work with individuals with disabilities can encourage them to discuss the roots of stereotyped thinking and ways of shaping new responses from others. Opportunities to role-play effective responses, to discuss ways of breaking down stereotyped thinking with others who share similar experiences, and to analyze the effects of one's behaviors can be useful to individuals who feel that they are being compartmentalized because of a personal characteristic. Chapter 13 presents specific strategies that professionals may use to help people who are blind or visually impaired become more comfortable in approaching issues related to human differences, and methods for attempting to change attitudes in the society at large are discussed later in this chapter.

HISTORY OF SOCIAL RESPONSES TO VISUAL IMPAIRMENT

Social attitudes toward differences among individuals at different times and places reflect economic changes and variations in religious teachings, political trends, and cultural values. This section briefly describes the history of social attitudes toward visual impairment. It should be noted that the discussion does not take into account the wide variations in social responses to disability that have existed in every period of history.

Responses to blindness have varied widely among cultural groups at different periods and at different socioeconomic levels. Nevertheless, trends in these responses have been notable over time. Changes in social perspectives can be viewed as a spiral that is variable within a period but broadens over time as changes take place in values, media, technology, and medical techniques. Tuttle and Tuttle's (1996) model of historical change, adapted from a model originally proposed by Lowenfeld (1975), describes historical changes in five periods that reflect varying societal perspectives on visual impairment: separation, protection, self-emancipation, education, and assimilation.

Separation

The first period was characterized by separation of people who were blind or visually impaired in many preliterate cultures. In subsistence cultures, disabilities were commonly regarded as undesirable, mainly because it was believed that people with disabilities could not contribute to the economic support of a community. In Sparta, blind babies were left to die in the mountains, and Athenians abandoned disabled infants in clay pots by the roadside. Some groups, such as the Serbian Wends, killed elderly members when they could no longer contribute to the support of the community (Koestler, 1976).

Protection

The second period, protection, began in Western cultures with the spread of Judaism and, later, Christianity. A dominant belief during this period was that citizens should assist and support dependent members, and for this reason the emphasis was on the physical care of blind people. Thus, church-supported institutions, which sometimes housed blind persons with people who had a variety of other disabilities, including mental illness, were often established. These institutions were charitable rather than rehabilitative, and their existence implied that blind people were incapable of contributing to society.

Religious communities also perpetuated some long-standing stereotypes about people who were blind. The concept that blindness is connected with a behavior of an individual or his or her family reflects a simplistic attempt to explain something that is often unexplainable, but it was reflected in religious books, such as the New Testament, which presents examples of blindness denoting helplessness, foolishness, pitifulness, and sinfulness (Monbeck, 1973).

In societies that responded protectively, some of the responsibility for support of blind citizens was eventually shifted to city or national governments. The first state-supported institution for blind citizens was established in Paris in 1254 to house 300 Crusaders who were blinded by the Turkish sultan during the political conflicts of the Seventh Crusade.

Although protectiveness was the predominant philosophy between A.D. 500 and 1600, it was by no means universal. The Egyptians viewed blindness as a treatable condition and developed medical treatments for the eyes. Many Eastern cultures began to identify work roles for their blind members (Koestler, 1976). There are undoubtedly countless other examples of constructive approaches toward integrating blind people into specific cultures that were not recorded before reading and writing were common.

Self-Emancipation

The third period, self-emancipation, emerged during the 17th and 18th centuries. Recognition that blind people could be employed and could contribute to society emerged early in China, Korea, and Japan, where traditional jobs for blind workers were identified as early as 200 B.C. (Vaughan, 1998). In these countries, blind people were often fortune-tellers, musicians, masseurs, and storytellers. In China and other eastern countries, work roles were supported by the establishment of guilds of blind people that created standards for professions and trained new workers in the skills they would need to be employed (Vaughan, 1998).

In European countries, some individual blind people achieved success in professions like music (Friedrich Dulon), law (Nicholas Bacon), and mathematics (John Gough) (Tuttle & Tuttle, 1996). Their success was due to their own initiatives, rather than to any formal educational or career opportunities, and they were exceptional. At that time, the typical blind person received no education and either resided in an institution or remained at home, assisting with household tasks.

Education

The fourth period, education, began in the West with the establishment of the Institute for the Blind in Paris by Valentin Haüy in 1784, followed by additional schools for blind children throughout the Western world. Although these schools were generally viewed as offering opportunities for blind students to learn, the disadvantages of separate placement were recognized from the beginning of formal education, and some insightful individuals envisioned a day when there would be other educational options.

One such individual was Johann Wilhelm Klein, an Austrian educator who recommended in 1845 that the education of blind children should be "transplanted into the families and into the local schools" and questioned the existing system: "Why should [blind children] be removed from their homes and placed in costly institutions that accommodate scarcely the sixtieth part of those who are in need of an education?" Klein (1845/1981, p. 165) questioned. He proposed that teachers be sent for training to the schools for the blind and then returned to their communities to teach groups of blind children.

During this period, there was further movement toward government-based services, rather than only services supported by churches or charitable agencies. This issue was discussed at the Vienna Congress of Teachers of the Blind in 1873, where a resolution was passed to recommend that governments assume responsibility for building schools for young children who were blind (Lowenfeld, 1981). In the United States, governmental responsibility for schools for blind children was evident in that the majority of these schools were operated by states' welfare authorities (Koestler, 1976). The increasing availability of education for some blind students eventually led to the movement toward equal participation of blind people in society—the fifth period.

Assimilation

In the 20th century in the United States, people who were visually impaired and their advocates worked to achieve integration and social equality—the goal of the final period, assimilation. Today, most American students with visual impairments are educated in their own communities, and all states now support rehabilitation and vocational preparation that fosters the entry of adults who are visually impaired into the job market. Federal legislation, such as the Americans with Disabilities Act of 1990, has brought issues of equality to the attention of the public.

Perhaps one impetus for the move toward more inclusive approaches in rehabilitation was Scott's (1967) *The Making of Blind Men.* In this book, Scott described the paternalism and control that were perpetuated by some agencies on people who were blind and increased the awareness of consumers of these agencies' services and professionals about the risks of separate services, such as patronizing approaches or encouragement of dependency. Strong consumer organizations, such as the American Council of the Blind, the National Federation of the Blind, and the National Association for Parents of Children with Visual Impairments, as well as organizations of professionals who are visually impaired, have advocated for more consumer-driven rehabilitation systems.

The periods of historical change just described tend to reflect the views of Western cultures. Because economics and social changes drive services to visually impaired individuals, elements of all five trends can be found today in different parts of the world. China, for example, established jobs and social roles for blind people earlier than most other countries, but the autonomy of blind workers was threatened under the Cultural Revolution of the 1960s and 1970s. Modern China has continued to develop programs for people with disabilities, with the goal of promoting the economic interests of the country (Vaughan, 1998). In a Mexican village described by Gwaltney (1970), social protection was still evident in the 1960s. Because blind people were thought to be protected by God, begging was an acceptable occupation for blind villagers, and children were expected to lead blind members of the community when these people wanted to travel.

Although the laws of many countries now recognize the rights of people with visual impairments to full access to those societies as citizens, true assimilation has yet to be achieved. Unemployment rates for blind people continue to be significantly higher than those of the general population. New technologies have created different standards for all workers, providing the tools of access to visually impaired people but creating a more competitive, rapid-production workplace for all employees. Access in social and leisure activities is still far from a reality, but more and more individuals in more areas of the world are coming to believe that people with visual impairments are entitled to full participation in society.

VISUAL IMPAIRMENT AND OTHER STATUS VARIABLES

People who live in a media-dominated society, such as the United States, often assume the mindset of the majority culture.

Given the variations in cultures, socioeconomic levels, and religious beliefs in the United States and throughout the world, however, this expectation is simplistic. Although the spiral of trends in attitudes toward visual impairment has become broader over time, it encompasses more persons than in the past, and understanding individual responses to visual impairment is more complex. This section discusses current views of visual impairment in the context of other factors and characteristics that affect individuals' statuses in a society.

Because people with visual impairments are as diverse as any other cross section of individuals, they encounter the same wide variety of responses to themselves as would anyone else. However, the people they meet may attempt to reconstruct their other characteristics—race, ethnicity, physical appearance, gender, values, and spiritual beliefs—according to stereotypes. That is, for people who are unaccustomed to visual impairment, that characteristic may appear to be the critical one, and their stereotypes about blindness may override the influences of individual variations that are more familiar to them. For example, people may believe that a woman is submissive because of her blindness, not because of her acculturation, or that a man is angry because of his visual impairment, not because his father taught him that behavior. People who are visually impaired face an additional challenge in both integrating the multiple influences on their self-identities and insulating their identities from the public assumption that visual impairment is their predominant characteristic.

In the past, it was often assumed that there was a connection between a family's behavior and the birth of a child with a disability. When people became blind as adults, it was assumed that they were somehow responsible for their blindness. Although this belief is less common in literate cultures, it is still widely held in some contemporary cultures, often self-contained cultures that are seeking explanations for seemingly inexplicable occurrences.

Comparisons with Other Stigmatized Groups

People with disabilities and others who are affected by stigma share some common experiences. All are vulnerable to other people's stereotypical thinking about them that is based on lack of experience and misinformation. Most stigmatized groups, including cultural and ethnic minorities, women, disabled individuals, and gays and lesbians, may be economically disadvantaged by their status. This disadvantage may be compounded when a person from such a group has more than one characteristic that is viewed stereotypically. For example, French (1994) described the barriers to appropriate medical and social services experienced by many disabled individuals from minority groups. She also noted that it is often presumed that members of particular ethnic groups are more likely to have particular disabilities, such as mental illness.

The effects of stereotypical thinking about people with visual impairments are different from those about other groups, however. One difference, previously mentioned, is the apparent social acceptability of certain responses toward people with visual impairments, which makes it more difficult to identify or to object to stereotypical responses from others. Another difference is the fact that, in contrast with most other stigmatizing conditions, people can acquire disabilities, including visual impairments, at any point in their lives. Thus, people with disabilities may find themselves struggling with conflicts in their own beliefs about disability that were formed before they were members of the affected group.

The support provided by families to disabled people and members of other stigmatized groups also varies. Whereas people from religious and ethnic minorities are typically members of families who have similar characteristics, the family members of people with disabilities and those who are gay or lesbian usually are not. Being atypical within one's family means that there are no adult relatives who can describe their own experiences with the particular status, so the individual must search outside the family for such connections.

Comparisons with Other Disabling Conditions

Grouping individuals into broad categories may reinforce stereotyped perceptions of the group and may minimize variations within groups. Frequently, people with disabilities are described as if disability is their most defining feature, without regard to their diverse lifestyles, cultural and family backgrounds, talents, and interests and the functional implications of their disability. Perhaps their only common experience is the misunderstanding by nondisabled individuals and social institutions.

The assumption of a common ground among disabled individuals can have an impact on the delivery of services. The "dual schools" operated in some states for students who are deaf or hearing impaired and those who are blind or visually impaired are examples of such categorical thinking. Although the motivation for such schools may be economic efficiency, the combination defies logic. Blind and deaf students have disabilities that require widely disparate adaptations, and they are more different in their educational needs than any randomly selected group of disabled or nondisabled students could be. Yet the assumption that "sensory impairment" implies shared needs has motivated many states to cluster services for students who need different educational adaptations.

The common assumption that people with disabilities have more positive attitudes toward people with other disabilities is not supported by research. Ravaud, Beaufils, and Paicheler (1987) reported less agreement among students with disabilities than among nondisabled students about the attributes of others with disabilities. Fitchen, Robillard, Judd, and Amsel (1988) reported studies that both validated and refuted this concept. They believed that methodological differences in studies accounted for this variation, but noted that "the students are caught between adopting the prevailing views of the majority and adopting the civil rights movement's ideology" (p. 180). The fact that many people with disabilities had a negative view of disabled individuals may also reflect the unconscious internalization of stereotypes in juxtaposition with a belief in one's own uniqueness and departure from the stereotype.

Blindness and visual impairment have connotations for society as a whole that make them more feared and yet more respected than other disabilities. These stereotypes tend to magnify an individual's abilities, so that an average student is viewed as brilliant if he or she is blind or a willing worker who is blind is seen as dedicated and remarkable for simply doing the job.

The historical advocacy of visually impaired individuals for their own needs has often separated them from other groups of disabled people. Tax deductions; preferential legislation such as the Randolph-Sheppard and the Wagner O'Day acts; and commissions for the blind in some states have provided stronger support for individuals with visual impairments than is provided to those with other disabilities. This separation reinforces the idea that visual impairment is different from other disabling conditions. Although this idea may result in better services, it may also reinforce the stereotype that people who are blind or visually impaired are somehow homogeneous. Visually impaired individuals have their own distinctive needs, but they also share a common cause with those who have other disabilities—the need to break down the solid barrier of stigma.

Multiple Stigmatizing Characteristics

Responses to individuals who have several stigmatized characteristics may reflect both overlapping and conflicting perspectives. When a person has several status characteristics, such as membership in a minority ethnic group, homosexuality, or a disability, his or her social status will vary, depending on the combination of characteristics. Landrine, Klonoff, Alcaraz, Scott, and

Wilkins (1995) described this situation as "multiple jeopardy"; that is, high status in more than one area results in increased advantage, whereas low status in two or more areas results in increased disadvantage. Since disability is considered a low variable by society as a whole, the combination of having a disability and being female, a member of a racial minority, or a lesbian may increase the negative effects of the other characteristic, whereas the combination of having both high- and low-status characteristics may tend to cancel each other out.

The greater the number of uncommon characteristics a person has, the less likely the person is to be discriminated against on the basis of any one of them. For a blind person who is a member of any other group that typically experiences discrimination, this likelihood makes it difficult to connect discrimination to a single status variable. Perhaps this is partly due to the conflicts presented for an individual who has stereotypical concepts about a variety of status variables. Will the person assume, for example, that an African American man who is blind is helpless because of his blindness, or is aggressive and violent on the basis of the racial stereotype of black men? Ironically, the simultaneous presence of both negative and positive stereotypes can dissolve the impact of the stereotypes because to resolve the conflicting assumptions, others are forced to regard the person who is their target as unique.

For a person who is marked by several low-status variables, the most liberating response may be to attempt to reshape social assumptions to create a new identity that is based on his or her differences. Thomson (1997) discussed such a "reassimilated identity" in the central character of Lorde's (1982) book, *Zami: A New Spelling of My Name*. Zami is an overweight African American woman with a visual impairment, whose "extraordinary body disqualifies her from the restrictions and benefits of conventional womanhood, freeing her to create an identity that incorporates a body distinguished by its markings—some painfully inflicted, some congenital—of her individual and cultural history" (p. 241). Thomson noted that this change in perspective has only recently become possible, with new political forces that recognize the value of differences. For those who can appreciate the changing paradigm, an individual like Zami, who embodies a number of uncommon traits, becomes a celebration of diversity.

CHANGING ATTITUDES TOWARD VISUAL IMPAIRMENT

Although stereotypical thinking is a strong mode of control, it can be altered. The first step in changing inaccurate and stereotypical perceptions is to provide information. Because the root of stereotypical thinking is the overgeneralization of a characteristic to a group of individuals, changing that thinking involves introducing more accurate information as well as making the reactor aware of his or her stereotyped perspective. The mass media, with their ability to control information, can be a powerful source of attitudinal change.

The Media

The print and broadcast media have both perpetuated and dissolved stereotypical concepts about disability. Films about blindness that were made between 1920 and 1950 generally presented one-dimensional perspectives on blindness or visual impairment: Blind characters were portrayed as either evil or as the epitome of perfection or saintliness, and the films' resolution was usually restoration of sight. More recent films have presented blind characters who are more realistic and multidimensional. However, blind characters still tend to be included primarily to represent an image of blindness. One example is the film, *Scent of a Woman,* the story of an embittered military man who became blind in adulthood. Despite the many accolades it received, the film presents a dilemma to people who are blind and their advocates. The main character is rigid and harsh, and so is his response to blindness. Viewers who are unfamiliar with blindness may assume that anger is typical of blind people, rather than a characteristic of one man's behavior.

The message that blindness or visual impairment is incidental and ordinary has not been widely communicated in films, and most visually impaired characters are depicted because they are blind or visually impaired. The message of normalcy will be conveyed only when films include characters whose blindness or visual impairments are secondary and who participate in telling stories that are not about their impairments.

Paradoxically, journalists and television broadcasters often perpetuate a stereotype merely by deciding to feature stories that focus on people who are blind or visually impaired. Most newspapers include such stories because the persons described in them have done something that is perceived as remarkable or have been victims of a crime. Although these are also the focuses of many newspaper articles about nondisabled individuals, readers may overgeneralize the images of superhero or victim when blindness is unfamiliar to them.

There have been improvements in the media's recent attempts to depict disability realistically. Accurate descriptions of an individual's abilities with balanced attention to the implications of disability can educate the public, and the mention of blindness or a visual impairment as secondary to the main purpose of the story can present it as just one characteristic. Some journalists and broadcasters adhere to the concept of "person first" language, identifying the disability only after the noun that names the person—for example, "the schoolteacher who is blind," rather than "the blind schoolteacher." However, the question of whether the creation of rules about language will defuse or reinforce a stereotype has not been resolved. Journalists and broadcasters, like the general public, are caught between the use of lengthy phrases like "persons who are blind" and the use of the more natural phrase, "blind people." There is no evidence that restructuring language alters attitudes, and journalists and broadcasters continue to use words that they believe will attract public attention to their stories.

The mass media can have a powerful effect on attitudes toward disability. Journalists and broadcasters can help to dissolve stereotypical thinking about people with disabilities by following these principles:

- A news story should provide factual information that is based on the experiences of real people with disabilities and their individual variations. An accurate description of the disability should be included in the text and should not comprise an entire headline.
- Any advocacy efforts should include individuals with the disability themselves, not just people who support or contribute to the efforts.
- Individuals with disabilities should be depicted in visible roles in the media, including television and radio broadcasting. The talents of reporters, such as National Public Radio's John Hockenberry who uses a wheelchair, or Deborah Kent, a journalist who is blind, convey a strong message about the capabilities of people with disabilities.
- An individual with a disability should not be described as representing the entire population of people with that disability. In most cases, such phrases as "the blind" or "the deaf" should be avoided because they erroneously imply that all people with that disability have a common experience.

Contact with Disabled Individuals

Although images portrayed in the mass media are powerful, they are distant from real experience. Having direct contact with individuals who have disabilities is a stronger influence on people's long-term attitudes, both positive and negative. Although it is often assumed that such direct contact naturally promotes more positive attitudes, research suggests that this is not always the case (Horne, 1988; Makas, 1993). Even though frequent contact with individuals who have disabilities decreases people's discomfort, it does not ensure that nondisabled people will develop positive attitudes toward these individuals.

Increased contact with people who have a particular characteristic does not ensure positive attitudes, but long-term contact, paired with accurate information, is generally an effective catalyst for change. Makas (1993) emphasized that people developed positive attitudes toward individuals with disabilities when increased contact was paired with a variety of other conditions, including status, pleasantness of interaction, intimacy, and length of the relationship. Horne (1988) cited studies that described both negative and positive attitudes that resulted from contact under various conditions. When contact was paired with the provision of information in these studies, positive attitudes occurred more frequently, although not universally.

Changes in attitude have been facilitated by the movement toward the greater inclusion of people with diverse characteristics in education, recreation, employment, and community activities that has allowed the public to have increased contact with them. In addition, information is more readily available to the general public about the causes of disabilities, which can reduce misunderstanding, and about ways to interact appropriately with people who have disabilitites, which can increase the comfort level of interactions.

Accurate Information

Along with more positive images in the media and greater positive contact with individuals with disabilities, the more widespread availability of accurate information can influence the public's attitudes toward disabilities. Efforts need to be made to replace false information with accurate representations of the causes and impact of disabilities. Folklore is filled with false information about disabilities, much of it family and cultural beliefs that are unconsciously assimilated during childhood. Wagner-Lampl and Oliver (1994) mentioned a variety of false beliefs about the causes of blindness, including excessive crying, sleeping with wet hair, practicing witchcraft, and wearing rubber boots at the wrong time or place. These beliefs are often communicated to young children by their families, and they may have a subtle but powerful impact on adults' responses to disabilities. Because such beliefs are often unconscious and long standing, changing them requires regular exposure to new information. Only information about the nature and effects of disabilities will allow people to think of them as common characteristics of people, not phenomena that are caused by an individual's behavior.

Formal Efforts to Change Attitudes

To be successful, such formal efforts should do the following:

- Include planned opportunities for several periods of contact over time and encourage active participation and response by those whose attitudes are being affected.
- Allow participants to meet people who share a common characteristic (such as a visual impairment) but who have broad individual variations. Include the experiences of people with various degrees of vision, occupations, ethnic backgrounds, and ages.
- Describe differences in individual functioning; for example, why some people choose to use canes or dog guides and others do not.
- Describe ways to facilitate interactions with people who are blind or visually impaired and have the participants practice them. These ways can include discussions of appropriate and inappropriate terminology; strategies for offering assistance, when appropriate; and resources for additional information on individual variations among people with visual impairments.
- Limit simulations of blindness or visual impairments to

short periods and have the participants perform a task that they can accomplish successfully. Wrapping a small package, opening a jar or bottle, sorting silverware, or tying shoelaces are examples of familiar tasks that will reinforce the role of tactile learning. Activities, such as walking around in unfamiliar areas, are likely to leave participants anxious and overwhelmed and hence to reinforce the idea that blindness is terrifying.

◆ Identify the benefits to a society of the inclusion of people with disabilities and acknowledge their individual variations, including the economic and social implications.

DE-EMPHASIZING DISABILITY

Although stereotypical thinking is still a dominant force in the formation of social attitudes, there is evidence that people can move beyond it toward greater understanding and acknowledgment of individual variations. Negative or inaccurate attitudes about people who are blind or visually impaired can be dissolved by providing accurate information that emphasizes individual variations and de-emphasizes the influence of blindness or visual impairment as a status variable. Perhaps the most important factor in attitudinal change is the increasing social participation of capable blind and visually impaired individuals who can communicate their experiences in performing the tasks of daily life.

The purpose of this book is to provide an expanded view of how individual variations, such as culture, gender, religion, and language, shape the separate personalities of people who are blind or visually impaired, just as they do for people without disabilities. The rich experiences gained by a society that values differences are a clear benefit. People with disabilities, including those with visual impairments, have greater freedom to contribute to their communities when others view their abilities and interests as more important than their disabilities.

REFERENCES

Fichten, C., Robillard, K., Judd, D., & Amsel, R. (1988). Students with physical disabilities in higher education: Attitudes and beliefs that affect integration. In H. Yuker (Ed.), *Attitudes toward persons with disabilities.* (pp. 171–186). New York: Springer.

Fichten, C., Robillard, K., Judd, D., & Amsel, R. (1989). College students with disabilities: Myths and realities. *Rehabilitation Psychology, 3,* 243–257.

French, S. (1994a). Dimensions of disability and impairment. In S. French (Ed.), *On equal terms: Working with disabled people* (pp. 17–34). London: Butterworth-Heinemann.

French, S. (1994b). Working with disabled people from minority ethnic groups. In S. French (Ed.), *On equal terms: Working with disabled people* (pp. 176–189). London: Butterworth-Heinemann.

Gold, M. (1975). Vocational training. In M. Gold, *Marc Gold: Did I say that? Articles and commentary on the try another way system* (pp. 167–174). Champaign, IL: Research Press.

Gwaltney, J. (1970). *The thrice shy.* New York: Columbia University Press.

Hannah, M. (1988). Teacher attitudes toward children with disabilities: An ecological analysis. In H. Yuker, (Ed.), *Attitudes toward persons with disabilities* (pp. 154–170). New York: Springer.

Horne, M. (1988). Modifying peer attitudes toward the handicapped: Procedures and research issues. In H. Yuker, (Ed.), *Attitudes toward persons with disabilities* (pp. 203–222). New York: Springer.

Klein, J. W. (1981). Guide to provide for blind children the necessary education in the schools of their home communities and in the circle of their families. In B. Lowenfeld, *Berthold Lowenfeld on blindness and blind people: Selected papers by Berthold Lowenfeld.* New York: American Foundation for the Blind. (Original work published 1845.)

Koestler, F. (1976). *The unseen minority: A social history of blindness in the United States.* New York: American Foundation for the Blind.

Landrine, H., Klonoff, E., Alcaraz, R., Scott, J., & Wilkins, P. (1995). Multiple variables in discrimination. In B. Lott & D. Maluso (Eds.), *The social psychology of interpersonal discrimination* (pp. 183–223). New York: Guilford Press.

Longmore, P. (1997). Conspicuous contribution and American cultural dilemmas: Telethon rituals of cleansing and renewal. In D. Mitchell & S. Snyder (Eds.), *The body and physical difference* (pp. 134–158). Ann Arbor: University of Michigan Press.

Lorde, A. (1982). *Zami: A new spelling of my name.* Trumansburg, NY: Crossing Press.

Lowenfeld, B. (1975). *The changing status of the blind from separation to integration.* Springfield, IL: Charles C Thomas.

Lowenfeld, B. (1981). 100 years ago: The Vienna Congress of teachers of the blind. In B. Lowenfeld, *Berthold Lowenfeld on blindness and blind people: Selected papers by Berthold Lowenfeld* (pp. 169–179). New York: American Foundation for the Blind.

Makas, E. (1988). Positive attitudes toward disabled people: Disabled and nondisabled persons' perspectives. *Journal of Social Issues, 44,* 49–61.

Makas, E. (1993). Getting in touch: The relationship between contact with and attitudes toward people with disabilities. In M. Nagler (Ed.), *Perspectives on disability* (pp. 121–136). Palo Alto, CA: Health Markets Research.

Monbeck, M. (1973). *The meaning of blindness: Attitudes toward blindness and blind people.* Bloomington: Indiana University Press.

Murphy, R. (1995). The body silent in America. In B. Ingstad & S. Whyte (Eds.), *Disability and culture* (pp. 140–158). Berkeley: University of California Press.

Preston, P. (1994). *Mother father deaf: Living with sound and silence.* Cambridge, MA: Harvard University Press.

Ravaud, J., Beaufils, B., & Paicheler, H. (1987). Stereotyping and intergroup perceptions of disabled and nondisabled children: A new perspective. *The Exceptional Child, 34,* 93–106.

Schmelkin, L. (1988). Multidimensional perspectives in the perception of disabilities. In H. Yuker, (Ed.), *Attitudes toward persons with disabilities* (pp. 127–137). New York: Springer.

Scott, R. A. (1967). *The making of blind men.* Hartford, CT: Connecticut Printers.

Stovall, C., & Sedlacek, W. (1981). *Attitudes of male and female university students toward students with different physical disabilities* (Research Report No 10–81). College Park: Maryland University Counseling Center. ERIC Document Reproductory Service No. ED 220 762.

Thomson, R. (1997). Disabled women as powerful women in Petry, Morrison, and Lord: Revising black female subjectivity. In D. Mitchell & S. Snyder (Eds.), *The body and physical difference* (pp. 240–266). Ann Arbor: University of Michigan Press.

Tuttle, D. W., & Tuttle, N. R. (1996). *Self-esteem and adjusting with blindness: The process of responding to life's demands.* Springfield, IL: Charles C Thomas.

Vaughan, C. E. (1998). *Social and cultural perspectives on blindness.* Springfield, IL: Charles C Thomas.

Wagner-Lampl, A., & Oliver, G. (1994). Folklore of blindness. *Journal of Visual Impairment & Blindness, 88,* 267–276.

Yuker, H. (1988). The effects of contact on attitudes toward disabled persons: Some empirical generalizations. In H. Yuker (Ed.), *Attitudes toward persons with disabilities* (pp. 262–274). New York: Springer.

Multiple Dimensions of Identity: Individuals with Visual Impairments

Madeline Milian

The way to help the blind . . . is to understand, correct, and remove the incapacities and inequalities of our entire civilization.
—Helen Keller (1913, p. 40)

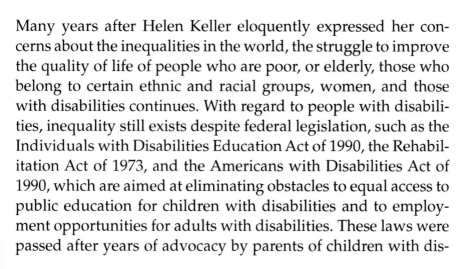

Many years after Helen Keller eloquently expressed her concerns about the inequalities in the world, the struggle to improve the quality of life of people who are poor, or elderly, those who belong to certain ethnic and racial groups, women, and those with disabilities continues. With regard to people with disabilities, inequality still exists despite federal legislation, such as the Individuals with Disabilities Education Act of 1990, the Rehabilitation Act of 1973, and the Americans with Disabilities Act of 1990, which are aimed at eliminating obstacles to equal access to public education for children with disabilities and to employment opportunities for adults with disabilities. These laws were passed after years of advocacy by parents of children with disabilities, adults with disabilities, and individuals and organizations working with and in support of people with disabilities.

Given this situation, educators and rehabilitation professionals who work with individuals who are blind or have low vision need to continue to work to improve educational and rehabilitation services. But the ability of many professionals to be effective advocates and agents of change is compromised by limited knowledge and understanding of the multiple dimensions—the different facets of identity—that define all people, including those with visual impairments, and how these dimensions influence the educational and rehabilitation needs of students and clients. The term *multiple dimensions* is used to refer to the diversity found in each person—a diversity that is based on gender, race, age, ethnicity, class, religious beliefs, disability status, and sexual orientation (Banks & McGee Banks, 1997).

This chapter introduces a number of concepts that are relevant to the discussion of diversity and explains how they relate to education and rehabilitation. A main goal of this chapter is to help educators and rehabilitation professionals understand the centrality of diversity in their daily work with individuals who are blind or visually impaired so that their practices can become more sensitive to the many attributes that define students and clients.

A number of beliefs or assumptions about diversity have guided the selection of areas that are included in this chapter:

1. Although the experiences of living with and adjusting to blindness or low vision are influenced by an individual's understanding of and experiences with visual impairments, these experiences are interpreted by each individual according to his or her cultural, gender, social, and religious attributes.

2. Individuals with visual impairments benefit from developing identities that encompass their multiple dimensions, including race, ethnicity, gender, class, disability, religious affiliations, and sexual orientation. These identities allow membership in a number of groups that share common

concerns and can offer the type of support that family members or professionals may be unable to provide.

3. It is essential for educators and rehabilitation professionals to facilitate and support the development of these multiple dimensions by designing programs that encourage and value these multiple dimensions and group memberships.
4. Educators and rehabilitation professionals need to be aware that their beliefs, thoughts, and expectations reflect their own cultural values and that these values influence their views and treatment of blind or visually impaired students and clients who come from different groups.
5. When working with diverse student or client groups, educators and rehabilitation professionals need to examine their own prejudices and stereotypes about members of diverse backgrounds to avoid situations that could lead to unintended discriminatory acts.

The author's beliefs and rationale for addressing the multiple dimensions of individuals with visual impairments have been informed by the work of many authors in the fields of disability research (Brown, 1994; Groce & Scheer, 1990; Linton, 1998; Nagler, 1993); self-esteem and blindness (Tuttle & Tuttle, 1996); social psychology and research on racial identity (Phinney, 1990; Tatum, 1997); minority groups with disabilities (Braithwaite, 1990; Gill, 1985; Longmore, 1987; Wertlieb, 1985); and multicultural education (Banks & McGee Banks, 1997; Nieto, 1996; Sleeter & Grant, 1994). However, it has been her personal involvement and professional work with individuals with visual impairments that have provided the impetus for the author to address these issues seriously and share some concerns and suggestions with other professionals.

DEVELOPING AN IDENTITY

One may question why it is relevant to address the question of identity and how this question may be related to teachers and rehabilitation professionals' daily work with students and clients who are blind or visually impaired. Although there are many reasons why professionals in education and rehabilitation need to be concerned and aware of the process of identity formation, only two general reasons are mentioned here. First, professionals need to understand the process and its implications, so they can develop programs that are responsive to their students and clients. Second, professionals need to understand their own identities, so they can reflect on the conflicts they may experience in their work with students and clients who come from different social, racial, religious, or ethnic groups and those with different sexual orientations. Given the increasing frequency with which professionals encounter students and clients from diverse backgrounds, a general understanding of the complexities of identity development will facilitate the work of clients and professionals and allow them to understand the apprehensions that are typically felt as the result of new experiences.

Erikson (1968, p. 22) stated that the question of identity is hard to grasp because it is a "process 'located' *in the core of the individual* and yet also *in the core of his communal culture,* a process which establishes, in fact, the identity of those two identities." Therefore, one cannot separate personal growth and communal change. He explained that

> identity formation employs a process of simultaneous reflection and observation, a process taking place on all levels of mental functioning, by which the individual judges himself in the light of what he perceives to be the way in which others judge him in comparison to themselves and to a typology significant to them; while he judges their way of judging him in light of how he perceives himself in comparison to them and to the types that have become relevant to him. (p. 22)

Erikson further explained that the process of identity formation is always changing. Adolescence is a particularly important part of this process because at this time adolescents begin to observe and reflect on the self and pose questions that influence their decisions on future occupations, religion, and other belief systems.

Two points require some clarification. First, despite the strong connection between personal and group identity, a series of studies (Spencer, 1982, 1985, 1987; cited in Banks, 1995) found that African American children can distinguish between their personal and group identities; that is, they can develop high self-esteem at the same time that they are aware of white bias. Second, although adolescence is a critical time in the process of forming an identity, studies have shown that young children are aware of racial differences by age 3 and have internalized society's attitudes toward African Americans and whites (Banks, 1995). The early work of Allport (1954) also indicated that young children may not understand the significance of group membership until they are 9 or 10, but develop ethnic identification and in-group loyalties much younger in life. The notion that young children in elementary schools are unaware of group differences and that blind children, in particular, do not notice group differences because they cannot see them are unfounded. Clearly, blind children are able to learn about other things they cannot see. They hear descriptions of others; touch others in the playground; hear voices and may notice differences in speech patterns; and, most important, are exposed to conversations about individual differences at home and on television.

Tatum (1997), reinforcing Erikson's (1968) notion of identity, explained that one's identity is shaped by individual characteristics, family dynamics, historical factors, and social and political contexts. With regard to the development of a racial identity, she suggested that one's racial identity is mediated by other characteristics such as gender, age, social class, sexual orientation, physical condition, and religion—a process similar to that of developing a personal identity. Likewise, the onset of visual impairment will also cause people to reevaluate their identity and to accept the visual impairment as one of their attributes (Tuttle & Tuttle, 1996). Those who have difficulty incorporating this new attribute into their individual identities and those who focus on the visual impairment as their determining attribute have problems adjusting to their new situation. This notion of how identity is shaped by outside forces reinforces the importance of understanding that the messages that students and clients receive from the mass media and from the people they come in contact with influence how they view themselves as people with individual characteristics that may be different from those of the dominant group.

Multiple attributes are not additive; rather, they interact with each other to shape the way people interpret the world and develop affinities. The intersection of these multiple dimensions defines people's identification and leads them to create alliances with different social and political causes. It also places many people in either advantaged or disadvantaged positions. For example, a young white man who is blind may be part of the advantaged group because of his age, race, and gender, but will be placed in the disadvantaged group because of his disability. On the other hand, an elderly middle-class African American woman who is blind may be placed in the disadvantaged group because of her age, gender, race, and disability, but may be in the advantaged group because of her middle-class status. Hanna and Rogovsky (1993) studied the status of African American women with physical disabilities and discussed the importance of exploring the interactions of their different status variables and the consequences for services for individuals with disabilities. They stated that "there is reason to believe that medical, rehabilitation, and other professionals are not independent of their culture" (p. 156).

In discussing multiple identities, Tatum (1997) explained that the part of one's identity that others notice becomes the focus of one's own attention and sets one apart as the "other" in the group. Personal attributes, such as race, ethnicity, gender, religion, sexual orientation, socioeconomic status, age, and physical or mental ability, can define people as "other." In a classroom that is not integrated on the basis of ethnicity and disability, the only blind Latino student will be much more aware of these two dimensions than in a classroom in which other students also have visual impairments or are Latinos.

It is important for teachers and rehabilitation professionals to recognize and acknowledge both their own and their students' and clients' multiple dimensions. These dimensions define people as individuals and members of communities and shape the educational and rehabilitation needs of students and clients and the services that professionals design and deliver. Ignoring these dimensions leads to culturally insensitive practices that are counterproductive to educational and rehabilitative goals.

VISUAL IMPAIRMENT AS A DIVERSITY FACTOR

Each person with a visual impairment has a different experience related to the onset of the visual impairment, the cause of the visual impairment, and the degree of vision loss. Some individuals may have always been visually impaired, others may have gradually lost their vision, and others may have experienced a sudden change in visual functions. Some may have stable conditions and visual functioning, while others may have fluctuating vision. In short, the experience of being visually impaired differs from person to person because of the diverse nature of low vision and blindness. One person with a visual impairment may be easily identified because of his or her use of a cane, visual aids, or a dog guide, while another will not be recognized as visually impaired until a situation occurs that indicates that the person needs assistance with visual information or a mobility-related skill. Indeed, it is sometimes difficult to find people with visual impairments who share the same experiences with blindness or low vision. This is more likely to be the case for those who have low vision than for those who are totally blind. The visual variability found in the population of those with visual impairments requires a highly individualized approach, rather than a global approach that attempts to take everyone's needs into consideration. Consequently, professionals in the field of education and rehabilitation need to take the notion that no two visually impaired students or clients are alike as a guiding principle in the way they approach their interactions with students or clients and their families.

Tuttle and Tuttle (1996) discussed how the degree and stability of vision influence the adjustment process and how an individual must come to accept blindness or low vision as one of his or her defining personal attributes before adequate adjustment can take place. Because of the diversity in etiology, onset, and ranges in functional vision, it may be difficult for individuals with visual impairments to find others who share the same visual concerns. However, patterns of similar educational, social, emotional, medical, or employment concerns can be found in groups of children, adolescents, and adults with visual impairments that can be shared with others who are experiencing vision loss. In this regard, educators and rehabilitation professionals can connect students and clients with other visually impaired children or adults who can be sources of friendship or guidance. These connections offer entry into a new community—that of individuals with visual impairments.

The common experiences shared by those who are visually impaired may constitute part of what researchers on disabilities have identified as the culture of disability. The following section presents some of the arguments about whether a culture of disability exists that can embrace all disability groups.

THE CULTURE OF DISABILITY

Disability studies have challenged the notion that disability is primarily a medical category and have reframed disability as a designation with primarily social and political significance (Linton, 1998). As Groce and Scheer (1990) suggested, disability can define and limit options for social, economic, and legal parity, but most of the problems of people with disabilities stem from the larger society. Therefore, one of the main aims of disability studies is to demonstrate that the status and roles given to those with disabilities are the product of social and political process, not the inevitable results of having a disability. Among the concepts that are widely discussed in the literature on disability studies are the oppression experienced by individuals with disabilities; the minority status given to those with disabilities; the power of language that is used to describe people with disabilities; and the inclusion of the study of disability in the humanities and liberal arts curricula, rather than the predominant practice of discussing disability only in applied fields, such as special education and rehabilitation (Brown, 1994; Charlton, 1998, Linton, 1998).

Brown (1994), who is a strong supporter of the notion of a culture of disability, provided a definition that was suggested by a participant in his study on the status of the disability culture: "First it is the filter through which we people with disabilities experience the world (shared experiences, & thoughtfully developed concepts). [Second, it is] our expression of ourselves in writing, words, art, etc. as well as organizations" (p. 12).

The concept of a disability culture has been contested by some people with disabilities and some persons in various academic disciplines. Brown suggested that the disagreement about the existence of a disability culture may be rooted in the definition of culture and the traditional roles that people with disabilities have been assigned in society. As he explained, the typical definition of culture includes a common language, ritual traditions, and the transmission of cultural traits through the family. If this definition of culture is accepted, the probable conclusion is that there is no culture of disability.

Linton (1998) also pointed out that anthropologists have not adequately studied disability or the experiences of people with disabilities. She stated that in disability groups, identification typically does not take place until adolescence or adulthood; consequently, culture is primarily transmitted from adult to adult. Therefore, the intergenerational framework traditionally used by anthropologists to understand the transmission of culture may not be conducive to the study of disability culture.

In addition, some individuals with disabilities may fear identification with a disability group because its status has been so denigrated that it may threaten their social goals. In other cases, family members may discourage their disabled children or adolescents from socializing with others with disabilities to avoid being identified with a group that has been traditionally marginalized. Brown believes that the case is not one of people rejecting the notion of disability culture, but rather one of misunderstanding it. The interpretation of the traditional meaning of culture leads to difficulties accepting a disability culture. Brown prefers to use a culture definition that refers to "a totality of socially transmitted behavior patterns, arts, beliefs, institutions, and all other products of human work and thought characteristic of a community or population" (p. 79). He argues that people with disabilities transmit their ways from one generation to the next, and when this does not occur is the result of oppression or stigma that prevents it.

Regardless of the controversy over the existence of a disability culture and the degree to which such a culture can include all those with disabilities, one can conclude that the contributions of individuals with disabilities have been minimized, if not excluded, from history and that people with disabilities share similar experiences on the basis of whether they were either born with a disability or acquired it some time during their lives. Although these experiences are not always the same, they tend to reflect similar themes of rejection, exclusion, pity, and contradictions. The following examples, specific to blindness, are illustrative of these experiences.

In a study of the experiences of adults with disabilities (Phillips, 1990), one participant, Kelly, who lost her vision at age 12, reported:

> One thing that happened after I went blind is that I tended to lose a lot of friends. . . . And I felt terrible. I felt like a real freak. I just felt that nobody liked me and that nobody wanted me around. My family and the people around me taught me to be ashamed of the way I looked and to hide. [After the surgery] I was really encouraged to wear dark glasses, and I was taught to think of myself as

being ugly, and to hide behind my glasses. I think those images still haunt me. (p. 852)

Kelly said that after attending a university with an active group of students with disabilities, she was finally able to discard her dark glasses and liberate herself from the shame she felt about being blind.

Paul, who has been legally blind since birth, told of his difficulties with dating and the reactions of his dates' parents:

> It got rougher in junior high school when dating became a big thing, because, you just didn't want to date a blind person. And even if you could get a girl to go out with you, she'd be ridiculed by all her girlfriends. Once, I got this girl to go out with me. The father informs me when I get into the house that "No daughter of his is going to date anyone who is less than a whole man." And he says to me, "You are not leaving the house with my daughter." And I said, "That's fine with me," and we sat down and watched TV all evening. He didn't like it. Then, I've had girls get embarrassed and walk away from me in restaurants. Yeah, my dates! This is all high school. As I got to college people tended to grow up. (Phillips, 1990, p. 852)

These stories are not unique; many adults with visual impairments can recall similar experiences. All these situations are the product of the negative perceptions that those who are sighted have created about people who are blind or have low vision, rather than the outcome of the disability itself. Whether or not these types of shared experiences are indicative of a disability culture, they seem to fit the criteria of minority-group status.

MINORITY-GROUP STATUS OF PEOPLE WITH DISABILITIES

A number of researchers have used a minority-group model to describe the status of people with disabilities. Wirth (1970, p. 34) defined a minority group as "a group of people who, because of their physical or cultural characteristics, are singled out from others in the society in which they live for differential and unequal treatment, and who therefore regard themselves as objects of collective discrimination." Fine and Asch (1993) applied Dworkin and Dworkin's (1976) definition of a minority group, which included the elements of differential power, differential and pejorative treatment, and group awareness, to people with disabilities. They contended that these criteria apply to people with disabilities, although not all people with disabilities have developed a minority-group consciousness.

In her analysis of the commonalities and differences between people with disabilities and other minority groups, Wertlieb (1985) found that, like other groups of minorities, people with disabilities are rejected and stigmatized by the larger society because of a physical characteristic that is perceived as undesirable and, as a result, are socially isolated and discriminated against in employment and educational opportunities. In addition, both groups are perceived of as having inferior levels of ability, and hence represent social liabilities and often experience role strains when they join the dominant group because of conflicts between personal and group expectations. They are also generally evaluated in terms of group membership, which leads to their being stereotyped and their individuality being ignored; have experienced educational segregation and have had to fight for their right to obtain equal opportunities in education; and often exhibit a more external locus of control that the rest of the population.

With regard to the differences between people with disabilities and those from other minority groups, Wertlieb (1985) explained that members of other minority groups are not characterized by the physical limitations that sometimes restrict certain groups of people with disabilities from physical activities. Furthermore, unlike racial and ethnic minority groups, people with disabilities do not share the same status as their relatives and thus do not receive the same type of family support against the prejudice and discrimination they often experience. Whereas members of racial, ethnic, and religious minorities are often encouraged by their families to take pride in their unique characteristics and to maintain their groups' values, traditions, and customs, people with disabilities frequently have to join organizations if they want to develop a sense of pride in their disabilities. In addition, the undesirable traits that are sometimes ascribed to other minority groups are thought to be voluntary and are often accepted by the majority, but overt expressions of hostility toward people with disabilities are typically not considered socially acceptable because the general public frequently exhibits behaviors that are guided by overconcern and protectiveness for those with disabilities. Finally, the general public does not usually fear that large groups of people with disabilities will move into their neighborhoods or take over desirable business locations, as they do racial and ethnic minority groups. However, the housing problems experienced by people with disabilities and the discomfort of able-bodied neighbors toward those with disabilities cannot be ignored.

Asch and Sacks (1983), who examined the autobiographies of 15 women and 10 men who were blind, found similar patterns of minority-group indicators in the experiences of these blind people and those of other marginal people. Some examples include the realization by those who had lost their vision in childhood or adolescence that their visual problems made them objects of pity, derision, hostility, or exclusion; the concern of those who became blind in adulthood about remaining connected to important people in their lives and making new friends; the fear and rejection that these blind people experienced from members of the opposite sex because of their blindness (which may have been party responsible for the fact that only 6 of the 15 women were married); and discrimination in schools, jobs, restaurants, and banks.

It is unrealistic to suggest that all the problems that people who are blind or have low vision experience are the result of prejudice and discrimination. Some activities or professions may be foreclosed to them because of their visual limitations. Moreover, personal acceptance of blindness and the development of a healthy self-concept are essential components of a successful and productive life. However, the importance of social forces and their role in the success or failure of individuals with visual impairments in educational, professional, and personal endeavors must also be recognized, given the long history of differences in power and status between those in the dominant group and those in minority groups.

MULTICULTURAL EDUCATION

The concept of multicultural education can provide a frame of reference to assist professionals who work in school districts and rehabilitation settings that are defined by diversity and social complexities in analyzing and improving their goals as professionals. This discussion refers not to some narrowly defined practices of multicultural education, such as the use of cultural artifacts like food and music in professional practice, but to the broader practices that can be used to improve services for all children and adults, including those with visual disabilities.

Nieto (1996, p. 307) described multicultural education as

> a process of comprehensive school reform and basic education for all students. It challenges and rejects racism and other forms of discrimination in schools and society and accepts and affirms the pluralism (ethnic, racial, linguistic, religious, economic, and gender, among others) that students, their communities, and teachers represent. Multicultural education permeates the curriculum and instructional strategies used in schools, as well as the interactions among teachers, students, and parents, and the very way that schools conceptualize the nature of teaching and learning. Because it uses critical pedagogy as its underlying philosophy and focuses on knowledge, reflection, and action (praxis) as the basis for social change, multicultural education promotes the democratic principles of social justice.

According to Sleeter and Grant (1994), the five goals of multicultural education promote

- the strength and value of cultural diversity,
- human rights and respect for those who are different from oneself,
- alternative life choices for people,
- social justice and equal opportunity for all people, and
- equity in the distribution of power among groups.

This definition and the goals of multicultural education can be used to help individuals who are visually impaired to understand the multiple dimensions of their identity and to provide services that are culturally relevant to these individuals and their family members.

Some in the field of disability studies (Linton, 1998) have argued for the inclusion of people with disabilities in the discipline of multicultural education and contended that disability is not considered within the larger discussion of diversity. This is an area that should be of interest to those in special education, rehabilitation programs, and general education programs from kindergarten through high school. Although many teacher preparation programs have courses related to the needs of special education students, these courses typically focus on required state competencies, laws and regulations in special education, and techniques for working with these students. These courses often treat disability in isolation from other human dimensions or sociopolitical concerns, whereas required courses in multicultural education tend to concentrate on issues related to race and ethnicity, class, and gender and ignore issues of disabilities or treat them in a superficial manner. Hence, future professionals generally have to integrate the information they obtained in disability-specific and multicultural education courses when they work with individuals with disabilities from diverse communities—a task that would challenge even the most capable experienced professionals.

Educators and rehabilitation professionals need to challenge and reject racism and other forms of discrimination in schools and rehabilitation settings; reconstruct curricula and professional practices to take into consideration the multiple dimension of students or clients, communities, schools, families, and professionals; and promote social justice. Given that individuals with visual impairments can be frequent targets of exclusion and discrimination, the goals of multicultural education can offer guidance for professional practices and lead to more productive educational and rehabilitation environments.

CONCLUDING THOUGHTS

The importance of understanding the multiple dimensions that define individuals and how these dimensions intersect may seem overwhelming to many professionals in the field of blindness who encounter many challenging situations. Some may ask: How do I find the time to learn about the individual attributes of my students and clients? How can I change my curriculum to reflect the culture of my students? How can I become more knowledgeable about cross-cultural communication? or How do I become a better advocate for my students and clients? Conversely, others may wonder if it is their role as educators and rehabilitation professionals to get involved in areas that appear, at least on the surface, to be disconnected from individuals' disabilities.

Although many of these questions can be answered only in specific teacher-preparation or in-service training courses, the most critical point is to view multiple dimensions as the norm. In other words, professionals need to consider differences between themselves and their students or clients not as barriers, but as a common and expected part of professional life. If they do so, they will no longer view their role as dealing solely with visual impairment, but will collaborate with other professionals to understand how the various attributes of students and clients significantly contribute to the education and rehabilitation process. In addition, professionals will no longer have a model or ideal student or client that they use as the "norm" from which to compare all others. Instead, they will accept the notion that all individuals with visual impairments are different and hence that a variety of approaches are needed. Finally, they will no longer see visual impairment as the defining factor in a person's life, but as one of many factors.

In a world where diversity is viewed as ordinary (Higgins & Coen, 2000), professionals, students, and clients will navigate their multiple dimensions through social networks that will be built on shared affinities and will link members of diverse groups working on a common cause, all aware of their individual dimensions, respected for what they bring to the group, and cognizant of their social responsibilities to communicate and collaborate across many groups to achieve a common goal. As Helen Keller stated in 1913: "[T]he blind man, however poignantly his individual suffering appeals to our hearts, is not a single, separate person whose problem can be solved by itself" (p. 38). Indeed, individuals with visual impairments are part of a social and cultural community. Professionals need to understand those social and cultural communities if they want to be effective advocates for their students' and clients' educational and rehabilitation needs and rights.

REFERENCES

Allport, G. W. (1954). *The nature of prejudice.* Cambridge, MA: Addison-Wesley.

Asch, A. , & Sacks, L. H. (1983). Lives without, lives within: Autobiographies of blind women and men. *Journal of Visual Impairment & Blindness, 77,* 242–247.

Banks, J. A. (1995). Multicultural education: Historical development, dimensions, and practice. In J. A. Banks & C. A. McGee Banks (Eds.), *Handbook of research on multicultural education* (pp. 3–24). New York: Macmillan.

Banks, J. A., & McGee Banks, C. A. (Eds.). (1997). *Multicultural education: Issues and perspectives* (3rd ed). Needham Heights, MA: Allyn & Bacon.

Braithwaite, D. O. (1990). From majority to minority: An analysis of cultural change from ablebodied to disabled. *International Journal of Intercultural Relations, 14,* 465–483.

Brown, S. E. (1994). *Investigating a culture of disability: Final report* (National Institute on Disability and Rehabilitation Research, Project No. H133F30010). [Available from the Institute on Disability Culture, 2260 Sunrise Point Road, Las Cruces, NM 88011].

Charlton, J. I. (1998). *Nothing about us without us: Disability oppression and empowerment.* Berkeley: Univ. of California Press.

Dworkin, A., & Dworkin, R. (Eds.). (1976). *The minority report.* New York: Praeger.

Erikson, E. H. (1968). *Identity: Youth and crisis.* New York: W. W. Norton.

Fine, M., & Asch, A. (1993). Disability beyond stigma: Social interaction, discrimination, and activism. In M. Nagler (Ed.), *Perspectives on disability* (pp. 49–62). Palo Alto, CA: Health Markets Research.

Gill, C. J. (1985). The family/professional alliance in rehabilitation viewed from a minority perspective. *American Behavioral Scientist, 28*(3), 424–428.

Groce, N., & Scheer, J. (1990). Introduction. *Social Science and Medicine, 30*(8), v-vi.

Hanna, J., & Rogovsky, E. (1993). On the situation of African-American women with physical disabilities. In M. Nagler (Ed.), *Perspectives on disability* (pp. 149–159). Palo Alto, CA: Health Markets Research.

Higgins, M., & Coen, T. (2000). *Streets, bedrooms and patios: The ordinariness of diversity in urban Oaxaca.* Austin: University of Texas Press.

Keller, H. (1913). *Out of the dark.* New York: Doubleday.

Linton, S. (1998). *Claiming disability: Knowledge and identity.* New York: New York University Press.

Longmore, P. K. (1987). Uncovering the hidden history of people with disabilities. *Reviews in American History, 15,* 355–364.

Nagler, M. (1993). The disabled: The acquisition of power. In M. Nagler (Ed.), *Perspectives on disability* (2nd ed., pp. 33–36). Palo Alto, CA: Health Markets Research.

Nieto, S. (1996). *Affirming diversity: The sociopolitical context of multicultural education* (2nd ed.). White Plains, NY: Longman.

Phillips, M. (1990). Damaged goods: Oral narratives of the experience of disability in American culture. *Social Science and Medicine, 30,* 849–857.

Phinney, J. S. (1990). Ethnic identity in adolescents and adults: Review of research. *Psychological Bulletin, 108,* 499–514.

Sleeter, C. E., & Grant, C. A. (1994). *Making choices for multicultural education: Five approaches to race, class, and gender* (2nd ed.). New York: Macmillan.

Tatum, B. D. (1997). *Why are all the black kids sitting together in the cafeteria? And other conversations about race.* New York: Basic Books.

Tuttle, D. W., & Tuttle, N. R. (1996). *Self-esteem and adjusting with blindness* (2nd ed.). Springfield, IL: Charles C Thomas.

Wertlieb, E. C. (1985). Minority group status of the disabled. *Human Relations, 38,* 1047–1063.

Wirth, L. (1970). The problem of minority groups. In M. Kurodawa (Ed.), *Minority responses: Comparative views of reactions to subordination* (pp. 34–42). New York: Random House.

PART II

Ethnic and Racial Diversity

CHAPTER 3

African Americans with Visual Impairments

Lila Cabbil
and Moniqueka E. Gold*

Megan is a precocious girl who is extremely friendly and has excellent verbal skills. Her mother remembered an occasion when Megan was 4, when the family went out to eat at a local restaurant. As a waiter approached to seat them, Megan turned to her mother and asked, in an urgent tone, "What color am I?" Muffling a gasp, Megan's mother looked at her husband.

The family followed the waiter to the table in silence. Megan patiently waited until they were seated and then repeated, "I said, 'What color am I?'" Both parents rattled off compliments, such as, "You're a beautiful sugar-cookie brown," "You're luscious chocolate brown," "You're like the yummy chocolate Easter Bunny," and "You're daddy's dark brown sugar." Undaunted, Megan asked: "Does that mean that I'm black? But I don't want to be black!" Megan said desperately. Her father said, "I'm black, and I'm happy about it. What's the problem, Megan?" "They talk mean about black people and they don't like them. I don't like them either," Megan explained.

Later, Megan's mother shared the frustration and hurt that she felt on hearing her daughter express such pain about her

---

*With the assistance of Desiree Cooper.

racial identity. The mother said, "It was so hurtful; here was a 4 year old who was not able to see prejudice, yet it is so powerful that she could feel it even at that age. It hurt her so much that she didn't want to be who she is. It presented yet another challenge to us as parents, a challenge to help build her racial self-esteem. It's been hard work, and I'm still working it out. I don't know if it will ever be over. I have had some positive results: otherwise I would be depressed."

African Americans with visual impairments are learning to overcome the ramifications of being African American in a society that has never completely embraced their culture. There are many similarities in the stigmas and inequities experienced by African Americans and by people with disabilities, including visual impairments. First, both groups have been excluded from the mainstream of American life for different reasons, and they both share an underprivileged status (Alston & Russo, 1994). For centuries, people with disabilities were shunned from society and treated as outcasts who did not have the same rights as other humans, and African Americans have experienced negative responses from society, simply because of their skin color.

Second, neither African Americans nor people with disabilities are expected to perform well in school. As a result, both groups have learned to deal with being excluded simply because of their membership in a minority group. Being excluded because of their race is commonplace for African Americans. Being an African American with a visual impairment is yet another story that has even more complex implications.

This chapter explores the two major cultural factors that contribute to the underlying strength of the African American family: religious beliefs and family kinships. Because empirical research on African Americans with visual impairments is limited, the authors developed a framework for investigating issues that are relevant to the social contexts in which African American families that include members with visual impairments develop coping skills. Finally, the authors discuss the educational implications of these issues for working with African Americans with visual impairments.

DEMOGRAPHICS

As of 2000, African Americans were the largest ethnic minority group in the United States, constituting over 35 million of the estimated population of over 275 million. Furthermore, it has been projected that out of the total estimated population of 337,814 million in 2025, 47,089 million will be black (U.S. Bureau of the Census, 2000) and that ethnic minority children will represent 41 percent of all U.S. children by 2030 (Arcia, Keyes, Gallagher, & Herrick, 1993).

The incidence of disability is more prevalent among Africa Americans than among any other ethnic group in the United States (Alston & Turner, 1994). Among white Americans, 8.4 percent have disabilities, and among African Americans 14.1 percent do (Marshall, 1987). With regard to visual impairment and blindness, of the estimated 4.3 million persons who are blind or visually impaired (Tielsch, Sommer, Witt, Katz, & Royal, 1990), "African Americans are twice as likely to be visually impaired as are whites of comparable social status" ("Vision and Hearing," 2000, p. 4).

The majority of African Americans with visual impairments (53 percent) reside in the South, the highest percentages living in central cities and nonfarm communities (Giesen et al., 1995). According to the United Way of America (1987), visual impairments among minorities increased during the 1980s and will increase further.

African American men, women, and children who are blind or visually impaired learn to cope with their disabilities through a cultural framework that differs from the mainstream culture in significant ways. To be an effective service provider for students who are both visually impaired and African American, professionals must not only understand the disability but learn as much as possible about the cultural context to respect and appreciate the African American heritage. By encouraging cultural pluralism and cultural sensitivity, they can avoid compounding any feelings of discrimination or oppression.

HEALTH AND VISUAL IMPAIRMENTS

The greater prevalence of visual impairments among African Americans may be attributed to three factors:

- lack of accessibility to adequate health care
- employment in occupations that are more likely to be physically demanding
- genetic predispositions toward conditions that can result in visual impairments (such as glaucoma, hypertension, and diabetes)

Access to Health Care and Occupational Risks

A higher incidence of visual impairment among African American newborns and infants is due, at least in part, to the rising cost of and lack of affordable health care. In 1995, inadequate prenatal care varied from 5.7 percent for white mothers to 23 percent for African American mothers. Those who were most likely to receive no prenatal care were young mothers and African American mothers.

Low socioeconomic status and poverty are the main reasons for the lack of access to preventive health care. According to the U.S. Bureau of the Census (1999), 33.3 percent of African American families had incomes below the poverty level in 1998, and 40.4 percent of African American children were living in the nation's poorest families (42.8 percent under age 6). Widespread poverty is a considerable barrier to adequate nutrition and health care, which increase the likelihood that African American children may suffer from a panoply of visual impairments, including blindness. Furthermore, since many African Americans do not have access to high-paying jobs, they may attempt to obtain employment in occupations that are physically demanding and therefore present more opportunities for injuries.

Genetic Predispositions

Visual impairments are often attributed to conditions that have genetic predispositions and that are more prevalent among African Americans, including sickle-cell anemia, glaucoma, hypertension, and diabetes. The prevalence of diabetes among African Americans is approximately 70 percent higher than among whites. Diabetic retinopathy is associated with high blood pressure and poor control of blood sugar levels and increases a person's tendency to develop cataracts (Orr, 1998). Consequently, African Americans are more likely to lose vision from retinopathy, cataracts, and glaucoma. African Americans have a five times greater risk for glaucoma than do whites, and their rate of blindness resulting from glaucoma is six times greater. Almost 6 percent of those over age 40 (the typical age of onset) are reported to have the condition.

As previously stated, individuals with diabetes are at higher risks of developing glaucoma. The danger of this disease is that it often progresses without pain or other obvious symptoms. For African Americans who avoid or cannot afford routine physical examinations and are prompted to get medical care mainly by crises, the disease may be well advanced before it is diagnosed. With diseases like diabetes, preventive medicine is critical to the prevention of blindness. Yet, especially in urban areas, where there is a concentration of the destitute and working poor, all but emergency medical care is often financially out of reach. It is common, then, for these families to seek medical care only when their symptoms become critical, increasing the chances that these individuals may develop vision-related complications.

A number of other factors may also influence health-management styles among African Americans. For example, the belief that a condition is not life threatening; the belief in prayer and spiritual healing; the high cost of medication, which leads some patients to cut pills in half or reduce the prescribed number of pills they take per day; and high levels of stress that may lead individuals to ignore dietary restrictions when they interfere with the opportunity to gain satisfaction from food.

AFRICAN AMERICANS AND VISUAL IMPAIRMENT

Although African Americans differ in skin color from the majority of people in the United States, it may be assumed that they otherwise experience the same effects of a visual impairment on their self-esteem as do most people with visual impairments. However, there is a dearth of literature on African Americans with visual impairments. Like others with visual impairments, African Americans must deal with the perceptions of sighted people that they are unable to work and play independently. Perceptions of helplessness because of visual impairments may be a source of frustration and may lead to feelings of inadequacy. Not being able to live up to the expectations of society may lead to feelings of inferiority that could lower self-esteem. These negative experiences may slowly chip away at self-confidence and feelings of self-worth (Gold, 1998).

African American Families

Among African Americans, the family has traditionally been extremely important, and traditional family values act as a buffer in dealing with negative life events (Rogers-Dulan & Blacher, 1995). The family structure has become an important component in the consideration of how African American families deal with having children with visual impairments.

African American families have been both criticized and applauded for their characteristics. A number of strengths of African American families are important to discuss, including distinctive coping strategies; religious beliefs that allow families to survive traumatic events, such as the onset of a visual impairment; religious supports for overcoming negative stereotypes and discrimination; and the support of kinship groups or extended family members.

The traditional nuclear family, consisting of a husband (the breadwinner), the wife (the homemaker), and their offspring was long considered the family norm. Today, however, it is no longer typical, since there are many other family forms. Furthermore, it is essential to recognize that a family system may be functional even though it differs from the traditional concept of the nuclear family structure (Boyd-Franklin, 1989).

Among African Americans, it is not atypical for single mothers to be the heads of households, who are responsible for both child rearing and earning the families' incomes. It is also not uncommon for families to be matriarchal, meaning that the mothers are the dominant figures even if the fathers are present. This role may have evolved from slave times, when the men were taken away from their families and sold, leaving the mothers to head the households (Dickerson, 1995). Perhaps the matriarchal family should be viewed as matrifocal, meaning the mother is the center of family without necessarily dominating it. In this family structure, the women in the family—the mother, sisters, and daughters—work together to rear the children and support the family.

Religious Connectedness

No matter how the flexible roles of family members are interpreted, religion or some type of spiritual orientation is a critical aspect of most African American families. It is through religion that African Americans give positive meaning to and cope with stressful events in their lives, as do many people with visual impairments (Erin, Rudin, & Njoroge, 1991). African American families seem to demonstrate more religious connectedness than do white families—a connectedness that goes back at least to the days of slavery, when African Americans sang spirituals in the fields as they were busy with their crops. Historically, African Americans have lived with high degrees of stress and anxiety caused by the stigma of being a "minority" and consider religion a social support system, which aids in coping with the daily stressors of life.

A larger majority of African Americans say that they belong to a specific church or religion, compared to Americans in general. In fact, the black church is one of the few institutions that African Americans look upon without suspicion and anger. This affinity for the church can be traced back to the abolition movement, when religious dissenters rebuked the institution of slavery, organized the Underground Railroad, and used the Bible to educate enslaved Africans. Using the Bible at church was often the first opportunity many enslaved Africans had to learn to read. Some believe that the black church is an outgrowth of a more ancient spirituality that has its roots in African culture.

Today, the black church still attempts to fulfill many of the basic needs of the African American community and, as Turner and Alston (1992) noted, is an extension of the extended family. It tends to be the center of political and social life as well as of religion, and is often the means by which resources are made available to the poorest communities. In many African American communities, is not uncommon for the black church to engage in employment training, economic development, and social services. The black church is also a place where worshipers not only pray together, but feel accepted and cared about and are considered significant no matter what their socioeconomic status, abilities, or level of functioning.

Through its religious teachings, the black church assists African Americans who have disabilities and their families to cope. For example, religious beliefs emphasize a positive outlook on the future and a shared faith that one's burdens will diminish and conditions will improve. This religious doctrine reflects a philosophy of concentrating on abilities and skills and refraining from a preoccupation with limitations or disabilities.

The black church also gives its members the opportunity to

build self-esteem and to establish a positive identity. In adition, through its programs, families whose members have disabilities can receive child care, food assistance, clothing assistance, financial support, and connections with additional resources.

The three African American parents of children who are visually impaired who were interviewed reflected the importance of their religious beliefs in coming to terms with their children's disability. One mother, Patricia, commented:

> I need the Lord to guide me. My family has a strong foundation in God. My spiritual stability gives my family stability. When we found out Donna had a vision problem, my first reaction was Lord, what am I gonna do? I knew that God would never give me more than I could bear, not more than my child could bear. We just treat her like the other children. That is how she knows she is not different, . . . she is our special gift from God.

Another parent stated:

> Finding out our daughter was blind was hard on us. We did not know anyone blind, so we felt so lost. My husband reminded me of a song our child sings at church, which says, "You can't tell me God won't make a way," and from that day forth I never worried about my child's abilities or what other people would consider her disabilities. She is now a junior at a small Baptist College in Tennessee. So yes, my faith gave me an inner peace to deal with her vision loss, but it opened my eyes to seeing so much more than I had before.

Tanisha, the mother of an elementary-age child with low vision, said:

> I feel black people were spiritual, and that goes back to slavery days. As a people, we have learned to rely on God because we know we have no one else to rely on. I have been raised to go to church. It gives me harmony and inner peace, and it helps me cope with the daily stressors of first being black and then having a child with some vision problems.

In contrast to the mainstream community, which increasingly segregates the church from all other aspects of everyday life, in the black community the black church is a powerful influence. Therefore, service providers should view the black church as a partner in reaching and training individuals with disabilities.

Kinships Groups and the Extended Family

The support of kinship groups has also contributed to the strength of the African American family. The belief that it helps when a whole village raises a child is still strong in the African American community.

The notion of kinship in the African American family is not the same as the mainstream concept of the nuclear family. For many African Americans, kinship is not limited to blood relationships, nor is it defined by geography. Strong kinship bonds exist between people who do not even live in the same households, and between "invented families," including neighbors and friends (Billingsley, 1974). Among African Americans, it is customary for people who have no genetic relationship to refer to one another as "brother" and "sister." Similar life experiences, such as a shared sociocultural and political past and shared hope for the future, have forged functional kinship bonds among many African Americans.

Strong social support systems may distinguish African American families who are able to cope with various problems from those who are unable to cope (Alston & Turner, 1994). These social supports among family members contributed to the strength needed when dealing with the stressors of life (Hanline & Daley, 1991). Hence, "traditional family life remains the one viable option for Black Americans of all socio-economic strata because it is less subject to the vagaries of race than any other institution in American life" (Staples, 1985, p. 1011). Kinship bonds or extended family members are a great source of emotional and social support that is essential for handling the stresses of having a family member with a disability.

Grandmothers are important members of extended African American families. In 1989, 1.2 million African American children were reported to be living with their grandparents (Dickerson, 1995). Some 30 years ago, Jackson (1970) found that African American grandmothers were more likely than African American grandfathers to be actively involved with grandchildren, to be the favorite grandparents, and to maintain relationships with their children. Hale (1982) compared African American and Caucasian grandmothers and found that African American grandmothers lived closer to their grandchildren than did Caucasian grandmothers and were more likely to care for their grandchildren and other nonrelated children for an extended amount of time. Grandmothers provide a great deal of support for child rearing and the coping strategies that families use whenever stress or trauma arises. McWilliam, McGhee, & Tocci (1998) reported that although most African American families typically depend on the extended family members, they especially depend on maternal grandmothers to assist with child rearing.

The greater community also exerts an influence on the responses to an individual's disability. When it is believed that a person loses his or her vision because of the sins of prior generations, an individual cannot be blamed for his or her own disabilities. Instead, the community often integrates the person into daily life, accepting the person and his or her disability as "the way it was meant to be." It is not considered proper to place people with disabilities in the care of institutions unless absolutely necessary. As a result, African American families who have family members with disabilities often find themselves embraced by their communities, yet shut off, either economically or culturally, from institutions that have resources to offer them.

LANGUAGE AND COMMUNICATION STYLES

A culture is a set of shared values and characteristics. Although no two individuals learn the same way or at the same pace, culture and ethnicity add another dimension to the learning environment, and professionals must take cultural differences into account if they are to establish communication and trust with clients of different cultures.

One way in which the African American culture is different from the Euro-American culture is that it has a shared communication system. Language and communication vary according to many factors, of which ethnicity is just one. Consequently, it is important that others learn to appreciate the variations in communication by many African Americans.

DeVeaux has indicated that African American men tend to have deeper and heavier voices than do men in the majority population (personal communication, June 1997). Thus, when they raise their voices, it may sometimes seem that they are upset, when they are not. In addition, African Americans sometimes use a dialect or nonstandard form of English (also referred to as African American vernacular) when in a relaxed environment with other African Americans. This dialect is like a shortened form or an abbreviated code of the English language, so that meanings may not be understood by others outside the community. For example, "Your outfit is FAT" means that "your outfit looks good"; "You are my boy" means "You are my friend or buddy," and "I got yo' back" means "I support you" (Ogbu, 1999).

The term *Ebonics* has been used to describe the type of language, or dialect, spoken by some African Americans. In 1996, the Oakland School District, in Oakland, California, proposed using Ebonics as a language of instruction to help African American children bridge the gap between Ebonics and standard English (Haynes, 1996; Lacey, 1997). The proposal was not approved, and this movement has since lost much of its momentum. In most African American families, children are taught standard English through modeling, but they may also use the African American vernacular at home and among friends and relatives.

It is important for service providers to learn to appreciate the many cultural differences in the African American community.

Once students and clients realize that there is interest in learning about their world, they may come to trust professionals and feel that their culture is worth learning. Understanding the dialect, expressive content, and language patterns of African Americans is similar to adjusting to the languages and accents of those who speak languages other than English.

The oral tradition of communication is integral to African American communication styles and learning preferences and is consistent with African Americans' tendency to be people oriented. African American men and women also have communication styles that contradict mainstream notions of appropriate gender roles; that is, African Americans view a range of behaviors that whites would categorize as either specifically masculine or specifically feminine as appropriate for both sexes. The masculine traits include aggressiveness, independence, self-confidence, nonconformity, and sexual assertiveness, and the feminine traits include nurturance, emotional expressiveness, and a focus on personal relationships.

THE MINORITY WITHIN THE MINORITY

Within the African American community, there are minorities within the minority as a result of the variety of skin colors and hues among African Americans (Neal & Wilson, 1989; Porter, 1991, Seltzer & Smith, 1991). What is considered attractive is often framed by colorism, which is defined as stereotypical attributions and prejudgments based on skin color (Okazawa-Rey, Robinson, & Ward, 1987). Given that color consciousness is rooted in social, political, and economic conditions that existed during slavery, colorism is often manifested as a preference for lighter skin tones over darker ones. Porter (1991) found that a lighter skin tone symbolized physical attractiveness and fostered a sense of sameness.

The concept of sameness within the African American community is even more complex for African Americans with albinism. Oculocutaneous albinism is any congenital condition that causes a reduction or lack of pigmentation in the skin and hair, as well as in retinal and iris tissue (Bishop & Inderbitzen, 1996), and causes a moderate-to-severe visual impairment. African Americans with oculocutaneous albinism may have skin color that varies from tan to fair or translucent, a different color and texture of hair (blond), and hair that is either finer or coarser than other members of the family who do not have albinism (Vander Kolk & Bright, 1983).

African Americans with albinism are often discriminated against by members of their own culture with darker skins because of the differences in their physical attributes. The National Organization for Albinism and Hypopigmentation ("African Americans with Albinism," 1996) reported that some African Americans said they have been accused by other African Americans as trying to pass as white because their skin is so fair. During the early 20th century, African Americans with albinism were often ostracized from people in their community, and today in many parts of Africa, people with albinism are avoided, treated as taboo, and considered bad luck and evil. Nevertheless, as was mentioned earlier, African Americans with visual impairments are still perceived more positively if their skin (hue) is lighter than if they have darker (ebony) skin.

African Americans with albinism often have to deal with feelings of unconnectedness to their families and low self-esteem because of both their visual impairments and the differences between their skin color and that of their immediate family members. These types of experiences were described by one young woman with albinism:

> Life is full of conflicts and oxymorons when you are a Black person with albinism like me. I used to wake up every morning and look, in the mirror, and think about all the decisions I had to face. The way people wear their hair says something about them. Like everything else in the way they present themselves it makes a statement. For me, it was a real dilemma: whether I relaxed or

straightened my hair, or whether I wore it in corn rows or braids, there was the possibility that others would think I was trying to pass for something I was not. Why worry about what others think? I generally don't. But sometimes I am still a little self-conscious and consider public reaction when I walk out onto the street.

Clothes are important too. How about speech? I used to wonder if I should talk in slang or speak like an Oxford professor. Still I look in Black magazines and notice that the make-up in the ads is not my shade. The people don't look like me. In fact, no one looked like me, on TV, in the movies, anywhere. When you have albinism and especially if your family is not Caucasian, you have to contend with all sorts of funny notions people have about you, such as: "You are adopted", "Your mother did not take enough vitamin D", "You are mixed . . . the result of inbreeding", "You have a sickness that robed [sic] you of your color . . . something that is catching", "You are or will become deaf, blind, or retarded", "You can see in the dark", and it goes on and on. You have to deal with all sorts of zany questions: "Were you born that way?", "Is there a cure?", "How long will your [sic] live?" As you grow older, you hope that the future world is better than the one you left behind with your childhood (Small, 1998, quoted in Gold, 1998, p. 1).

IMPLICATIONS FOR PROFESSIONAL PRACTICE

Although African American people may share a culture, they are all individuals who have different backgrounds and different experiences and thus have a variety of learning styles. Given this basic concept, this section presents some general recommendations for service providers to keep in mind to be able to provide educational services to African Americans with visual impairments in a way that respects their heritage and does not compound negative stereotypes.

All people have their own values, biases, and prejudices. Therefore, the first step when working with people from a different ethnic group is to become aware of the cultural values, biases, and prejudices that influence one's perspectives, judgments, attitudes, and behaviors, as well as previous experiences with the African American culture (whether personally or via the media). With the history of oppression and racial discrimination in this country, service providers must first get in touch with their individual feelings, values, and biases regarding the African American culture and educating African Americans with visual impairments. Since all people typically interpret others according to similarities and differences in their cultural references, awareness and self-examination are necessary for eliminating unconscious biased behaviors.

The following suggestions provide some guidelines for professionals who work with African American students and clients.

Get to know the African American culture. Ask thoughtful, caring questions that will help you become sensitive to and appreciative of the culture. Show students how you care by asking them or their family members questions that you may have about the culture. Holding cultural fairs, having open class discussions about culture, and inviting multicultural speakers, including African Americans who have visual impairments, to address a class, are ways to enhance cultural understanding.

Do not make assumptions about the abilities of students or clients. It is critical to remember that all people can learn. False assumptions that are due to the lack of or limited experiences with or sensitivity to the African American culture may hamper our perceptions and influence relationships with students or clients. Preconceived notions about the limited abilities of certain students or clients can damage their self-esteem and limit their opportunities.

Refrain from compounding the internalized oppression of African Americans. Because compounding the internal oppression of African Americans often happens on an unconscious level, it is probably the most difficult recommendation to implement. Think about how materials, lectures, and examples are being received by African American students or clients. Are the examples culturally sensitive to them? Are you unconsciously sending messages of superiority or inferiority? For example, telling students to have their mothers sign permission slips implies that all families have mothers who are the primary caregivers. For children who are being raised by grandparents, these assumptions reinforce the feeling that the extended family is not the "acceptable" or "correct" family type.

Defuse feelings of distrust and cynicism first by validating the feelings, then encouraging the open expression of the feelings, and finally by helping students develop a plan of action to deal with the feelings. Given their history in the United States, African Americans often have a deep-seated distrust and cynicism toward institutions. This distrust and cynicism may be demonstrated by destructiveness toward self, family, and/or community, by the failure to keep appointments, and by noncompliance with prescribed regimens. Be prepared to deal with such feelings head on by encouraging open dialogue; enlisting the opinions of leaders in the African American community; and being open minded and flexible, not defensive and inflexible.

Maintain a philosophy of inclusiveness and full integration to cultivate and nurture self-esteem, self-confidence, and self-worth. Recruit personnel from the African American community to work with all aspects of service delivery. To see African Americans as role models and as competent, respected citizens in schools can help build a sense of self-worth among students who are a minority within the minority. The cultural competence of all staff can be enhanced through the resources of staff sharing. Pay attention to the images of African Americans portrayed in books, magazines, brochures, calendars, photographs/pictures, audio tapes, mailings, and other types of information utilized and disseminated by the program. Are the images stereotypes? Are African Americans included? If so, do they represent the diversity among African Americans, their lifestyles, roles, and contributions to American life?

Encourage an atmosphere that is not judgmental and fosters mutual respect between professionals and African American students or clients. By creating an air of mutual respect, one can develop and maintain open communication. Open communication leads to growth and information sharing about expectations, needs, and goals. It can be facilitated by being patient when a person of African American descent is communicating, especially if the person is attempting to translate slang or transition from using slang or a dialect to using standard English. African Americans are often treated as if they are incompetent or receive condescending looks or even resentful remarks if they cannot verbally express their feelings, needs, or desires by demonstrating an effective command of the English language.

Use all available resources, including the black church, which can be an important entrée into the black community. Consider starting an outreach program in the church or enlisting the services of the church to help you identify people who are visually impaired. Religious leaders can be enlisted to support or endorse the implementation of an intervention/treatment plan. The support needed for transportation, socialization, supportive role models, and other resources may develop from connecting and networking within the black church or local religious organizations.

Embrace the resources of kinship groups or the extended family. Strong social support systems, such as kinship groups and extended family systems, distinguish African American families who are able to cope with the stressors associated with having children with visual impairments. The role flexibility within kinship groups provides more opportunities to network with family members and to provide the services that will best meet the special needs of the children and their families. Taking advantage of the wealth of knowledge that extended family members have about the children with visual impairments in the families, such as about postnatal history, limited experiences, and personal likes and dislikes, can assist professionals in providing individualized education or rehabilitation programs.

These suggestions are provided to assist educational and rehabilitation professionals in beginning to address the specific cultural aspects of their work with African American students or clients with visual impairments and their families. They lay the foundation of what is known and provide a glimmer of what needs to be expanded for the effective delivery of services.

CONCLUSION

This chapter has examined the issues faced by many African Americans with visual impairments. It identified religious connectedness and kinship groups and extended families as the two major factors that assist members of the African American family to accept and face the challenges that are often encountered when a family member has a visual impairment. Being a minority within the minority, African Americans with visual impairments continue to experience the double whammy of racism and discrimination because of their visual status. Recommendations have been provided in an attempt to guide professionals as they develop programming that facilitates individual learning needs, cultural awareness/sensitivity, dignity, and independence. Understanding the values, customs and historical perspective of students and clients is the first step to providing effective programs.

REFERENCES

African Americans with albinism. (1996). [On-line]. Available: http://www.albinism.org/publications/

Alston, R. J., & Russo, C. J. (1994). *Brown v. board of education* and the Americans with Disabilities Act: Vistas of equal educational opportunities for African Americans. *Journal of Negro Education, 63,* 349–357.

Alston, R. J., & Turner, W. L. (1994). A family strengths model of adjustment to disability for African American clients. *Journal of Counseling & Development, 72,* 378–383.

Arcia, E., Keyes, L., Gallagher, J. J., & Herrick, H. (1993). National portrait of sociodemographic factors associated with the underutilization of services: Relevance to early intervention. *Journal of Early Intervention, 17,* 283–297.

Billingsley, A. (1974). *Black families and the struggle for survival: Teaching our children to walk tall.* New York: Friendship Press.

Bishop, J. A., & Inderbitzen, H. M. (1996). Peer acceptance and friendship: An investigation of their relation to self-esteem. *Journal of Early Adolescence, 15,* 476–489.

Boyd-Franklin, M. (1989). Five key factors in the treatment of black families. *Journal of Psycho-therapy and the Family, 6,* 53–67.

Dickerson, J. J. (1995). *African American single mothers.* Thousand Oaks, CA: Sage.

Erin, J. N., Rudin, D., & Njoroge, M. (1991). Religious beliefs of parents of children with visual impairments. *Journal of Visual Impairment & Blindness, 85,* 157–162.

Giesen, J. M. and others. (1995). *Participation levels of African Americans in the profession of blindness services: Views of service providers* (ERIC Document Reproduction Service Number ED 391 264).

Gold, M. (1998). *The effects of the physical features associated with albinism on the self-esteem of African American youth with albinism.* Doctoral dissertation, Peabody College, Vanderbilt University, Nashville, TN.

Hale, J. (1982). *Black children: Their roots, culture, and learning styles.* Provo, UT: Brigham Young University Press.

Hanline, M. F. & Daley, S. E. (1991). Family coping strategies and strengths in Hispanic, African-American and Caucasian families of young children. *Topics in Early Childhood Special Education, 12,* 351–366.

Haynes, V. D. (1996, December 20). Ebonics: Schools want black English as 2nd language: California district seeks federal funds for Ebonics. *Chicago Tribune* [On-line]. Available: http://www2.nau.edu/~jmw22/ChicagoTribune122096.html

Jackson, J. J. (1970). Kinship relations among urban black. *Journal of Social Behavioral Sciences,16,* 1–13.

Lacey, M. (1997, January 24). U.S. Senate panel grills officials on Ebonics policy. *Los Angeles Times* [On-line]. Available: http://www2.nau.edu/~jm22/LATimes124.html.

Marshall, S. (1987, October). Fighting for their rights. *Ebony,* pp. 68–70.

Neal, A. M., & Wilson, M. L. (1989). The role of skin color and features in the black community: Implications for black women and therapy. *Clinical Psychology Review, 9,* 323–333.

Ogbu, J. (1990). Beyond language: Ebonics, proper English and identity in a Black-American speech community. *American Educational Research Journal, 36,* 147–184.

Okazawa-Rey,M. Robinson, T. L., & Ward, J. V. (1987). Black women and the politics of skin color and hair. *Women & Therapy, 6,* 89–102.

Orr, A. L. (1998). *Issues in aging and vision: A curriculum for university programs and in-service training.* New York: American Foundation for the Blind.

Porter, C. (1991). Social reasons for skin tone preferences of black school-age children. *Journal of American Orthopsychiatric Association, 61,* 149–154.

Rogers-Dulan, J., & Blacher, J. (1995). African American families, religion, and disability: A conceptual framework. *Mental Retardation, 33,* 226–238.

Seltzer, R., & Smith, R. (1991). Color differences in the Afro-American community and the differences they make. *Journal of Black Studies, 21,* 279–286.

Staples, R. (1985). Changes in black family structure: The conflict between family ideology and structural conditions. *Journal of Marriage and the Family, 47,* 1005–1013.

Tielsch, J. M., Sommer, A., Witt, K., Katz, J., & Royal, R. M. (1990). Blindness and visual impairment in an American urban population: The Baltimore Eye Survey. *Archives of Ophthalmology, 108,* 286–290.

Turner, W. L., & Alston, R. J. (1992). The role of the family in psychosocial adaptation to physical disabilities for African Americans. *Journal of the National Medical Association, 86,* 915–921.

United Way of America (1987). [On-line]. Available: http://www.united way.org

U.S. Bureau of the Census. Projections of the resident population by race, Hispanic origin, and nativity. (2000). [On-line]. Available: http://www. census.gov/population/www/projections/natsum-Ts.html

U.S. Bureau of the Census. (1999, October 4). Poverty 1998 (on-line). Available: http://www.census.gov/hhes/poverty/poverty/98/table5.html

Vander Kolk, C., & Bright, B. (1983). Albinism: A survey of attitudes and behavior. *Journal of Visual Impairment & Blindness, 77,* 49–51.

Vision and hearing. (2000, September 19). Chap. 28 in *Healthy people 2010: Conference edition* (pp. 1–17) [On-line]. Available: http://Web.health.gove/ healthypeople/Document/html/Volume2/28Vision.htm#Toc47205229

CHAPTER 4

Asian Americans and Pacific Islanders with Visual Impairments

Carol Yumiko Love

Patty, a young Asian American college student, strongly identi-
fies with her Asian American community while maintaining contact with her Asian roots. She is sensitive to the changes that are
occuring in Asia, specifically in Hong Kong, as attitudes and the
social structure change to reflect a greater sensitivity to the provision of accommodations for persons with disabilities. Born and
raised in the United States, Patty has a strongly supportive family. Patty represents just one facet of the diverse group of Asian
Americans, particularly in her perspective on having a visual impairment. Patty has congenital left hemianopia. She accesses information via auditory media (tapes, readers) and uses a cane for
mobility purposes.

This chapter presents an overview of information on the diverse
population of Asian Americans and Pacific Islanders, including
background information, family values, and beliefs about health
and disability issues, and includes excerpts from interviews of
individuals with visual impairments and recommendations for
professionals who work with Asian Americans and Pacific
Islanders with visual impairments and their families. In consid-

ering these factors, readers need to keep in mind the ethnic and cultural diversity that exists among and between these various groups. It is hoped that the essences of the traditions and world-views presented here will lead professionals to collaborate and establish working relationships with these families.

DEMOGRAPHICS

Asian Americans and Pacific Islanders are one of the fastest-growing ethnic minority groups in the United States (Chan, 1992; Pang, 1995; U.S. Bureau of the Census, 1999). By 2020 Asian Americans and Pacific Islanders are expected to represent 19.7 million people, 6.1 percent of the total U.S. population (U.S. Bureau of the Census, 1999). Asian Americans and Pacific Islanders encompass a large expanse of land, cultures, nations, and languages and thus constitute a highly diverse ethnic group.

As a population, Asian Americans and Pacific Islanders are ethnically and culturally diverse and include numerous cultural groups with origins in the Asian continent and the Pacific Islands. The continent of Asia is divided into the specific regions of South Asia, Southeast Asia, and East Asia (Epanchin, Towsend, & Stoddard, 1994). South Asia includes Bangladesh, Nepal, Pakistan, and India; Southeast Asia includes Myanmar, Thailand, Laos, Cambodia, Vietnam, the Philippines, Indonesia, Singapore, and Malaysia; and East Asia includes Japan, Korea, Hong Kong, Taiwan, and China. The Pacific Islands region is comprised of thousands of islands, most of which are archipelagos, including Polynesia, Micronesia, the Marshall Islands, the Samoa Islands, and the Mariana Islands; the notable islands are Samoa, Guam, Fiji, Tonga, Tahiti, and Hawaii.

The major groups of Asian Americans and Pacific Islanders in the United States are (from the largest to the smallest) Vietnamese Americans, Chinese Americans, Japanese Americans, Filipino Americans, Asian Indian Americans, and Korean Americans. There are also numerous other smaller groups.

According to the U.S. Bureau of the Census (1998, 1999), about

55 percent of Asian Americans and Pacific Islanders in the United States live in the West, many in metropolitan areas. The states with the largest groups of Asian Americans and Pacific Islanders are (from the largest to the smallest number of residents) California, New York, Hawaii, Texas, New Jersey, Illinois, Washington, Florida, Virginia, and Massachusetts. Six out of 10 Asian Americans and Pacific Islanders were born in foreign countries, notably China, the Philippines, and Vietnam.

The average Asian American and Pacific Islander family has 3.17 persons, compared with 2.58 persons in the average white household. In 1997, there were about 2.2 million Asian American and Pacific Islander families, 80 percent of whom were representing married-couple families. The children in these families (under age 18) were more likely to live with both parents (84 percent) than were the children in non-Hispanic white families (77 percent). In 1997, Asian Americans and Pacific Islanders had the highest proportion of college graduates among persons aged 25 years and older (42 percent), and the median age of Asian Americans was 31 years (U.S. Bureau of the Census, 1999).

Asian Americans and Pacific Islanders had the highest median household income ($43,276) in 1997 (U.S. Bureau of the Census, 1998), probably because of the larger number of workers per family in the workforce and the higher levels of educational attainment, since the incomes of individual family members were not statistically different from those in white households. Among workers aged 16 and older, 38 percent of Asian American and Pacific Islander men and 32 percent of women were employed as professionals (such as engineers, managers, teachers, lawyers, dentists, and reporters). Approximately 603,426 businesses were owned by Asian Americans and Pacific Islanders in 1997, mainly Chinese, Koreans, and Asian Indians.

HISTORICAL BACKGROUND

The major ethnic groups of Asian Americans and Pacific Islanders immigrated to the United States primarily for economic opportunity, higher education, family reunification, and a higher standard of living and because of political turmoil in their native countries (Chung, 1996). The order of immigration of these groups (from the past to the most recent) is as follows: Hawaiians, Chinese, Japanese, Korean, Filipinos, Asian Indians, Vietnamese, and other Southeast Asians (Akamatsu, 1993). Many Pacific Islanders, Chinese, Japanese, Asian Indians, and Koreans came to the United States to find better-paying jobs, advance more quickly up the economic ladder, and gain economic security. Many Southeast Asians, Vietnamese, Laotians, Cambodians, and Hmong came primarily because of political turmoil in their native countries and have gained more political stability, greater economic security, and greater freedom than in their homelands. After settling in the United States, individuals or families may undertake a second migration to different states because of such factors as "better jobs, family reunification, familiar climate, and well-established [Asian] communities" (Chung, 1996, p. 78).

Hawaii

In the late 1800s, many Japanese, Filipinos, Koreans, and Chinese immigrated to Hawaii to work on the sugar cane plantations (Takaki, 1994). Because of the harsh conditions on these plantations, some laborers worked on them only until their contractual agreements were fulfilled or broke their labor contracts (Takaki, 1994); these laborers typically left for another island of Hawaii or for California. Even with the demands of the plantation labor camps, the number of Asian immigrants was significant, and many stayed in Hawaii (Takaki, 1994).

Pacific Islanders

Pacific Islanders include Polynesians, Micronesians, and Melanesians, and Polynesians include Hawaiians, Samoans, Tongans, and Tahitians (U.S. Department of Commerce, 1993). Micronesians include the large group of Guamanians, also known as Chamorros, and Melanesians are mainly from Fiji. One of the main reasons for Pacific Islander immigration is the pursuit of higher education (U.S. Census Bureau, 1999). Approximately one-third are employed in such jobs as sales, technical, and administrative support. Additionally, this ethnic group is well represented in a variety of positions in the labor market (from managerial and professional to laborers). Pacific Islanders did not "technically" immigrate to the United States. In the 1800s and 1900s, the United States enforced colonial expansion (conquest of the Philippines and annexation of Hawaii in 1898). Many of the early Pacific Islanders were farm laborers (Arkamatsu, 1993).

Chinese

Chinese immigration to the United States occurred during a time of great economic opportunity—the California gold rush—and simultaneous political, social, and economic unrest in China about 1849 (Nakanishi & Rittner, 1996). This group of immigrants traditionally formed strong ethnic communities or enclaves, such as Chinatowns, wherever they lived. The Chinese Exclusion Act of 1882, which specifically blocked the immigration of Chinese persons, was enacted because of the shortage of work for the U.S. citizen labor force. As economic competition grew, Chinese laborers were willing to accept lower wages. The act was renewed until 1943 (Wong & Chang, 1992). Chinese immigrants have worked in a variety of jobs, including farm laborers, restaurant workers and owners, laundry workers and owners, and business owners. The increased Chinese immigration in early 1990 was the result of the reversion of Hong Kong to Chinese sovereignty (from British). The new immigrants tend to be either unskilled laborers or upper-middle class professionals (with not much range in between) (Chan, 1992).

Japanese

In the late 1800s, Japanese first came to Hawaii as plantation laborers (Takaki, 1995). Later, they went to California, where they worked in canneries, as farm laborers, and railroad workers. During World War II, President Franklin D. Roosevelt signed Executive Order 9066, which forced persons of Japanese ancestry into relocation camps as potential security risks and deprived them of equal protection under the law, along with their rights of due process (Takaki, 1995). At that time, Japanese lost property, businesses, and other possessions. By the end of WWII, many of the internment camps were closed, but the official closure by the U.S. government came in 1974 (Chan, 1992). The Civil Liberties Act of 1988 provided a formal apology for Executive Order 9066, and in October 1990, survivors began receiving redress monies (Chan 1992). Today, the Japanese people represent a wide range of the general labor force, with the highest per capita income among Asian American groups (U.S. Bureau of the Census, 1999). Japanese immigration has decreased over the years in large part because of the need for labor and economic expansion of post-WWII Japan (Takaki, 1995).

Koreans

Koreans immigrated to Hawaii, along with many other Asian ethnic groups who were recruited to work on plantations. They fled their country for economic reasons and because of the occupation by Japan in the early 1900s (Nakanishi & Rittner, 1996). Many Korean women were often "war brides," who came to live in the United States following World War II and the Korean War. Among Asian American groups, they have the highest rate of self-employment (Chan, 1992). Many are owners of small businesses (e.g., convenience stores, markets, manicure salons, and gas stations).

Filipinos

Initially, Filipinos were recruited in the early 1900s to work on plantations in Hawaii (Nakanishi & Rittner, 1996; Takaki, 1994). Plantation life was arduous, and the Filipinos faced open discrimination. During World War II, many Filipinos enlisted in and supported the U.S. war effort. Filipino women also came to the United States after World War II as war brides. Many of these immigrants are well-educated people who are seeking higher wages in the United States. Many immigrants in the healthcare profession (e.g., doctors, pharmacists) face difficulties in obtaining U.S. licenses because of strict regulations. Many Filipinos are turning to self-employment.

Asian Indians

In the early 1900s, Asian Indians immigrated to Washington State to work in the lumber mills or railways and to California to work on farms (Takaki, 1995). They did not form tightly knit ethnic communities while in the United States (Takaki, 1995). With the change in quota regulations after the 1965 Immigration Act, greater numbers of immigrants from southern Asia began to appear. Initially, many immigrants were farm laborers. The new immigrants are highly educated people from cities. Asian Indians, especially Pakistanis, are highly visible, and many are entrepreneurs (Takaki, 1995).

Southeast Asians

Ethnic groups that have immigrated to the United States from Southeast Asia include Vietnamese, Laotians, Cambodians, Hmong, and ethnic Chinese (Chung, 1996). Many of these immigrants were refugees who fled their native countries because of political repression, war, and economic upheavals in the 1970s. Large Southeast Asian groups can be found in California, New York, Washington, and Minnesota (Takaki, 1995). This ethnic group is extremely heterogeneous and represents a wide range of professions, from unskilled to highly skilled professionals (Chan, 1992).

Vietnamese

The Vietnamese are the largest group of Southeast Asians to immigrate to the United States. Vietnam was controlled by China for hundreds of years, but in the late 1800s, it and much of the rest of Southeast Asia became a French colony. From 1940 to 1945, Japan occupied Vietnam. In 1954, the French withdrew their control over Vietnam, and it was partitioned into North Vietnam and South Vietnam. In 1961, the United States began actively supporting South Vietnamese anti-Communist forces in their civil war against the North Vietnamese. By the time the United States withdrew its last advisors in 1975, a generation of Vietnamese had grown up with a U.S. influence. Near the end of its involvement, the U.S. government helped thousands of Vietnamese refugees immigrate to the United States. This war also involved Laos and Cambodia, resulting in similar immigration of refugees from these countries. After 20 years of war, Vietnam was officially unified in 1976.

Two waves of Vietnamese refugees fled to the United States. The first wave occurred from 1975 until 1977, after the fall of Saigon at the end of the Vietnam War. The first wave of refugees were members of an elite class who had some command of English and/or French, were well educated, and had been exposed to Western or urban culture. The U.S. government supported these immigrants with sea- and airlifts out of Saigon. The second wave of refugees, who came between 1978 and 1980, differed from the first in that they were of agrarian background, had little command of English, and were not well educated.

LAOTIANS

During the political turmoil of the Vietnam War, many Laotians fled their country to Thailand. The Thai government forced these refugees into camps with substandard living conditions (Chung, 1996). In about 1986, the Thai government allowed refugees to immigrate to the United States.

CAMBODIANS

Cambodia may be the oldest of the Southeast Asian countries (Chung, 1996). It remained relatively unchanged for thousands of years, until the first century C.E. (Chung, 1996). At that time, there was a strong Indian influence in religion and the society. After the late 1800s, Cambodia came under French rule and remained a French colony until 1953. Cambodians fled their country in three waves as refugees. The first wave of refugees, who came to the United States about 1975, consisted of governmental officials and well-educated professionals. The second wave fled about 1978, when Vietnam invaded Cambodia. The third wave, who came about a year later, included governmental personnel, rural dwellers, and well-educated persons.

HMONG

The Hmong, who have their ancestral roots in Siberia, eventually immigrated to China. Persecuted by the Chinese for not conforming to the Chinese way of life, the Hmong were forced to become migratory for many years. They eventually settled in the mountainous regions of Southeast Asia, where, isolated for several generations, they built and strengthened their ethnic community (Chung, 1996). In the 1970s, many Hmong refugees fled to the United States because of political turmoil in Southeast Asia.

FAMILY VALUES AND BELIEFS

Given the many differences among the groups of Asian Americans and Pacific Islanders, there is also a wide variation in the values and beliefs of families who belong to these cultural and ethnic groups. Family values and beliefs may be influenced by such factors as country of origin, length of residence in the United States, religious background, and socioeconomic status (Pang, 1995).

Typically, in Asian American and Pacific Islander families, there are strict roles that define each family member (Chung, 1996). Some Asian American and Pacific Islander families, such as the Japanese, Chinese, Filipino, and Koreans, usually follow a patrilineal hierarchy (Chung, 1996; Nakanishi & Rittner, 1996). In the immediate family unit, consisting of a father, a mother, and children, the father is usually in charge of the household, as the bread-winner, ultimate decision maker, and disciplinarian. The mother may be engaged primarily in child rearing and negotiating relationships among family members, and the children are expected to be obedient to the mother and father. Multiple generations may live within a household or in close proximity. Age often plays an important role, with greater status designated to elderly family members. The higher the person's status in the family, the greater the input on decision making and advice (Chung, 1996).

In line with the patrilineal hierarchy is the importance accorded to male heirs and lineage (Chung, 1996). Sons are often considered to have a higher status than daughters and to be responsible for caring for their aging parents.

Other Asian American and Pacific Islander families, such as Vietnamese and Laotians, may follow a matriarchal hierarchy. Still other ethnic groups may follow a hierarchy ordained by a community or village. Yet another system of family organization may be a collective society, in which the organization is attributed to social status of the family within the community (Chung, 1996).

The family is considered more important than the individual in general. Individuals make personal sacrifices to protect and defend their families' honor (Nakanishi & Rittner, 1996). The roles of family members are strictly defined, and members usually include aunts, uncles, grandparents.

Important family decisions may be made by significant family members, family members and a religious leader, or family members and a significant community leader. Besides the issue of who is involved in the decision-making process, another crucial factor is who makes the final decision.

Many Asian American and Pacific Islander families place great value on and emphasize academic achievement, socioeconomic status, and household income (Nakanishi & Rittner, 1996). These values can cause conflict for children, who experience the pressures of having to succeed in any task they attempt and feel frustrated when they fail. Asian American parents also put pressure on their children to "get along with others, to be sensitive and considerate of others, to reciprocate favors, to be circumspect about criticisms, and to avoid behaviors which could be interpreted as hostile or aggressive" (Nakanishi & Rittner, 1996, p. 95). These types of expectations had an effect on Tommy, a Vietnamese boy who was visually impaired:

Tommy, a 14 year old who is visually impaired as result of nystagmus and myopia, immigrated with his family from Vietnam when he was 12. He recently considered joining a Vietnamese gang because his friends are members, he wants to gain a sense of kinship with persons of similar ethnic background, and he feels misunderstood by the "white culture" and his parents. Tommy stated that he does not enjoy school and has difficulty with reading and math activities. He has been prescribed eyeglasses, but prefers not to wear them because he thinks they make him look "dumb." He added that he may have a "learning problem."

Tommy believes that his teachers and his parents place "lots of importance on academics, like getting all A's, staying in school. School is hard, and I don't see why I need it. My one friend has a lot of money, and he only went up to the fifth grade. People have the idea that Asians are supposed to be smart. That hurts me when I get bad grades and stuff."

According to Tommy, his teachers and parents set high standards for him academically, socially, and morally. When he does not achieve these high standards, he is chastised or punished. He refers to himself as an "outcast" or a "rebel" and feels a kinship with friends he has made in a local Vietnamese gang. Many of these gang members share similar views with Tommy about failure. In addition, Tommy has not been given career guidance or counseling and does not know what he would like to do with his life.

Some Asian American and Pacific Islander families consider it important for their children to learn cultural customs, traditions, and beliefs, so the children can observe them and pass them on to their children (Nakanishi & Rittner, 1996). When children are young, family members instill in them the significance of heritage, language, and moral values. As the children grow older, the family's influence may lessen and outside influences may have a greater impact.

The major religions observed by Asian Americans and Pacific Islanders are Confucianism, Taoism, and Buddhism (Cheng, 1995; Chung, 1996). Other religions include Christianity, Islam, and Hinduism. Confucianism teaches the importance of a defined social class system, the family, and education (Spector, 1996). Taoism teaches the importance of allowing life to balance itself and for the individual not to interfere with this balance (Cheng, 1995). Buddhism stresses the importance of the cycles of life and for the soul to work through these cycles to reach Nirvana (Nakanishi & Rittner, 1996). Many of these religious beliefs place more emphasis on spirituality than on the acquisition of material possessions. Other qualities that are stressed are patience, humility, selflessness, and self-discipline (Nakanishi & Rittner, 1996; Spector, 1996).

In addition, some Asian American and Pacific Islander families may practice ancestor worship by making special offerings and performing rituals in homage to their ancestors (Chung, 1996). In this practice, emphasis is placed on the link between persons who are living and those who have passed on to the afterlife.

In sum, Asian Americans and Pacific Islanders traditionally view their families as the foundation for developing their value and belief systems. From birth, their children are brought up to revere, respect, and honor their families (Chung, 1996), who often include mothers and fathers, as well as extended family members and/or members of a cultural community. To work effectively with Asian American or Pacific Islander families, it is essential for professionals to respect and pay attention to these values. The following suggestions will help establish effective communication paths for supportive relationships (Hyun & Fowler, 1995; Pang, 1997):

- Discuss with the family members who would be a good interpreter, since personal matters may be discussed during meetings. The interpreter should be proficient in the family's primary language and in the professional's language, sensitive to the family's culture, and aware that the content of the meeting is confidential. Sometimes the family may ask a leader from the cultural community to be the interpreter. (Selecting appropriate translators is discussed in more detail later in this chapter.)
- Determine who is the primary caregiver in the family. This person will most likely become the link for items that require follow-through at home. Making several observational visits in the home or asking about daily routines (such as eating and sleeping patterns) can help determine the family member who is the primary caregiver.
- Determine who is the decision maker in the family. It is important to obtain the cooperation of the decision maker to facilitate meeting the goals and objectives for the student or client.
- Discuss the time and location of each meeting with the family.
- Discuss with the family who will be attending each meeting. In doing so, encourage the parents to invite persons who would help support them: friends, religious or community leaders, or other relatives.
- Ask the family if they have any transportation concerns or if they need child care to attend a meeting.
- Address family members by their titles and surnames (e.g., Mr. Hwang, or Miss Chen), not by their first names.
- Obtain clarification from parents or family members regularly.
- Develop and use good listening skills.

◆ Avoid direct eye contact.

◆ Avoid touching objects in the family's home. Some items may be considered sacred or part of religious custom.

◆ Learn and use simple words in the family's primary language.

◆ Asian American or Pacific Islander students, often labeled by others as the "model minority," may feel pressure from family members or teachers to excel academically. Expectations from others may be unrealistic or not compatible with an individual student's actual achievement level or personal expectations. It is important for the professional to be aware of this family dynamic and to be sensitive in their explanations to parents about a student's progress.

◆ Have all written communications translated into the family's primary language before they are sent to a student's or client's home.

◆ Some families may need information provided verbally, rather than in writing. Ask each family whether this is the case for him or her.

◆ Do not assume that because family members do not display a great deal of outward emotion they do not care about their child's or family member's needs or do not have concerns about or expectations for their child or other family member. Some Asian Americans or Pacific Islanders may be shy and sit quietly and may not readily respond to questions asked by professionals. Furthermore, in some cultures, the professional is seen as an authority figure, and it may be unheard of to question, discuss, or disagree with an authority figure.

The key to understanding family dynamics and logistics is often to establish cross-cultural communication with the family. That is, the professional must carefully observe and listen to family members and answer their questions before he or she asks them questions for further clarification.

BELIEFS ABOUT HEALTH AND DISABILITY

Asian Americans and Pacific Islanders adhere to a variety of philosophies to explain the causes of diseases or other conditions. In some of these philosophies, the focus is on the environment or nature, which is often given humanlike qualities, such as breathing, feeling, seeing, and having a spirit. Furthermore, harmony between nature and the body is respected and even revered, and the presence of a disease or condition is considered to upset this harmony or balance (Spector, 1996). In other philosophies, the physical manifestations of diseases or disabling conditions are viewed as signs of fate or Karma (Chung, 1996). Yet another view is that illness is a result of misdeeds or acts the person has committed against nature or another person. However, belief in these traditional views of the cause of diseases or disabilities does not mean that Western medicine is shunned. In large concentrated clusters of ethnic communities (e.g., Chinatown, Little Tokyo) many traditional practitioners coexist, literally next door, with highly trained Western practitioners. Dialogue between these two types of practitioners will enhance the services provided by each and should be encouraged. The following section explains some traditional views of healing and disability held by Asian Americans and Pacific Islanders.

Healing

Some Asian American and Pacific Islander families may utilize one or more traditional methods of dealing with health and disability issues. It is important to remember that not all families of this population deal with these issues in the same way. For some families, length of residence in the United States may be an important factor in determining how they will respond to treatment and other services (Hyun & Fowler, 1995; Pang, 1995).

One traditional method of healing is wearing or carrying amulets or charms, which may contain pictographs, words, or letters to ward off evil spirits or may be made of a particular material that imparts magical powers to its owner (Chung, 1996; Spector, 1996). Some Asian Americans and Pacific Islanders believe that inanimate objects, such as amulets, as well as animate objects, have a soul or spirit. Amulets may be Chinese or Japanese characters painted on strips of paper that are then worn, hung over a doorway, or carried in a purse. Chinese jade is sometimes carved into charms that are worn to provide health, good luck, and safety. Cambodians, Laotians, and Hmong children may wear strings that have been tied with special prayer knots; these strings are seen as the link between the person and his or her ancestors.

Other traditional methods of healing are the following (Chung, 1996; Spector, 1996):

- A healer—a person who is trained to use a specific healing technique or method—may be called in.
- Moxibustion, which may be practiced by Southeast Asians, is the use of special suction cups and heat on various parts of the body to draw out toxins from the body.
- Acupuncture, practiced by Chinese or Japanese people, is the use of special needles placed on particular points of the body for healing.
- A special diet, consisting of certain foods or combination of foods, may be prescribed for person who is sick.
- Specific herbs may be used in the diet for medicinal purposes; expert herbalists are common in the Chinese culture.
- Massage may be used by a trained expert to apply pressure to a part of the body that needs healing.
- Prayers may be offered by a variety of religious experts (mainly Christian or Buddhist) to promote healing.
- Offerings at shrines may be made in different forms by a family or family member to promote healing.

Attitudes Toward Disability

Attitudes toward persons with disabilities, including visual impairment, are extremely varied among Asian Americans and Pacific Islanders. Some groups view a congenital disability or birth defect as a sign that the mother, while pregnant, committed an offense against family members, others, or ancestors (Chung, 1996). Others may believe that such disabilities are caused by the pregnant woman eating certain foods or failing to avoid certain circumstances. As a result, many groups consider pregnancy as a time of caution, prevention, and safety for women. Traditionally, since many groups viewed birth defects as shameful, family members did not discuss this topic.

Some Asian Americans and Pacific Islanders hold specific culturally stereotypic beliefs about persons who are blind or visually impaired.

The following example of Lisa and her parents shows how such traditional views may be altered:

Lisa, a 5 year old who is totally blind as a result of retinopathy of prematurity, was born in the United States. Her parents immigrated to the United States from Taiwan seven years ago to pursue graduate degrees at a local university. Lisa attends kindergarten at a local school for blind students. Lisa's parents moved to this area so Lisa could attend this school and receive specialized services in braille. Her parents were initially unsure of what expectations they should have for Lisa's future, as well as for the present. They want her to attend a private school for the remainder of her schooling and to have specialized services provided by an itinerant teacher of students with visual impairments. They stated: "Since immigrating to the United States and having Lisa, who has a vision problem, our views of persons with disabilities has really changed. Our parents were very upset about Lisa's condition, but now they see how she can become independent and receive much help from the specialized training at the school for the blind. They are more optimistic. We are more optimistic about her future and want the best for her."

Lisa's parents and relatives' more positive outlook is due to influences in their community, their length of residence in the United States, and their adoption of Western customs and values.

The belief that certain jobs are specifically "tailored" for persons with visual impairments may be yet another cultural stereotype held by Asian Americans and Pacific Islanders. For example, some persons from Japan and Korea believe that only a person who is blind can be a masseur or masseuse on the assumption that the senses other than sight are enhanced in persons who are blind. In Thailand, persons who are blind or visually impaired are vendors of lottery tickets because it is thought that they bring good luck to the buyers (P. Sumranveth, teacher of students with visual impairments, personal communication, October 10, 1997).

As with illness, some Asian Americans and Pacific Islanders believe that disability is a result of the person's own misdeeds, as in the following example:

Melinda, age 35, who is totally blind as a result of glaucoma, immigrated to the United States from the Philippines six years ago. When she first arrived in the United States, Melinda lived with a relative largely because she was unsure of how to earn a living in her new home. She did not realize that this relative would treat her so differently from her upbringing and lifestyle by preventing her from acting independently. A friend of this relative, who was also Filipino, told Melinda, "No matter how many showers you take, you'll still be dirty." Melinda interpreted this statement to mean that this friend believed that her blindness was the result of some irreparable offense she had committed. She quickly realized the importance of moving out and living on her own.

Other Asian Americans and Pacific Islanders may have more positive attitudes toward persons with disabilities.

Melinda says that her mother, a social worker in the Philippines who had experience working with persons who were blind or visually impaired, has been a major influence in her life. Her mother has required Melinda to have the same responsibilities and expectations for independence as her other children. As an adult, Melinda has been actively involved in organizations for persons who are blind. When she was still in the Philippines, she was appointed by the government to represent the blind women's organization and attend a conference in the United States.

Additional factors that typically affect attitudes toward persons who are blind or visually impaired are the type of visual impairment, prognosis of the medical condition, amount of remaining vision, age of onset, and family support (Tuttle & Tuttle, 1996). These factors should also be considered by professionals who work with family members of Asian Americans or Pacific Islanders who are blind or visually impaired. In the following example, a woman is faced with emerging family conflict (son's diagnosis) as well as realistic expectations (daughter's expectations).

Augustine, aged 56, was born and raised in the United States. Her ethnic background is Hawaiian and Swedish. Augustine believes that her family's difficulty in dealing with her visual impairment is not due to cultural or familial beliefs. Her son has difficulty talking to her about aspects of her visual impairment because he was recently diagnosed with the same condition. In contrast, her daughter is "very hard on me. That's actually been the best thing. She expects me to do things for myself."

Many factors contribute to a greater awareness of and sensitivity toward persons with disabilities in families. Some change-inducing factors may include familial attitudes, exposure to other cultural ideas, exchange of information with other service providers, and exposure to real-life situations that support positive outcomes (Ratliff, 1996).

Implications for Professionals

It is important for professionals who work with Asian American or Pacific Islander students or clients with visual impairments to develop an understanding of the families' beliefs about disability by conducting many observations of or informal interviews with various family members. Family members may have varying levels of understanding of service delivery processes like the setting of goals and objectives for a student's Individualized Education Program, depending on their participation and the types of barriers they have encountered along the way. It is important for the professional to prepare families by sharing prior information, especially before meetings (e.g., annual review, initial assessment) or special events (Hyun & Fowler, 1995).

Developing an understanding of how the family views illness or disability (by collecting personal information from various family members) will help to provide a foundation on which the professional can decide how to better relate information on goals and objectives for the child/family member who has a disability. In setting up a plan for working with a student or client who is blind or visually impaired, the professional needs to keep in mind the suggestions for establishing effective communication with Asian American and Pacific Islander families. In addition, the following suggestions will help the professional take a family's attitudes toward disability into consideration when establishing goals and objectives for the visually impaired individual:

- ◆ Goals and objectives should be discussed and developed with family members, as well as with the student or client, when appropriate, to ensure that outcomes are culturally acceptable.
- ◆ Goals and objectives should be written in "clear nonintrusive language" (Hyun & Fowler, 1995, p. 27) and should be in the family's primary language. Words and phrases used in the goals and objectives should be understood and used by family members.
- ◆ Goals and objectives may have to be reviewed and dis-

cussed frequently in informal meetings with family members. It is important to reevaluate goals and objectives when they are not being followed by family members, since family members may not consider particular goals or objectives to be important. At the initial meeting, family members may not have voiced their concerns about the goals and objectives out of respect for the professional.

Professionals should also note:

- Goals and objectives established in the school setting may not necessarily be carried over to the home setting. For example, the teacher may expect the student to speak up and ask many questions. This behavior may not be viewed as important or appropriate in the home.
- In teaching the student or client specific behaviors may have to be explicitly modeled, for example, teaching the individual how to respond when asked, "How are you?" or explaining what it means if someone says, "Excuse me."
- Explaining and modeling specific follow-through routines and practices in the home may also be necessary. (Hyun & Fowler, 1995). For example, the term *self-feeding* may have a variety of meanings, so the professional will have to determine (with family members) how and when this will be conducted—meal times? snack times? with finger foods? and so on.

For goals and objectives to be implemented, it may take several observations of the family's daily home routines and informal interviews with family members. The professional should be flexible and work toward helping family members understand the goals or objectives.

OTHER ISSUES FOR PROFESSIONALS

For work with Asian American and Pacific Islander families whose children have visual impairments, professionals and researchers have made some basic suggestions to help support and empower the families. Just as no two families are alike, there are widely diverse characteristics among Asian American and Pacific Islander families. Factors that may influence familial beliefs and how members respond to their children with visual impairments include the length of residence in the United States, educational level, beliefs about persons who have disabilities, association with their own ethnic communities, religion, socio-economic status, ways of dealing with health issues, and attitudes toward child rearing (Hyun & Fowler, 1995; Pang, 1995). The greater the length of residence in the United States, the greater the chances that the family has been exposed to Western influences on their ideals, concerns, and ways of dealing with issues.

Ethical Issues

Ratliff (1996) discussed ethical concerns that may surface when working with families from diverse cultures. Although Ratliff discussed these concerns specifically in relation to the health care professions, concerns will surface in a variety of situations in which there are cultural differences between families and professionals. These ethical concerns include informed consent, paternalism, issues of care, and respect.

Informed consent means that people who agree to treatment have received accurate, specific information about their diseases or conditions and various alternative forms of treatment and their side effects and benefits. It can include the provision of directions for medication dosages, information on conditions, and descriptions of procedures in the person's preferred language.

A professional's paternalistic attitude toward persons of different cultures is often manifest as benevolence, the provision of scanty or no information, or the failure to provide information in the client's or student's primary language because the professional knows what is best for the client or student. A professional with a paternalistic attitude believes that only the dominant culture is important or valid and minimizes the importance of supporting people from other cultures. One can see how paternalism is often closely linked to issues of informed consent. The professional may not actively seek alternative methods for conveying information to the individual, such as having material translated or providing an interpreter. In addition, the traditional values held by some Asian Americans and Pacific Islanders of respect for elders or professionals may reinforce the paternalistic attitudes of professionals.

Issues of care include access and quality. It is important for persons from diverse cultures to have access to high-quality services on a variety of levels. Points to consider are the geographic location of a professional office, the time of day when services are provided, and the child care needs of the family during office hours. Furthermore, some professionals chastise family members when they seek services "too late." Care must be taken to provide high-quality services to family members at the time they ask for assistance, not to blame them for waiting until the conditions are advanced.

The last ethical issue is respect. Respect involves traveling the two-way street of education. That is, for services to be provided respectfully, the professional must be open to learning about the family's culture and respecting the family's decisions, even if those decisions do not conform to the professional's recommendations. The professional also needs to give the family time and practice to learn about the dominant culture and how services provided by professionals can parallel the family's viewpoints.

Key strategies that may help professionals develop a sensitive awareness of and enhance their work with families include the following:

- ◆ View each family as unique (Hyun & Fowler, 1995). Families are as heterogeneous within ethnic or cultural groups as are other groups. What works for one family may not work for another.
- ◆ Become a lifelong learner about your own culture and other

cultures (Hyun & Fowler, 1995). The path to learning about a culture is long and involves a variety of learning tools, including interviewing people of other cultures, watching videotapes or films, attending conferences, reading articles or books; and participating in cultural activities.

◆ Explore your own attitudes and beliefs about another culture by asking yourself: "When I was growing up, what did my family say about people from different cultures?" (Hyun & Fowler, 1995, p. 26). Myths about a particular cultural group may surface, and the exploration of these myths will be meaningful.

An important consideration in working with Asian Americans and Pacific Islanders is the myth of the "model minority" (Chun, 1995; Pang, 1995; Takaki, 1989). Although many Asian Americans and Pacific Islanders have been successful in education and business, some have not. This stereotype can be a particular problem for students who do not succeed, who do not understand the connection between education and advancement in the United States, and who rebel against authority.

Communication Issues

As was noted earlier, communication is a crucial element in working with families from culturally diverse backgrounds. Modes of communication by some Asian Americans and Pacific Islanders may include nonverbal cueing and the use of silence (Hyun & Fowler, 1995; Spector, 1996). Nonverbal cueing includes the avoidance of eye contact as a sign of respect, especially toward elders and professionals. Silence may also be a method of conveying respect, especially when used while listening to a speaker, or may convey disagreement, particularly when it occurs abruptly during an active verbal exchange. Gender may also be an issue, since some cultures believe that confidential information should be shared only between persons of the same gender (Chung, 1996).

Along with communication is the need to select appropriate interpreters. Interpreters should be selected on the basis of proficiency in the family's language and sensitivity to the needs of the family (Chung, 1996; Hyun & Fowler, 1995). Family members may feel uncomfortable with an interpreter who is insensitive to their cultural customs or who does not command their respect. Selecting and working with an appropriate interpreter can be difficult, however, because of the variety of dialects and languages spoken by Asian Americans and Pacific Islanders. Although children in Asian American and Pacific Islander families are often bilingual, speaking both English and their home languages, it is not appropriate to use them as interpreters for other family members (Chung, 1996).

Information on proficient bilingual translators can be obtained from a variety of sources (including churches, organizations in ethnic communities, administrative offices of school districts, family members, and the Internet). Be prepared to have a list of questions ready for the interpreter on the specific needs and demands of the task at hand. Also, ensure that the translator provides references and follow up by interviewing these references or others who have used the particular translator's services (Ratliff, 1996).

As was mentioned earlier, a number of practices help to ensure smooth communication with families (Hyun & Fowler, 1995; Spector, 1996):

- ◆ Have all written communication translated in the home language.
- ◆ Ask family members how they would prefer to be addressed. Some people prefer to be addressed only by their titles and surnames.
- ◆ Learn spoken greetings or key words in the home language to use with family members.
- ◆ Ask about the family's daily routines to ensure that services are scheduled at a convenient time for the family.
- ◆ Be patient.

- Implement changes that parallel positive family beliefs and practices.
- Periodically check on the family's understanding of its expectations for the child's progress or problems and concerns members may have—on an ongoing basis. Do not wait for a crisis to occur.

Preparation is the key to alleviating many problems that may prove to be hazardous to a professional's future working relationship with a family. Hyun and Fowler (1996) stressed the importance of including the family in planning critical elements to be included in a meeting before it is held. At that time, family members should be encouraged to express their opinions about the environment in which the meeting is to be held, time to hold the meeting, their child care needs during the meeting, persons to invite who offer support to the family, the number of persons that will be present at the meeting, and who the decision maker of the family is (Hyun & Fowler, 1996).

Educational Issues

Asian American or Pacific Islander cultures may have different attitudes toward education than does the mainstream culture. It is important for professionals to understand these differences so they do not misinterpret the students' behavior. Cheng (1995, cited in Pang, 1997) explained some Asian American and Pacific Islander values toward education this way:

- School and teachers are treated with formality. Thus, students will address their teachers and other professionals formally (such as Mr. Smith or Miss Lee) and will not use the professionals' first names when invited to do so.
- Teachers are treated as authority figures who are to be obeyed and respected. Students may not question, discuss, or argue with teachers, even if they believe the teachers are incorrect. Students must obey any request or command

made by their teachers, even at the expense of their personal value systems.

♦ Students may be expected "not to make waves" and to be cooperative. A student may hold some or all of the following beliefs: Do not call attention to oneself, do what the teacher says, get along with and help others, let others be first, and do not show off in front of the class.

♦ For some Asian American or Pacific Islanders, cooperation may mean sharing answers with others. This practice can cause conflicts with teachers who expect individual achievement and work.

♦ Some students are able to provide rote knowledge and facts, but have difficulty analyzing, applying, or synthesizing information.

♦ Some Asian American or Pacific Islander parents may view homework as a must. They believe that teachers who do not require homework are not doing a good job educating their children.

♦ Some Asian American or Pacific Islander students are expected to be obedient and compliant. Therefore, when they engage in rebellious behavior, teachers may be shocked and not know how to react.

♦ A stereotype that some teachers may have about Asian American and Pacific Islander students is that they do well in technical or scientific fields, such as mathematics. This stereotype may be compounded by the fact that some Asian American or Pacific Islander students are attracted to science or math because these subjects deal mainly with abstract ideas. In language-related courses, such as English or creative writing, students are required to express their personal feelings or thoughts, which can produce high levels of anxiety for some.

♦ Some Asian American or Pacific Islander parents may think that "elective courses" are irrelevant to their children's education. They may also not approve of or understand such ideals as exploration of self-esteem, independence, and creativity. In these cases, students may be advised to explain to parents why they are taking elective courses. Reasons might include "Because I am interested in learning more about a particular profession or vocation." Students can also conduct job search reports that are shared with parents as a rationale for taking the elective courses.

CONCLUSION

Although a laundry list of suggestions and tips can help professionals work with families from culturally diverse backgrounds, it is important to remember that no two families are alike. While one strategy may be effective with a particular family, it may prove disastrous with another. Therefore, flexibility and respect for a family's cultural values are a must. As Hyun and Fowler (1995, p. 28) emphasized: "Enthusiasm, openness, and willingness are the most important characteristics that support [a] meaningful partnership between professionals and culturally diverse families."

REFERENCES

Akamatsu, C. T. (1993). Teaching deaf Asian and Pacific Island American children. In K. M. Christensen & G. L. Delgado (Eds.), *Multicultural issues in deafness* (pp. 127–142). New York: Longman.

Chan, S. (1992). Families with Asian roots. In E. W. Lynch & M. J. Hanson (Eds.), *Developing cross-cultural competence: A guide for working with young children and their families* (pp. 181–257). Baltimore, MD: Paul H. Brookes.

Cheng, L. L. (1995). Service delivery to Asian/Pacific LEP children: A cross-cultural framework. In D. T. Nakanishi & T. Y. Nishida (Eds.), *The Asian American educational experience: A source book for teachers and students* (pp. 212–220). New York: Routledge.

Chun, K. (1995). The myth of Asian American success and its educational ramifications. In D. T. Nakanishi & T. Y. Nishida (Eds.), *The Asian American educational experience: A source book for teachers and students* (pp. 95–112). New York: Routledge.

Chung, E. L. (1996). Asian Americans. In M. C. Julia, *Multicultural awareness in the health care professions* (pp. 77–110). Boston: Allyn & Bacon.

Epanchin, B. C., Townsend, B., & Stoddard, K. (1994). *Constructive classroom management: Strategies for creating positive learning environments.* Pacific Grove, CA: Brooks/Cole.

Hyun, J. K., & Fowler, S. A. (1995). Respect, cultural sensitivity, and communication. *Teaching Exceptional Children, 28*(1), 25–28.

Nakanishi, M., & Rittner, B. (1996). Social work practice with Asian Americans. In D. F. Harrison, B. A. Thyer, & J. S. Wodarski (Eds.), *Cultural diversity and social work practice* (pp. 87–111). Springfield, IL: Charles C Thomas.

Pang, V. O. (1995). Asian American children: A diverse population. In D. T. Nakanishi & T. Y. Nishida (Eds.), *The Asian American educational experience: A source book for teachers and students* (pp. 167–179). New York: Routledge.

Pang, V. O. (1997). Caring for the whole child: Asian Pacific American students. In J. J. Irvine (Ed.), *Critical knowledge for diverse teachers and learners* (pp. 149–188). Washington, DC: American Association of Colleges for Teacher Education.

Ratliff, S. S. (1996). The multicultural challenge to health care. In M. C. Julia, *Multicultural awareness in the health care professions* (pp. 164–181). Boston: Allyn & Bacon.

Spector, R. E. (1996). *Cultural diversity in health and illness* (4th ed.). Stamford, CT: Appleton & Lange.

Takaki, R. (1993). *Strangers from a different shore: A history of Asian Americans.* New York: Penguin Books.

Takaki, R. (1994). *Raising cane: The world of plantation Hawaii.* New York: Chelsea House.

Takaki, R. (1995). *Strangers at the gates again: Asian American immigration after 1965.* New York: Chelsea House.

Tuttle, D. W., & Tuttle, N. R. (1996). *Self-esteem and adjusting with blindness* (2nd ed.). Springfield, IL: Charles C Thomas.

U.S. Bureau of the Census. (1998, April). *Census Bureau Facts for Features: Asian and Pacific Islander American Heritage Month: May 1–31* [On-line]. Available: http://www.census.gov:/Press-Release/ff98–05.html

U.S. Bureau of the Census. (1999, April). *Census Bureau Facts for Features: Asian and Pacific Islander American Heritage Month: May 1–31* [On-line]. Available: http://www.census.gov:/Press-Release/www/1999/cb99ff06.html

U.S. Department of Commerce (1993). *We the Americans: Pacific Islanders.* Washington, DC: U.S. Government Printing Office.

Wong, K. S., & Chan, S. (Eds.). (1998). *Claiming America: Constructing Chinese American identities during the exclusion era.* Philadelphia: Temple University Press.

C H A P T E R 5

Latinos with Visual Impairments

Madeline Milian
and Vivian I. Correa

Eight-year-old Cristina is Gloria and Julián Romero's first child. She was born in a small town in Mexico with a number of physical complications, including anophthalmia (absence of the eyeball) and facial malformations. After she spent three months in the hospital, the doctors asked the family to take Cristina home because there was nothing else they could do and suggested that it was better for her to die at home. At home, Gloria and Julián took turns supervising her day and night to make sure that she was still breathing. After a few months, Cristina started to improve and eventually started drinking milk. When Cristina's health was stable, Julián moved to the United States to earn money so he could help pay for the medical expenses.

When Cristina was 3 years old, she and Gloria reunited with Julián in the United States. Within a few months, Cristina started attending an early intervention program for students with visual

This chapter is dedicated to the memory of Luis Cardenas. His exemplary life as an advocate on behalf of visually impaired children and immigrants in the Denver community serves as an example of the contributions that people who are blind can make to society. Those who knew of his efforts will always remember him as an outstanding citizen and a caring human being.

impairments and underwent a series of reconstructive surgeries to enlarge her eye orbits to fit prostheses and repair other facial malformations. In addition to her initial medical problems, Cristina also experienced severe seizures that are now under control with medication. At the present time, Cristina's health condition is stable; however, her early problems resulted in cognitive and motor delays. She attends a special education class and receives itinerant services from a teacher of students with visual impairments. Two years ago, the Romeros added a boy to the family.

———————————

———————————

Lorenzo, a successful self-employed interpreter, who was born in Havana, Cuba, in 1958, is married and has an 8–year-old daughter. When he was 3 years old, the family moved to Miami, and shortly after moved to Colorado. When Lorenzo was 12, he was diagnosed with Type I diabetes. Since he had met other people with the disease, he understood its possible medical complications. He was also aware that diabetes could lead to blindness, and by the time he was 21, he had lost most of his vision. In his life so far, diabetes has also caused kidney failure that has required two transplants, three mild heart attacks, and the amputation of his toes. Lorenzo feels that blindness has been an inconvenience to him, but that some of his other health problems have been much more limiting to his life.

———————————

Within a few years, the Hispanic population, or Latinos as some of its members prefer to be called (the terms are used interchangeably here), will be the largest minority group in the United States. Certainly, the diversity within this population presents a challenge for educators who work with Latino students and clients because it is often difficult to make generalizations. Some of the factors that create this diversity are place of birth, generational status, race, language spoken, legal status, urban versus rural upbringing, education, and socioeconomic levels. Hence, the first rule when working with such a diverse population is the importance of understanding each individual child and family.

This chapter reviews the demographic, historical, socioeconomic, linguistic, and other characteristics of the population and presents data, when available, on the population of Latinos with visual impairments. In addition, it explores the cultural tendencies among Hispanic people, along with their implications for individuals with visual impairments and their families and the specific concerns of Latino families with members who are blind or visually impaired. The chapter concludes with recommendations for professionals who work with Latino students or clients who are blind or visually impaired.

DEMOGRAPHICS OF LATINOS IN THE UNITED STATES

One of the most dramatic shifts in U.S. demographics is the growing number of Hispanics in the population. The Hispanic population is expected to grow four times as fast as the rest of the population and to surpass the number of African Americans by 2005 (Robinson, 1998). One out of every 4 Americans will be of Hispanic descent by 2050, up from 1 in 9 in 1998. The Hispanic school-age population increased steadily, from 9.9 percent in 1986 to 12.3 percent in 1992 (National Center for Education Statistics, 1994).

In 1999, the Hispanic population in the United States included approximately 31.7 million people, or 11.7 percent of the total population, and consisted of the following groups: Mexicans (65.2 percent), Central and South Americans (14.3 percent), Puerto Ricans (9.6 percent), Cubans (4.3 percent), and other Hispanics (6.6 percent). Most Latinos, an estimated 91.2 percent, are white, and 5.6 percent are black. Hispanics live in every state of the nation, with the largest communities in California and Texas and the smallest communities in North Dakota and Vermont (National Council of La Raza, n.d.; U.S. Bureau of Census, 1997, 1999).

Overall, the Hispanic population in the United States is young and likely to live below the poverty level, to be unemployed, and to have lower levels of educational attainment than non-Hispanic whites. For example, although Hispanic children represented 15.7 percent of all children living in the United States in 1998, they constituted 28.5 percent of all children in poverty (U.S. Bureau of Census, 1999).

A comparison of the demographics of the general Latino population and of Latino families whose children have visual impairments reveals similar patterns, according to a study by Milian-Perrone (1994) and Ferrell's (1998) study of Project PRISM.[1] For example, the overall population increase among Hispanics in the United States is also prevalent in the Latino population with disabilities, including those with visual impairments. In 1991, Hispanic children represented 11.7 percent of all children living in the United States, while in 1998 the percentage increased to 15.7 (Montgomery, 1993; U.S. Bureau of Census, 1999). The information on ethnicity collected for Project PRISM (Ferrell, 1998) indicates that 15.8 percent of the young children who participated in this longitudinal study were Hispanic, roughly similar to their proportion of the total population. The largest number of Latino families of students with visual impairments in the Milian-Perrone study identified themselves as Mexicans, followed by Central and South Americans, Puerto Ricans, Dominicans, and Cubans (similar to the breakdown in the general population), and 13 percent of the families identified themselves as being of "mixed" Hispanic background, indicating that the members of these families came from more than one place of origin. Clearly, diversity exists even within Hispanic families. Information on family income in the Milian-Perone study confirmed the poverty experienced by many Hispanic families: 45 percent made less than $13,000 per year and only 5.5 percent made $50,000 or more.

---

[1] The Milian-Perrone study surveyed 183 Latino families of students with visual impairments to investigate families' perceptions about the schools their children attended and how schools involved them in school-family activities. Project PRISM examined the sequence and rate of development of 202 children with visual impairments ages birth to five years.

In addition, information on socioeconomic levels from Project PRISM indicated that the income levels of 80 percent of the Hispanic families in Ferrell's study were below the state median. The educational level of parents was also low, with 42.6% of the families having less than a high school education and only 9.3% having a bachelor's or advanced degree.

DIVERSITY IN THE HISPANIC COMMUNITY

With over 17 Hispanic subgroups in the United States, there is no common subculture of Hispanics. Robinson (1998) made a compelling case for studying the cultural and behavioral differences and commonalities among the major Hispanic subgroups, stating that it is important to speak of Hispanics not as one ethnic group but as many. Although the Hispanic subgroups share a common language (Spanish), there can be substantial differences among them in economic, educational, and geographic backgrounds. For example, Nicaraguan immigrants are mostly poor, rural, and young, averaging 26 years of age and nine years of schooling, whereas Houston's Mexican American population are mainly working-class residents of ethnic enclaves, even though 56 percent of them were born in the United States (Robinson, 1998). Both groups may have difficulty obtaining social and school services, but families from Nicaragua may face more of a challenge in finding out about and using the social resources available to them. Another example that can illustrate the diversity of Hispanics is the case of Cubans in the United States. As a group, Cubans have a much higher percentage of college graduates than Hispanics in general, 24.8 percent compared to 10.9 percent; and while 22.7 percent of Hispanic families live below the poverty level, this figure is only 11 percent for Cuban families (U.S. Bureau of Census, 1999). Differences in cultural values may also be found among subgroups of Hispanics. The following sections provide information on the political history and diverse immigration patterns of some of the largest Hispanic groups in the United States, using the categories identified by the federal government and the census.

Mexican Americans

Although *Mexican American* is the term frequently used to identify this subgroup, a variety of terms are also used, including *Mexicano, Chicano, Latino,* and *Hispanic.* The term *Mexican origin* is often used to distinguish those who were born in Mexico from those who were born in the United States. The term *Mexican Americans* is used in this section to refer to all persons who are of Mexican ancestry, as well as those of Spanish origin whose ancestors settled in what had been Mexican-owned territories before their annexation by the United States in 1848. The Mexican American population is highly diverse in that it includes many individuals who differ in their length of residence in the United States, physical appearance, language used, religious practices, educational level, place of residence, and economic status. The root of this diversity can best be explained by looking briefly at its history in the United States.

One of the major historical events associated with Mexican Americans was the Treaty of Guadalupe Hidalgo, signed in Mexico City in 1848, which officially ended the Mexican-American War. Under the terms of the treaty, all the Mexican territory generally north of the Rio Grande and Gila rivers was ceded to the United States, including the present areas of Arizona, California, Nevada, and New Mexico and parts of Wyoming and Colorado. Together with the annexation of Texas in 1845, the treaty added a significant number of people of Mexican origin to the United States. This subgroup differed from other Latino subgroups, including many Mexican Americans, in that they never immigrated to the United States but were annexed.

During the last half of the 19th century, the official count of Mexican Americans was less than 17,000 (McLemore & Romo, 1985). However, beginning in 1906, the number of Mexican immigrants began to increase dramatically because of the substantial number of documented and "nonstatistical" workers who arrived. These workers were encouraged to come to the United States because of the shortage of cheap labor created by the interruption of the flow of unskilled workers from Europe to the United States during World War I and the Bracero Program that was created to bring Mexican workers into the United States to ease the manpower shortage during World War II and that was later extended until 1964.

Central and South Americans

The subgroup of Central and South Americans is the most heterogeneous within the Latino population, since its members come from or can trace their origin to any of the Spanish-speaking countries in Central or South America. Members of this subgroup range from immigrants from poor rural areas in Nicaragua and El Salvador to those from more affluent urban areas in Columbia and Argentina. Because of its diversity generalizations about this subgroup are difficult to formulate and are of limited value.

Nevertheless, Central and South Americans have some common characteristics. First, many of them were driven out of their countries by political turmoil and civil war—experiences that created high levels of psychological stress among this population, particularly among the women (Salgado de Snyder, Cervantes, & Padilla, 1990). Second, unlike other groups of immigrants who came to the United States for political reasons who are given legally recognized refugee status when they entered the country, many members of this subgroup did not receive refugee status. Finally, many immigrants from Central America and South America came from rural areas where education was not available and hence tend to be poorly educated and lack the type of skills needed to compete in the workplace.

Puerto Ricans

Puerto Ricans first came to the mainland at the end of the 19th century, and the flow increased after residents of the island became U.S. citizens in 1917. Between 1945 and 1955, over 50,000 Puerto Ricans left the island each year in search of economic relief. During the first half of the 20th century, 90 percent of Puerto Ricans who came to the mainland ended up in New York City; later waves went to other parts of the Northeast or other places, such as Ohio, Illinois, and California (Zentella, 1988).

Unique to Puerto Ricans is their U.S. citizenship, which allows those who have the financial means to do so to travel back and forth freely and easily from the island to the mainland. This two-way flow of people between the island and the mainland, as well as the unsettled issue of Puerto Rico's status vis-à-vis the United States and the movements for statehood or national independence, differentiate Puerto Ricans from other Hispanic subgroups (Bennett, 1990). However, Puerto Ricans share with other immigrants and ethnic groups a history of colonial rule, cultural conflicts related to the pressures of Americanization, and racial discrimination.

Cubans

Cubans began to come to the United States in the latter part of the 19th century, and though their numbers were not large at that time, these early immigrants established the precedent and cultural foundation for the later waves of immigrants (McCoy & Gonzalez, 1985). The Cuban population in the United States grew gradually, mainly during periods of political instability on the island. A drastic and sudden change in the immigration pattern occured in 1959 after the Cuban Revolution. García and Otheguy (1988), modifying the work of Llanes (1982), recognized three large waves of immigration with three interludes between them.

The first wave began in January 1959 and ended in October 1962 with the Cuban missile crisis. These immigrants were mostly white, middle-aged, and well educated. From 1962 to 1965, most Cubans entered the United States through intermediary countries or arrived on the coast of Florida in small boats and rafts.

The second large wave of immigration began in 1965 and ended 1973. This wave was called the Freedom Flights Family

Reunification Program. This was a program that aimed at re-uniting families who already had a family member in the United States. The U.S. family member was the sponsor. It brought a more racially and socially heterogeneous group of Cubans, and while most were educated, there were many more members of the middle and working class (García & Otheguy, 1988). From 1973 to 1980, a smaller number of Cubans immigrated, mainly those who came through intermediary countries, ex-political prisoners, and family members of Cubans already in the country.

The third wave, known as the Mariel boatlift because the Cuban government allowed Cuban citizens to leave for the United States on boats from the harbor at Mariel, lasted only from April to September 1980. It brought a large number of young Cubans, blacks, single men, and unskilled manual labor-ers. Also, unlike previous Cuban immigrants who obtained refugee status on entering the United States, those who arrived in the third wave were given only "entrant" status (McCoy & Gonzalez, 1985). Since the Mariel boatlift, a small but continuous number of Cubans have entered the United States either through third countries or in small boats and rafts. However, the number of people coming in small boats and rafts drastically increased in the early 1990s when the Soviet Union abandoned its in-volvement in Cuba, creating political and economic isolation for the island. Today, Cubans continue to arrive on Florida shores in small boats and rafts; others come through an agreement be-tween the United States and Cuban governments that aims to re-strict illegal immigration (García, 1996). The United States em-bargo of Cuba, which began in 1961, has been cited as one of the reasons for the economic decline in the country (Barry, 2000; Gardfield & Santana, 1997).

Other Hispanics

The category of "other" Hispanics tries to account for Latinos who do not trace their origin to Puerto Rico, Mexico, Cuba, or Central and South America. By a process of elimination, this label includes Latinos who are from Spain or trace their origin to Spain, those from the Dominican Republic, and any others who identify themselves as Hispanic on census forms.

The Dominican community has a strong presence in New York City. Dominicans began to come to the United States in the mid-1960s as a result of political upheaval and continued to come in later years because of economic hardship (Gonzalez, 1991). Dominicans were the fastest-growing ethnic group in New York City in the 1980s, constituting the second-largest Hispanic group in that city. In the 1990s, they had the lowest income of any major racial and ethnic group in New York City, high unemployment rates (18.6 percent for women and 16 percent for men), and low educational attainment (61.5 percent of those aged 25 years or older do not have high school diplomas). In addition, 49 percent of Dominican families, versus an average of 25.6 percent for other New York City families, are headed by women (*Columbia University Record*, 1998; Ojito, 1997).

In summary, significant sociodemographic variables, historical factors, and differences in immigration patterns are found among Latinos living in the United States. These variables point to a highly heterogeneous population that functions at different levels socially, economically, and politically. The heterogeneity of the Latino population will continue to increase as a result of intermarriages within and outside Latino groups. In the future, it may not be easy to categorize Latinos according to their countries of origin. When working with members of the Latino community, professionals need to remember that students and clients from the same subgroup may function differently, depending on their socioeconomic and immigration histories.

LANGUAGE

Although many Latinos in the United States share a common language, Spanish, many others speak only English or speak "Spanglish" (a combination of Spanish and English), especially if they are not dominant in either Spanish or English (Robinson,

1998). Often, first-generation immigrants find it difficult to navigate the predominately English-speaking community, while third- and fourth-generation Hispanics may have never learned Spanish, other than some common words or phrases used in the homes of their elders. In addition, people who are fluent in both languages may move freely from one language to the other or combine the two by using Spanglish or by switching from one language to the other at different points in a conversation. For these reasons, assumptions about individuals' fluency in and use of English or Spanish are not recommended.

To illustrate the different levels of language use, the participants in Milian-Perrone's (1994) study of Latino children with visual impairments, 32.8 percent of the family members said they spoke only Spanish, 28.4 percent said they spoke Spanish better than English, 23 percent said they spoke English and Spanish equally well, 11.5 percent said they spoke English better than Spanish, and 4.4 percent said they spoke only English. In contrast, of the visually impaired children in these families, 41.5 percent spoke English and Spanish equally well, 15.3 percent spoke only English, and just 3.8 percent spoke Spanish.

Today, unlike in years past, maintaining the Spanish language is a priority for many Latino families. As Lorenzo explained:

> I was very lucky that my parents always kept our Spanish going. A lot of people who came from different countries did not want their kids to speak Spanish because they thought that it would actually hinder them and that people [would] discriminate against them for it. But [we were] the exact opposite; we always wanted to keep our culture and Spanish going, but knowing full well that [we] had to learn English.

Indeed, Lorenzo's fluency in both Spanish and English gave him the opportunity to own his own translating service.

Like the differences found in the English spoken in the United States, Australia, and England, similar minor differences exist in the use of Spanish depending on the country of origin. Table 1 lists some different words for the same concepts used by Mexicans and Puerto Ricans.

Service providers who are unaware of these differences may use a form of Spanish that confuses their students or clients. Moreover, some populations from Mexico and Central American countries speak indigenous languages as their first language and Spanish only as their second language. It is important for school districts and rehabilitation agencies to have a clear understanding of a family's dominant language so that services can be provided in ways that will be truly beneficial to individuals with visual impairments.

When families are Spanish dominant or speak an indigenous language, communicating with the predominately English-speaking community is challenging. The use of translators and interpreters is important and required, but schools and social services agencies with limited resources often do not provide these services. When translators are used, it is important to prepare them for conferences and meetings ahead of time. Lynch and Hanson (1998) presented an excellent guide to preparing translators and interpreters for work with families of children in schools.

Another factor to consider is that some Spanish-speaking individuals may not write and read Spanish. Therefore, providing written information in Spanish may not help them to obtain social and educational services unless the information is also provided or reviewed orally. Furthermore, for individuals who have low levels of literacy, it is important for professionals to provide the information clearly and not to use professional jargon and to treat these individuals with respect. Illiteracy is typically an indication of lack of educational opportunities, rather than low intellectual ability, and lack of educational opportunities is, unfortunately, common in Central and South America.

Interpersonal communication styles must also be considered when working with Hispanic individuals and families. For example, physical proximity, space, and eye contact are important

Table 1.
Differences in Spanish Terms Used by Mexicans and Puerto Ricans

English Term	Mexican Term	Puerto Rican Term
infant/baby	criatura	bebé
children	chiquillitos	nenes
little boy/little girl	chamaquito/chamaquita	niñito/niñita
baby's milk bottle	titi	bibí
fever	calentura	fiebre
cold or virus	gripe	catarro
she is sick	está mala	está enferma
to walk	andar	caminar
to cry	chiar or chillar	llorar
lollipop	paleta	dulce
medical insurance	aseguranza	seguro médico
bus	bus	guagua

features of communication with others. Hispanics are generally more comfortable with touch, direct eye contact, and a close space when communicating with other Hispanics, so that interactions with service providers who are not Hispanic may seem formal and impersonal to them. However, there is a diversity in communication styles among the Hispanic subgroups as well. For example, Mexicans often prefer a formal and literal style of communication with social work or school personnel, often addressing service providers by their surnames and using the formal case *usted* rather than the informal *tú*. In contrast, Puerto Ricans may be less formal and more open in their communication with community personnel, using the informal *tú* form for direct address in Spanish (Correa et al., 1997).

HEALTH ISSUES

It is important to review, if only briefly, some of the primary health care concerns and problems found in the Latino community, particularly because of the association among prenatal care, preventive health care, environmental conditions, health behaviors, nutrition, and health problems with the onset of disabilities. However, there is limited information on factors that influence the health status of the various Latino subgroups. Thus, studies are needed to examine the biological, socioeconomic, cultural, behavioral, and other differences among Latino subgroups to comprehend and improve the health status of these groups (Zambrana & Ellis, 1995).

Diabetes has been of special interest to professionals in the field of visual impairment because of its association with retinopathy. Diabetes is the leading cause of new cases of blindness in people aged 20–74, and each year 12,000 to 24,000 individuals lose their sight because of it (American Diabetes Association, 1997). Of the two major types of diabetes, Type I (in which the body does not produce any insulin) typically occurs in children and young adults and accounts for 5–10 percent of people with diabetes, and Type II (caused by the body's inability to make enough insulin or to use it properly) accounts for 90–95 percent of cases. In 1997, 15.7 million people in the United States (5.9 percent of the population), had diabetes. Because the prevalence of diabetes increases with age, however, about 18.4 percent of people aged 65 and older had diabetes that year. Although there is a higher incidence of Type I diabetes among whites than among other racial groups, Hispanics have three times the risk of developing Type II diabetes than do non-Hispanic whites and have a greater risk of developing complications from it (National Institute of Diabetes and Digestive and Kidney Disease, 1995; Vision and Hearing, 2000). In 1999, the National Diabetes Information Clearinghouse published a summary of findings based on five population studies that have investigated the incidence and progression of diabetes among Hispanics. This summary indicated that 1.2 million Hispanics were known to have diabetes, and 675,000 had diabetes but did not know it; 1 in every four Mexican Americans and Puerto Ricans, and 1 in every six Cubans over 45 years old has diabetes; being overweight or physically inactive are two risk factors that are present in the

Hispanic population; and that there is a higher incidence of eye and kidney disease in Hispanics than in non-Hispanic whites.

Another health problem found in the Latino population is a disproportionate rate of HIV infection. In 1998, Hispanics, who constituted 13 percent of the population, accounted for 20 percent of AIDS cases, and 23 percent of the children with AIDS reported to the Centers for Disease Control were Hispanic (National Institute of Allergy and Infectious Diseases, 2000a, 2000b). Factors that place Hispanics at a greater risk of HIV include intravenous drug use, multiple sexual partners, unprotected sexual intercourse, and the perceptions by heterosexual Hispanic men that they are not at risk (Zambrana & Ellis, 1995). Given the number of visual complications associated with AIDS, it is likely that professionals in the field of visual impairments, particularly those who work in geographic areas with large concentrations of HIV infection, will encounter students or clients whose vision loss is due to this disease.

Access to medical care and insurance are serious concerns for members of the Latino community, given that the ability to pay for health care determines the frequency with which medical services are used. Among the Latino subgroups, Central and South Americans and Mexican Americans have the lowest access to medical coverage, whereas Puerto Ricans have the highest (Angel & Angel, 1997). For Latinos over age 65, use of private health insurance ranged from 14 percent to 27 percent, depending on the subgroup, compared to 67 percent for non-Hispanic whites; the use of Medicare ranged from 19 percent to 29 percent, compared to 18 percent for non-Hispanic whites; the use of Medicaid ranged from 37 percent to 55 percent, compared to 13 percent for non-Hispanic whites; no access to any type of medical coverage ranged from 2 percent to 5 percent, compared to 1 percent for non-Hispanic whites (Angel & Angel, 1997).

Latinas have high birth rates and often bear their first children at a young age. For this reason, access to prenatal and postnatal care, which is essential for all women, is especially crucial for Latinas. According to the U.S. Department of Health and Human

Services (1991), among the various Latino subgroups, Puerto Rican women are the most likely to receive late or no prenatal care (17%), followed by Central American and Mexican American women (13%). In California, Mexican-born women are the least likely to begin prenatal care during the first trimester. Mexican immigrants face a number of barriers to access to medical care: low levels of education, low incomes, limited knowledge of English, stress related to being immigrants, and fear associated with being undocumented (Zambrana & Ellis, 1995). It is interesting, that although the rates of low birth weight among Latino infants are comparable to those among non-Hispanic infants, Latino infants are at a greater risk of being born prematurely. For example, in Project PRISM (Ferrell, 1998) 11 out of 28 Hispanic young children, but only 21 out of 112 non-Hispanic white young children, were identified as having retinopathy of prematurity, a complication of very low birth weight.

The difficulties faced by Hispanics in the health care system can lead to delays in referrals of those who are blind or visually impaired to agencies that provide appropriate services and consequently may result in a population that is inadequately served. Although teachers can refer school-age children to services, a medical facility is usually involved in connecting children under age 5 to early intervention services or elderly people for rehabilitation services. Public service announcements on Spanish radio and television stations about the availability of educational and rehabilitation opportunities for blind or visually impaired individuals and improved contact with facilities that provide medical care to low-income populations can be valuable means of delivering information to Latinos who are experiencing vision problems.

PERCEPTIONS OF DISABILITIES

Peoples' beliefs about the causes and treatment of illness and disability may vary across cultural and ethnic backgrounds, socioeconomic levels, religions, and localities, and variations in such beliefs exist within and among different Latino subgroups. Some Hispanic families have been found to hold folk beliefs about the causes of disabilities often associated with *el mal ojo* (evil eye), *sustos* (frights), *mal puestos* (evil hex), and *nervios* (nerves) (Guarnaccia, Parra, Deschamps, Milstein, & Argiles, 1992; Lynch & Hanson, 1998; Mardiros, 1989). Furthermore, some Hispanics use religious rites, such as prayer, pilgrimages to holy sites, vows, and indigenous healers like *curanderos* (healers) or spiritists for addressing or treating diseases or disabilities (Guarnaccia, et al., 1992; Lynch & Hanson, 1998; Mardiros, 1989; Trotter & Chavira, 1981).

Some authors caution, however, that more information is needed on the extent to which Hispanic families truly hold folk beliefs about disabilities and seek treatments that are alternatives to established biomedical, educational, and psychotherapeutic care for their children with disabilities. For instance, Skinner, Bailey, Correa, and Rodriguez (1999) found that the Hispanic families they studied generally did not use exotic treatments for or hold folk beliefs about causes of disabilities. Some families said that they knew of such folk beliefs but spoke of them as stories told by the elders of their communities or associated them with small enclaves of people living in certain rural parts of their native countries. Therefore, service providers need to be aware that most Hispanic families today subscribe to modern approaches to health care. When barriers to services exist, they may be related more to the fact that the services are not culturally responsive or are economically inaccessible than to families' exotic folk beliefs about disabilities.

The religious beliefs of Hispanic families are often integral to the families' perceptions of the causes of disabilities, as discussed in more detail later in this chapter. For example, some Hispanic families who are Catholic may believe that a child with a disability is a gift from God to special parents, whereas other families may believe that the child is sent as a punishment for a parent's sin (Skinner et al., 1999).

Understanding families' belief about disabilities gives service providers greater insight into the psychological coping strategies that families use in dealing with disabilities. For example, parents who believe that a child with a disability was born as a test from God of their personal strength may describe ways that they are coping and struggling to better themselves by increasing their sense of responsibilities, becoming better parents, sacrificing their own needs for the child's, eliminating the use of alcohol or drugs, or developing a stronger faith in God. Service providers may assist families by providing them with resources (such as a support group or church-related helpers) to help them reframe the event of disability in a way that may enhance the well-being of their members (Skinner et al., 1999).

CULTURAL FACTORS THAT INFLUENCE LATINOS

Some professionals who are not familiar with members of the Latino community may feel intimidated or even threatened by the thought of having to provide educational or rehabilitation services to visually impaired individuals who are not native English speakers and who may have traditional cultural values. Instead, professionals can view this experience as an opportunity to learn from a group of people who share a rich and interesting past and who, given their growing numbers, are becoming influential members of this society.

This section describes some of the major cultural influences that tend to shape Latino families and individuals. Given the wide variations among different groups of Latinos, as well as among individuals, these should be viewed as tendencies that apply to the culture at large, rather than specific descriptions that can be applied to particular individuals.

Family Dynamics and Values

The family plays a central role in virtually every Latino subgroup. Therefore, an examination of cultural values or tendencies that may be found in Latino families is essential for understanding the dynamics of the families of students and clients. So-tomayor (1991) described the Latino family as an interdependent and interactive kin network that allows for mutual and recipro-cal help among its members. The extended family is essential to the Latino family unit, and it transcends the typical consan-guineous and conjugal lines to include the *compadrazgo* ("copar-enthood") system, which extends responsibility for children's emotional and financial well-being to two additional adults—a *madrina* (godmother) and a *padrino* (godfather) (Vega, Hough, & Romero, 1983). This system gives Latino parents the opportunity to extend the status of relative to close friends or to elevate the family status of a relative by creating closer bonds to their child. Moreover, it enables the parents to share the responsibilities and joys of parenting with the *comadre* (comother) and *compadre* (co-father).

Frequently, the literature on Latino families has concentrated on specific subgroups, such as Mexican American families (see, for example, Delgado-Gaitán & Trueba, 1991; Vega et al., 1983) or Puerto Rican families (see, for example, Figler, 1992; Harry, 1992). However, Marín and VanOss Marín (1991) reviewed the literature and categorized some of the relevant cultural values that have been found among various subgroups: allocentrism, *simpatía*, familialism, power distance, personal space, time ori-entation, and gender roles.

The influence of these cultural values on the interactions be-tween Latino families and educational and other institutions should be of interest to professionals who work with families of students or clients who are blind or visually impaired. In the fol-lowing sections, cultural traits are examined in relation to their affect on family dynamics and interactions between families, schools, and professionals. It should be noted, however, that these cultural tendencies are given only as guidelines, since they are not present or do not exist with the same degree and inten-sity in every Latino, given the heterogeneous nature of the Latino population; thus, generalizations should be avoided be-cause they lead only to stereotypes.

ALLOCENTRISM

Allocentrism is a Latino cultural value that has also been referred to as collectivism. Allocentric societies emphasize the needs, objectives, and points of view of an in-group, whereas individualistic cultures emphasize personal objectives, attitudes, and values. In an ethnographic study of the way first-generation Latino children are reared by immigrant parents, Delgado-Gaitán and Trueba (1991), observed collective behaviors both among children and between parents and children. Parents verbally encouraged their children to work together and often modeled collective behaviors during their daily activities.

Evidence of collectivism was also observed in Tapia's (1992) study of motivational orientations in Puerto Rican and European American children aged 10–12. Motivational orientations were described as individualistic, cooperative, and competitive—in other words, whether a child showed preference for maximizing individual, joint, or relative gains, respectively. Tapia concluded that a cooperative motivational orientation predominated over a competitive orientation in Puerto Rican children.

SIMPATÍA

Simpatía stresses the importance of avoiding conflicts and promoting behaviors that foster pleasant social interactions and is most likely the result of the allocentric values of Hispanics (Marín & VanOss Marín, 1991). One is *simpático* if one is agreeable and nonconfrontational and respects others. For example, when recent Mexican and Central American mothers of infants were asked to participate in Lieberman's (1989) study, some unwilling mothers found it difficult to say no, so they agreed to participate but were never home when the visits were scheduled. By agreeing, the mothers not only displayed a positive behavior, but avoided a possible stressful social interaction. Lieberman also found that to form a relationship with the mothers, the members of the intervention team had to accept food, attend children's birthday parties, praise the mothers' dresses and new hairstyles, and converse with the mothers about topics that were dear to them. The families interpreted the team members' initial refusal to do these things as arrogance or contempt for them.

It is not uncommon to hear teachers of students with visual impairments share their confusion and frustration when Latino families agree, in meetings of Individualized Education Program (IEP) teams, to reinforce behaviors or to follow through with certain procedures, only to do so inconsistently or not at all. Although families may not follow through on behaviors or procedures because they do not know how to do so, they may also be exercising *simpatía*, that is, agreeing to comply with suggestions that may be incompatible with what they believe or that they are unable to do.

FAMILIALISM

Familialism (*familismo*), is also extremely important to Latinos (Abi-Nader, 1990; Anderson, 1989; Harry, 1992; Lieberman, 1989). This cultural value fosters strong identification with and attachment to the nuclear and extended families and feelings of loyalty, reciprocity, and solidarity among family members (Triandis, Marín, Betancourt, Lisansky, & Chang, 1982).

Case studies illustrate the personal meaning of familialism for Latino students. For example, in Abi-Nader's (1990) study of college-bound Latino high school students' motivations for achieving educational success, the influence of familialism was poignantly described by the students in statements such as these: "One of the most ideal things in life is to buy my mother a home" or "My wish is, I wish I could find my mother a house." These students were driven by the strong sense of reciprocity to their families and were using this value as a vehicle to achieve educational success.

In another case study, Nieto (1992) interviewed 10 successful high school students representing a variety of racial, ethnic, linguistic, and social class groups: Students were considered successful if they had developed both academic skills and positive attitudes about themselves and about the value of education. The comments of Marisol Martinez, a U.S.-born student of

Puerto Rican parents, about her family also demonstrate the value of familialism:

> They like school and they encourage you to keep going, you know. I think they're proud of us 'cause my sisters and brothers, they all have nice report cards; they never stood back, you know, and usually we do this for my mother. We like to see her the way she wants to be, you know, to see her happy. (Nieto, 1992, p. 126)

Harry (1992) conducted an ethnographic study of 12 low-income Puerto Rican parents whose children had been identified as either having mental retardation or a learning disability. Some participants thought that their families had been disgraced because they thought that some of the information included in the social history indicated that the children's difficulties were a result of immorality in the family. However, the value of familialism could also be responsible for positive outcomes, such as the acceptance of the child's disability. After analyzing the parents' comments, Harry concluded:

> An intriguing feature of this is the fact that, while a strong concept of group identity makes the whole group vulnerable, there is also a resilience created by the assumption of a group identity; that is, inasmuch as the individual may bring shame to the group, so may aspects of the group's identity serve to protect the individual. (p. 150)

It is possible that this cultural trait facilitates a natural network of support for Latino families and a structure for sharing emotional and financial success and failures with the immediate and extended family. For example, Lorenzo, who was introduced at the beginning of this chapter, had established himself in California when he was single. However, when his wife gave birth to their daughter, they decided to return to Colorado because they wanted their daughter to grow up with her grandparents and cousins. In doing so, Lorenzo and his wife expanded their family support unit.

POWER DISTANCE

Power distance may be defined as the perception of interpersonal power or influence between individuals. Marín and VanOss Marín (1991) suggested that Latinos are high power-distance individuals, in that they value conformity and obedience and support autocratic and authoritarian attitudes. Individuals may be perceived as powerful by others in a society because of inherent or inherited traits; therefore, those who are supposedly more intelligent or have greater wealth or education are perceived as more powerful.

Given the definition of power distance and its ramifications for social interactions among individuals, one can predict its influence on child-rearing practices and family-school relationships. For example, the Mexican and Central American mothers in Lieberman's (1989, p. 201) study strongly believed that "parents should be in charge, that disobedience and disrespectful behavior should not be allowed, and that good parents keep a tight hold on their child's expression of angry feelings." Although professionals in the field of special education encourage and expect family members, at least theoretically, to participate in the educational process as equal partners, the cultural tendencies of power distance as well as *simpatía* may prevent many Latino families, particularly low-income families who lack formal education, from participating as true equal partners in IEP meetings. When one's cultural tendencies discourage disagreement and encourage respect for authority, it may be unthinkable to disagree in front of people who one perceives to be more powerful.

In such circumstances, it is the professional's responsibility to provide families with resources that will facilitate their active involvement in educating their children with visual impairments. For example, Gloria Romero, the mother of Cristina who was profiled at the beginning of this chapter, has become an active and integral member of Cristina's educational team with the assistance of a bilingual parent advocate from the school district. She also credits the information she received at the preschool

Cristina attended as helping her to understand her rights as a parent of a child with a visual impairment. In fact, there have been occasions when teachers and administrators have described Gloria as a demanding mother who has unrealistic expectations for her child. It may be that professionals who are accustomed to interacting with more agreeable Latino families may not know how to react to the demands of Latinos who are knowledgeable and assertive.

PERSONAL SPACE

Another difference in the interactional styles of Latinos and members of other ethnic groups is personal space. Basing their ideas on the writings of Condon, Peters, and Carmen (1970) on the ways in which individuals from different cultures use, value, and share space, Chamberlain and Medinos-Landurand (1991) referred to this area as "proximity" and "touching." Marín and VanOss Marín (1991), citing the anthropological writings of Hall (1969), suggested that Latinos need less physical space than do non-Hispanic whites when interacting socially and that this physical closeness is perceived not as a violation of personal space, but as a sign of being demonstrative and responsive to the person with whom one is interacting.

The variation in preferences for personal space among different cultures and its implications for how people interact with each other have direct ramifications on the way some Latino families view non-Latino school personnel, and vice versa. For example, Latinos may view members of other ethnic groups as distant or impersonal because they prefer more personal space between speakers, whereas members of other ethnic groups may view Latinos as being too personal or emotional because they maintain less distance and display more affectionate gestures through touching. Families' perceptions of the school environment as nondemonstrative and emotionally distant could influence their willingness to participate in school-related activities. Similarly, non-Latino educators' discomfort in interacting with Latino families at a close physical distance may create friction between the educators and families that will thwart open communication.

TIME ORIENTATION

Attitudes toward time seem to vary across cultures, and cultural background can influence whether one is future oriented or present oriented (Marín & VanOss Marín, 1991). Future-oriented individuals emphasize planning, delayed gratification, punctuality, and efficiency, whereas present-oriented individuals are generally less able to delay gratification and plan for the future and place less emphasis on punctuality and efficiency.

Chamberlain and Medinos-Landurand (1991) and Marín and VanOss Marín (1991) suggested that Latinos are present oriented in that they have a flexible attitude toward time and place greater value on the quality of their interpersonal relationships than on the length of time these interactions require. This present orientation is important in the context of special education, since school personnel typically structure IEP meetings for limited blocks of time, which they believe contributes to the efficiency of the meetings. Latino families may be dissatisfied with the interactions in these meetings because of the inflexibility and rigidity in the time devoted to issues. Less experienced in using time efficiently, these families may not bring up all the concerns they have about their children's disabilities and IEPs within the allotted time.

GENDER ROLES

Traditionally, Latino men have been expected to be more dominant over women, whereas Latinas have been expected to be submissive, passive, selfless, and home centered (Ambert & Figler, 1992; Hines, García-Preto, McGoldrick, & Weltman, 1992). Women are therefore expected to assume caretaking roles in the family and men are more likely to assume financial responsibility for elderly parents, younger siblings, and nephews and nieces, as well as their wives and children. Gloria Romero, for example, is in charge of making all decisions related to

Cristina's education. She attends all IEP meetings and parent-teacher conferences; telephones school district personnel, when necessary; makes all doctors' appointments, and takes care of other issues related to the education and medical care of her children. Julián is responsible for the financial support of his immediate family in the United States, as well as for assisting their relatives in Mexico.

The gender-role values of the adults are likely to determine important child-rearing practices, such as discipline, and issues of authority and decision making by the adults. Delgado-Gaitán and Trueba's (1991) ethnographic study of children of immigrant Mexican and Central American families clearly illustrated incidents of different rules based on gender. For example, the authors stated that "while the parents saw the disparity between the amount of work performed by the girls and the boys, they believed that girls should remain at home while boys were allowed more freedom to leave the house." (pp. 69–70)

School personnel need to be sensitive when communicating with Latino fathers who hold traditional gender-role values, particularly if the fathers also have low incomes. Nicolau and Ramos (1990) explained that these fathers tend to avoid functions that can be viewed as "learning" activities, since these functions typically threaten their control and dignity or indicate that they have flaws or weaknesses. For example, if fathers are asked questions and do not know the answers, fathers may perceive their failure to respond as a reflection on them as the heads of their families.

It is important to note that perceptions of gender roles in most industrialized countries are going through a transition, since there are more families headed by women, more working couples, and increased advocacy for the rights of women. Naturally, social and economic factors create changes in the traditionally held gender expectations of Latinos, just as they do for other cultural groups, whether they are living in the United States or in their native countries.

Others Factors Influencing the Lives of Latinos

Two other important factors should be noted in considering the influence of Latino culture on clients and families. They are the impact of religion in their lives and the degree to which individuals have adapted to the new culture.

RELIGION

In Latino cultures, religion has considerable influence on the understanding of disabilities, how families accept and adapt to the birth of a child with a disability, and how the family changes thereafter. Many Latino families practice Catholicism, some in its traditional form and others in a form that has been shaped by African or Native American beliefs and practices. More recently, Hispanics in the United States and those still living in their native countries have joined other denominations such as Pentecostal and Baptist.

It is important to distinguish formal religion from informal or personal religion for Latino families. In a study of Puerto Rican and Mexican families of children with disabilities, Bailey, Skinner, Correa, and Arcia (1997) concluded that faith in God provided families with greater support in adjusting to having children with disabilities than did attending church. Although some families said that they went to church weekly, most said that they attended church less than once a month; the barriers to church attendance they noted included the lack of transportation and of child care at church for children with disabilities and the children's inability to participate and behave during the church services. Most of the families reported receiving much personal strength from their faith in God and often described their faith as central in coping with the day-to-day struggles of raising a child with disabilities. For example, a Puerto Rican mother said:

> I'll tell you something with all sincerity, I'm not a very religious
> person but I'm a very realistic person, but the relationship I have

with God is something different, very intimate and very personal. A lot of people think I am an imperfect person. A person is imperfect but this relation of mine with God is an intimate relationship and when I need to have that communication with God, I get away [*me alejo*] and I go into my room or I'll go for a walk to have that communication, like no other, and that's what I think makes me a Christian person, that intimate relationship with Him. I can go to church and listen to the pastor's preaching [*predicando*] and understand what he's preaching and sometimes through that preaching He [God] gives a message to a person. And as a Christian, if you have that communication [with God], then you will hear it and you'll know that it's for you and for those who are there listening. That intimate relationship is the only thing important in my spiritual life. (Bailey, Skinner, Correa, & Arcia, 1997)

Informal religion, such as personal communication with and praying to God appeared to be key in providing families with assistance in their day-to-day lives. A conversation with Gloria Romero, Cristina's mother, revealed that although she is not a practicing Catholic and does not think the Catholic Church has provided assistance for her, she views herself as a believer. She credited her strong faith in God with helping her accept Cristina's disabilities and giving her the strength to survive the difficult moments she has faced in her life. She tearfully spoke of Cristina's early years and the separation from her family in Mexico as extremely stressful times in her life when she needed to depend on her faith in God.

A conversation with a Puerto Rican single mother of a 4-year-old blind child with developmental delays also revealed how religion and belief in God provide families and individuals with a way of understanding disabilities. When asked whether her son's disabilities were a result of somebody wishing her wrong or an evil eye, she responded:

To me, the way I put it, my son come out the way he is because God is putting me to a test. That's the way—I mean, I used to go to church a lot. So that's how I see it. To see if I could survive. Either that or He is just teaching me a lesson 'cause maybe I did something wrong and He is trying to teach me the other side, you know, since [my son] can't see. So I can understand. I have a gift— that's how I put it. (Bailey, Skinner, Correa, & Arcia, 1997)

Although religious beliefs and their influence or the understanding and acceptance of disabilities is not limited to Latinos, it may be helpful to consider them as a factor that could explain possible within-group differences among Latinos. For example, one early study (Zuk, Miller, Bartram, & Kling, 1961) that measured mothers' acceptance of children with disabilities found high positive adjustment in Catholic families rearing children with developmental disabilities. A Latino family with strong religious beliefs will view the disability of their child on the basis of the teachings of their religion, while another Latino family will rely on factors not directly related to their religious faith to understand, accept, adapt, and deal with concerns related to the child's disability. In a study of religious beliefs of parents of children with visual impairments, Erin, Rudin, and Njoroge (1991) also reported the important role that religion played in coping and adjusting to the children's disabilities. The authors also cautioned that service providers should not feel uncomfortable when parents talk about their religious beliefs and practices and suggested that service providers become familiar with the views of different religions.

ACCULTURATION

Finally, although it is not a characteristic of the Latino culture per se, the concept of acculturation may be an important one in understanding the heterogeneity of the cultural tendencies displayed by members of the Latino population in the United States. Acculturation, as defined by Szapocznik, Scopetta, Kurtines, and Aramalde (1978), is the process of accommodating to a host culture by a member of a migrant culture. Acculturation involves the modification of the person's customs, habits, language usage, lifestyle, and value orientations. It progresses as a function of the length of time the person has been exposed to the host culture and of the age at which the person was first exposed to the new culture. Szapocznik et al. (1978) further divided this concept into the dimensions of behavioral acculturation and value acculturation. Behavioral acculturation is the gradual adoption of the language, customs, habits, and lifestyle of the new culture; value acculturation is the gradual adoption of the new culture's basic value orientation.

According to Leung (1988), acculturation results in four levels of adaptation to the new culture:

1. traditionalism—maintaining the values of the traditional culture
2. marginality—rejecting the old and not accepting the new culture
3. biculturation—integrating the two cultures
4. overacculturation—rejecting the traditional culture

Six factors have been identified that can influence the direction of acculturation: length of time in the host culture, proximity to the traditional culture, age, birthplace, gender, and intermarriage.

As individuals adapt to the new culture, a number of changes tend to take place, including the following (Berry, Kim, Minde, & Mok, 1987):

1. physical changes, such as housing, climate, and living conditions
2. biological changes, such as nutritional status, diseases, and intermarriage
3. cultural changes, such as alteration or replacement of political, economic, technical, linguistic, religious, and social institutions
4. changes in social relationships
5. physiological changes, such as behavioral changes and mental health status

The concept of acculturation facilitates the understanding of individual differences among Latinos. Professionals will better understand the students and clients they are working with when they can refer to the acculturation continuum to examine some of the behaviors that may be puzzling to them. Doing so will also assist them in developing services that may be more culturally appropriate for a particular student or client.

CONCERNS OF LATINO FAMILIES OF STUDENTS WITH VISUAL IMPAIRMENTS

It is expected that Latino families of students with visual impairments share many, or at least some, of the cultural tendencies and demographic characteristics of the general population of Latino families in the United States. One distinction is the presence of a visual impairment and the additional concerns it creates for the family. Milian-Perrone's (1994) study of Latino families with children with visual impairments identified a number of concerns from the family members' statements. (Although many family members used Spanish to express their concerns, these comments have been translated into English so they could be presented in this book.) Five categories of concerns are discussed next, including the child's future, the progress of the visual impairment, and safety issues.

The Child's Future

The parents' statements reflected their uncertainty about the obstacles that their children's visual impairments might present in completing their education, obtaining employment, finding partners, and raising families. Some representative comments included these:

> My concern is that in the future she will not be able to have a job and support herself.

My concern is that my child will not be able to achieve and maintain a middle-class lifestyle.

My greatest concern is that my son can advance in all areas and that he is able to complete his education, including attending the university.

What will his future be? What trade will he be able to learn? Will his visual limitation interfere with his ability to attend college? Will he have a family, or will he be rejected by women?

Educational Issues

The concerns expressed by family members in this area reflected their interest in and worries about their children's ability to learn, the quality of education provided by the schools, the resources available to educate children with visual impairments, placement issues, and necessary adaptations to support their children's education. The following are some of the concerns the parents expressed:

I feel the special education program my son is receiving does not function in a way that will help him to graduate from high school.

My concern is that every day the district continues to cut funding, and there will come the day the school will not receive the funding they need.

My greatest concern is that my child will not be able to read and write.

The education provided is very poor. One can't compare it to the education normal students receive. Students with visual impairments spend time doing fill-in-the-blank type work. Large-print books are ordered very late and students receive them months after the school year started.

Progression of the Visual Impairment

The parents shared their concerns about the status and progression of their children's visual impairments and the adjustments needed as vision decreases. Other comments reflected their interest in knowing about medical advances that may improve their children's vision or their inability to provide the type of medical care that could benefit their children's visual prognoses. Some of the concerns the parents mentioned included:

> My main concern is that his cataracts will come back.

> I worry that his myopia could advance, although the specialist assures us that he is going to get better.

> That my child will be completely blind one day and the difficulties this will bring for him and for me to adjust to his new stage. I think this will be very difficult and painful and I don't think I am ready for it.

> Anything new on current technology as far as operations to restore my son's sight.

> My concern is not having money to be able to consult with a good doctor.

Self-Sufficiency and Independence

The parents' responses under this category expressed their desire for their children to become independent and self-sufficient and their fears that this goal might not be realized. Some of the comments were as follows:

> My greatest concern is to be able to give her enough confidence so she can do more things for herself.

> I worry that my child will not be able to become self-sufficient and not be able to be on his own in society.

> I wonder about his independence and if he is going to be able to do without me. I mean, I'll always be behind him, but I would like to know that he will be safe and secure.

> My greatest concern as a mother is that my son can become self-sufficient and useful to society.

Although these parents mentioned that self-sufficiency and independence are important concerns, service providers who work with Latino students and clients often mention the apparent discrepancies between the families' and service providers' views of independence. Dean's (1998) study of Latino families' perceptions of their children's mobility program confirmed this discrepancy; whereas the families described independence in terms of education, work, and relationships with others, the service providers focused on the children's ability to travel independently. This discrepancy may be due, in part, to the different values held by parents and professionals. For example, while service providers may want to teach daily skills with the goal of supporting students when they become young adults and move away from home, family members may not approve of this goal because moving away from home means abandoning the family. Family members will support the teaching of daily living skills if they perceive them as helping the student or client contribute to the family by assisting with chores or teaching a younger brother or sister. Thus, families and professionals differ in the types of activities they associate with independence, rather than with the general concept of independence. In other words, Latino families also want their children to be independent but formulate the achievement of these goals in ways that are culturally acceptable to them.

Safety Issues

The parents shared their concerns about safety issues that might affect their children as a result of the visual impairments, such as possible accidents because of decreased vision or others' treatment of the children that could result in some type of injury. The following comments are examples:

> My greatest concern is that he'll get seriously hurt because he doesn't see something coming or doesn't see someone coming to attack him.

> The abuse of other children on my daughter because of her handicap.

> That he may get hit by a car because he might not see it.

> I worry that something will happen to her when she is not with us, or that someone will sexually abuse her.

In addition to the five main concerns just discussed, the parents raised two other concerns that are worth including: the possibility of future discrimination in education and employment because of the child's visual impairment and the need for the family, child, and society in general to accept the child's visual disability. These two areas were viewed as possible obstacles that could preclude children from maximizing their potential and making use of opportunities that would facilitate their full integration into society.

RECOMMENDATIONS FOR PROFESSIONALS

Some professionals who have lived in states with large populations of Latinos feel comfortable interacting with Latinos and are knowledgeable about their culture and language. Others who are not familiar with the Latino population need to take some steps to assist them in designing programs and communicating with students or clients and their families in a culturally sensitive manner. The following are some suggestions for professionals who are not familiar with the Latino population.

1. Refrain from making generalizations about a Latino sub-group that may not pertain to every individual in the group. Instead, emphasize the need for an individualized approach to special education and rehabilitation services for each family.

2. Obtain information about the origin of the population in a specific community. Are they new, or do they have a long history in the community? Which subgroup do they belong to, and is it the main subgroup in the community? What social organizations in the community can provide assistance to professionals in understanding the family or can provide services the family may need?

3. Become familiar with the immigration history of the individual family you are working with. Did the family come to the United States for political or economic reasons? How long have they been in the United States? Do they have a family support system? Are there members of the family who speak English?

4. As the first step in establishing a relationship with a family, especially a family that is new to a community and may be undocumented, connect them with agencies that can provide for their basic needs and relevant information on services.

5. Understand that many Latino families immigrate to the United States seeking better medical and educational services for their children with disabilities. However, in the United States, they often experience discrimination and frustration in obtaining services if the services are not provided in Spanish and in a culturally sensitive manner.

6. A professional who speaks only English and works with a family that speaks only Spanish may want to try some of the following suggestions:
   ◆ Bring an interpreter when visiting the family the first few times.
   ◆ Give the family written materials in both English and Spanish.

- ◆ Learn basic phrases that are applicable to the case.
- ◆ Purchase a good English–Spanish dictionary.
- ◆ Enroll in a Spanish class or purchase a Spanish language CD-ROM or audiocassette.

7. Encourage families with young children and who have limited English proficiency to continue using Spanish in communicating with their children. Telling stories to, conversing with, and reading to the children in Spanish will stimulate their cognitive development and improve their communication skills much more than will using limited English skills.

8. When puzzled by family members' actions or comments, ask someone who is more knowledgeable about the family and its culture to help interpret the situation.

SUMMARY

The continuing growth of the Latino population will require professionals in the field of special education and rehabilitation to develop skills that will facilitate their work with Latino students and clients who are visually impaired. Teacher preparation programs and school districts will need to initiate and sustain their efforts to prepare beginning and experienced teachers and rehabilitation professionals for work with members of the Latino community. In some cases, professionals will need to obtain resources and establish connections with others who are more experienced with Latino students and clients. The final goal is to offer educational and rehabilitation services that will provide opportunities for each student's or client's productive participation in his or her family and community.

REFERENCES

Abi-Nader, J. (1990). "A house for my mother": Motivating Hispanic high school students. *Anthropology & Education Quarterly, 21,* 41–58.

Ambert, N. A., & Figler, C. S. (1992). Puerto Ricans: Historical and cultural perspectives. In A. N. Ambert & M. D. Alvarez (Eds.), *Puerto Rican children on the mainland: Interdisciplinary perspectives* (pp. 17–37). New York: Garland.

American Diabetes Association. (1997). *Diabetes facts and figures* [On-line]. Available: http://www.diabetes.org/ada/c20f/html

Anderson, P. P. (1989). Issues in serving culturally diverse families of young children with disabilities. *Early Child Development and Care, 50,* 167–188.

Angel, R. J., & Angel, J. L. (1997). Health service use and long-term care among Hispanics. In K. S. Markides & M. R. Miranda (Eds.), *Minorities, aging, and health* (pp. 343–366). Thousand Oaks, CA: Sage.

Bailey, D., Skinner, D., Correa, V., & Arcia, E. (1997). *Religiosity in Hispanic families of children with disabilities.* Paper presented at the national Gatlingburg conference, Riverside, CA.

Barry, M. (January 18, 2000). Effect of the U.S. embargo and economic decline on health in Cuba. *Anals of Internal Medicine, 132,* 151–157.

Bennett, C. I. (1990). *Comprehensive multicultural education: Theory and practice* (2nd ed.). Boston: Allyn & Bacon.

Berry, J. W., Kim, U., Minde, T., & Mok, D. (1987). Comparative studies of acculturative stress. *International Migration Review, 21,* 491–511.

Chamberlain, P., & Medinos-Landurand, P. (1991). Practical considerations for the assessment of LEP students with special needs. In E. L. Hamayan & J. S. Damico (Eds.), *Limiting bias in the assessment of bilingual students* (pp. 112–156). Austin, TX: Pro-Ed.

Columbia University Record. (1998). *Dominicans are city's fastest growing, poorest group, says study* [On-line]. Available: http/www.columbia.edu/cu/record/record2020.22.html

Condon, E., Peters, J. Y., & Carmen, S. (1979). *Special education in the Hispanic child: Cultural perspectives.* Philadelphia: Temple University Teacher Corps Mid-Atlantic Network.

Correa, I. V., Skinner, D., Vazquez-Montilla, E., Reyes-Blanes, M., Ponte, R., & Rodriguez, P. (1997, January), *The Latino Family Research Project: Implications for early intervention and research.* Paper presented at the 1997 Symposium on Culturally and Linguistically Diverse Exceptional Learners, New Orleans.

Dean, T. (1998). Hispanic families' perception of orientation and mobility: Research brief. In E. Siffermann, M. Williams, & B. B. Blasch, *Conference Proceedings, The 9th International Mobility Conference: O&M Moving into the Twenty-First Century* (129–130). Atlanta GA: Rehabilitation Research & Development Center, Atlanta, VA Medical Center.

Delgado-Gaitán, C., & Trueba, H. (1991). *Crossing cultural borders.* Bristol, PA: Falmer Press.

Erin, J. N., Rudin, D., & Njoroge, M. (1991). Religious beliefs of parents of children with visual impairments. *Journal of Visual Impairment and Blindness, 85,* 157–162.

Ferrell, K. A. (1998). *Project PRISM: A longitudinal study of developmental patterns of children who are visually impaired (Final report).* (Field-initiated research H023C101, U.S. Department of Education, Office of Special Education and Rehabilitative Services). [Available from Division of Special Education, University of Northern Colorado, Greeley, CO 80639].

Figler, C. S. (1992). Puerto Rican families on the mainland: Stresses and support systems. In A. N. Ambert & M. D. Alvarez (Eds.), *Puerto Rican children on the mainland: Interdisciplinary perspectives* (pp. 299–327). New York: Garland.

García, M. C. (1996). *Havana USA: Cuban exiles and Cuban Americans in south Florida, 1959–1994.* Los Angeles, CA: University of California Press.

García, O., & Otheguy, R. (1988). The language situation of Cuban Americans. In S. L. McKay & S. C. Wong (Eds.), *Language diversity: Problem or resource? A social and educational perspective on language minorities in the United States* (pp. 166–192). New York: Newbury House.

Gardfield, R., & Santana, S. (1997). The impact of the economic crisis and the U.S. embargo on health in Cuba. *American Journal of Public Health* [On-line]. Available: http://www.usaengage.org/news/9701ajph.html

Gonzalez, D. (1991, September 1). Dominican immigration alters Hispanic New York. *New York Times,* pp. 1, 4.

Guarnaccia, P. J., Parra, P., Deschamps, A., Milstein, G., & Argiles, N. (1992). Si dios quiere: Hispanic families' experiences of caring for a seriously mentally ill family member. *Culture, Medicine, and Psychiatry, 16,* 187–215.

Hall, E. T. (1969). *The hidden dimension.* Garden City, NY: Doubleday.

Harry, B. (1992). *Cultural diversity, families, and the special education system: Communication and empowerment.* New York: Teachers College Press.

Hines, P. M., García-Preto, N., McGoldrick, R. A., & Weltman, S. (1992). Intergenerational relationships across cultures. *Families in Society, 73,* 323–338.

Leung, E. K. (1988). Cultural and acculturational commonalities and diversities among Asian Americans: Identification and programming considerations. In A. A. Ortiz & B. A. Ramirez (Eds.), *Schools and the culturally diverse exceptional student: Promising practices and future directions* (pp. 86–95). Reston, VA: Council for Exceptional Children.

Lieberman, A. F. (1989). What is culturally sensitive intervention? *Early Child Development and Care, 50,* 197–204.

Llanes, J. (1982). *Cuban-Americans: Masters of survival.* Cambridge, MA: ABT Books.

Lynch, W. W., & Hanson, M. J. (1998). *Developing cross-cultural competence: A guide for working with children and their families* (2nd ed.). Baltimore, MD: Paul H. Brookes.

Mardiros, M. (1989). Conception of childhood disability among Mexican-American parents. *Medical Anthropology, 12,* 55–68.

Marín, G., & VanOss Marín, B. (1991). *Research with Hispanic populations* (Applied Social Research Methods Series, Vol. 23). Newbury Park, CA: Sage.

McCoy, G. C., & Gonzalez, D. H. (1985). Cuban immigration and Mariel immigrants. In J. Szapocznick, R. Cohen, & R. Hernandez (Eds.), *Coping with adolescent refugees: The Mariel boatlift* (pp. 22–38). New York: Praeger.

McLemore, S. D., & Romo, R. (1985). The origins and development of the Mexican American people. In R. O. de la Garza, F. D. Bean, C. M. Bonjean, R. Romo, & R. Alvarez (Eds.), *The Mexican American experience: An interdisciplinary anthology* (pp. 3–32). Austin: University of Texas Press.

Milian-Perrone, M. (1994). *Family involvement and attitudes about school programs among Latino families of students with visual impairments.* Unpublished doctoral dissertation, Teachers College, Columbia University.

Montgomery, P. A. (March 1993). *The Hispanic population in the United States: Current Population Reports* (Series P-20, No.475). Washington, DC: U.S. Government Printing Office.

National Center for Education Statistics (1994). *Digest of Education Statistics 1994.* U.S. Department of Education, Office of Educational Research and Improvement. Washington, D.C.

National Council of La Raza. (n.d.) *Twenty most frequently asked questions about the Latino community* [On-line]. Available: http://www.clr.org/about/nclrfq.html

National Diabetes Information Clearinghouse. (April 1999). *Diabetes in Hispanic Americans* [On-line]. Available: http://www.niddk.nih.gov/health/diabetes/pubs/hispan.htm

National Institute of Allergy and Infectious Diseases (1997). *Minorities and HIV infections.* [On-line]. Available: niaid.nih.gov/factsheets/Minor.html

National Institute of Allergy and Infectious Diseases. (2000a, February). Backgrounder—HIV infection in infants and children [On-line]. Available: http://www.niidonih.gov/newsroom/simle/background.html

National Institute of Diabetes and Digestive and Kidney Disease. (1995). *Diabetes in America* (2nd ed.). Washington, DC: U.S. Government Printing Office.

Nicolau, S., & Ramos, C. L. (1990). *Together is better: Building strong relationships between school and Hispanic parents.* New York: Hispanic Policy Development Project.

Nieto, S. (1992). *Affirming diversity: The sociopolitical context of multicultural education.* New York: Longman.

Ojito, M. (1997, December 16). Dominicans, scrabbling for hope: As poverty rises, more women are heading households. *New York Times* (national ed.), p. C27.

Robinson, L. (1998, May 11). Hispanics don't exist. *U.S. News and World Report,* pp. 26–32.

Salgado de Snyder, V. N., Cervantes, R. C., & Padilla, A. M. (1990). Gender and ethnic differences in psychosocial stress and generalized distress among Hispanics. *Sex Roles: A Journal of Research, 22*(7–8), 441–453.

Skinner, D., Bailey, D., Correa, V., & Rodriguez, P. (1999). Narrating self and disability: Latino mothers' construction of identities vis-à-vis their child with special needs. *Exceptional Children, 65,* 54–63.

Sotomayor, M. (1991). Introduction. In M. Sotomayor (Ed.), *Empowering Hispanic families: A critical issue for the '90s* (pp. xi–xxiii). Milwaukee, WI: Family Service America.

Szapocznick, J., Scopetta, M. A., Kurtines, W., & Aranalde, M. A. (1978). Theory and measurement of acculturation. *Interamerican Journal of Psychology, 12,* 113–130.

Tapia, M. R. (1992). Motivational orientations, learning, and the Puerto Rican child. In A. N. Ambert & M. D. Alvarez (Eds.), *Puerto Rican children on the mainland: Interdisciplinary perspectives* (pp. 109–131). New York: Garland.

Triandis, H. C., Marín, G., Betancourt, H., Lisansky, J., & Chang, B. (1982). *Dimensions of familism among Hispanic and mainstream navy recruits.* Chicago: University of Illinois, Department of Psychology.

Trotter, R. T., & Chavira, J. A. (1981). *Curanderismo: Mexican American folk healing.* Athens: University of Georgia Press.

U.S. Bureau of the Census. (1997). *Estimates of the population of states by age, sex, race, and Hispanic origin: 1990 to 1996.* [On-line]. Available: http://www.census.gov/population/estimates/state/srh/srhus96.txt

U.S. Bureau of the Census. (1999, March). *The Hispanic population in the United States: Population characteristics* [On-line]. Available: http://www.census.gov/population/www/socdemo/hispanic/ho99.html

U.S. Department of Health and Human Services. (1991). *Health status of minorities and low-income groups.* Washington, DC: Government Printing Office.

Vega, W. A., Hough, R. A., & Romero, A. (1983). Family life patterns of Mexican-Americans. In G. Johnson Powell (Ed.), *The psychosocial development of minority group children* (pp. 194–215). New York: Brunner/Mazel.

Vision and hearing. (2000, September 19). Chap. 28 in *Healthy People 2010:*

Conference edition (pp. 1–17) [On-line]. Available: http://web.health.gov/healthypeople/Document/html/Volume2/28Vision.htm

Zambrana, R. E., & Ellis, B. K. (1995). Contemporary research issues in Hispanic/Latino women's health. In D. L. Adams (Ed.)., *Health issues for women of color: A cultural diversity perspective* (pp. 42–70). Thousand Oaks, CA: Sage.

Zentella, A. C. (1988). The language situation of Puerto Ricans. In S. L. McKay & S. C. Wong (Eds.), *Language diversity: Problem or resource? A social and educational perspective on language minorities in the United States* (pp. 140–163). New York: Newbury House.

Zuk, G. H., Miller, R. L., Bartram, J. B., & Kling, F. (1961). Maternal acceptance of retarded children: A questionnaire study of attitudes and religious background. *Child Development, 32,* 525–540.

C H A P T E R   6

Native Americans with Visual Impairments

Irene Topor

Before I was hired to teach adaptive physical education in the Chinle School District, I spent one week living in a hogan, which is the traditional Navajo home on the reservation in this area. The superintendent of the school district believed in having us become familiar with the culture by "living it." There were 14 other people and me. We prepared our meals by butchering sheep and cleaning the intestines. We tried a variety of foods that were unfamiliar to me. We hiked daily in a nearby canyon. Ms. Thomas, the superintendent, told us stories about the culture every day. She insisted that if we were to stay and teach her children, that we respect them and that we were in Chinle to learn their ways. She said that if we learned about their culture, we would "adjust" to one another. For example, we were told to play string games (making spiderwebs or cobwebs) or jump rope after the first snow, or we would be breaking tradition with tribal beliefs. Flying kites during the month of March was not acceptable, according to some of the clans on the reservation. I remember that only 3 of the 15 people stayed to work in the district after the weeklong orientation." (M. J. Martinez, personal communication, 1997)

As a teacher of exceptional students, Ms. Martinez is sensitive to the Native American traditions and culture that have continued for thousands of years and generations of ancestors. Historians and anthropologists have confirmed the existence of unique Native American societies through evidence found at religious and burial sites and pottery, clothing, and basketry discovered throughout the United States and other parts of the world. The materials and artifacts clearly support the idea that Native American people made use of the land and resources to accomplish much in the arts and sciences that equaled or exceeded the achievements of Europeans (Joe & Malach, 1998).

Service providers who are of other cultures need to understand the customs, beliefs, and communication styles of Native Americans to provide the best possible intervention and education to individuals in these unique cultures. This chapter presents an overview of the current demographics of Native Americans, including population, language, geographic distribution, and social and economic considerations. It then discusses what is known about the most common causes of eye disease in young and elderly Native Americans and finally the effect of Native American cultural beliefs and customs on the treatment of this small but diverse group of people with visual impairments.

Many of the references and much of the information presented here reflect the Native American experiences of the Southwest.

DEMOGRAPHICS
Geographic Distribution

Native American families live in every state and in most major cities. The 554 distinct tribal groups and villages found in the United States (Egan, 1998) have diverse cultures. They include the "woodland" Indians of the Northeast, Pueblos of the Southwest, Seminoles of the Southeast, Menominees and Chippewas in Wisconsin, Eastern Cherokees in North Carolina, Choctaws in Mississippi, Creeks in Alabama, and several tribes that scattered along the northern, southern, and eastern coasts. In addition, there are coastal communities of the Northwest and Eskimo/ Aleut tribes in the Arctic.

The federal government recognizes all these tribes, or nations, as sovereign entities, with the right to make their own laws enforced by various degrees of power. These nations cover 56 million acres, 314 reservations, and about 1.5 million people living on or near tribal land, less than 1 percent of the overall population of the United States, spread over slightly more than 2 percent of the land (Egan, 1998; Indian Health Service [IHS], 2000). The remainder of the estimated 2.4 million Native Americans in 2000 live in urban and suburban areas (U.S. Bureau of the Census, 1999b). Native Americans are a significant rural population, especially in the West, where about half the people live on or near reservations. The vast majority of these are in rural and remote areas (Seekins, 1997).

Population

The once-dominant Native American population was reduced from slightly less than 1 million people in 1750 to 250,000 in 1890 (Thornton, 1990) because of disease and warfare. Epidemics, such as typhus and small pox, killed a substantial number of Native Americans. In addition, Native Americans were captured by both European and Native American enemies, sometimes slaughtered, and often enslaved.

The introduction of alcohol had a depopulating effect on the Native American tribes. In the late 17th century, Native American leaders recognized that traders from other areas were offering alcohol to their people and pleaded with the colonial leaders to curb the spread of alcohol. Many native societies were destroyed by the quest for alcohol. As Thornton (1990, p. 66) noted, "Alcohol loosened the Indian's hold on his land. Treaties were signed 'under the influence,' an abuse that fueled Indian-white conflict throughout the colonial period and beyond."

The population of Native Americans has rebounded since the

late 19th century. According to the U.S. Bureau of the Census (1999a, 1999c) there are about 2.4 million Native Americans in 2000, up from 2.1 million in 1990 and 1.4 million in 1980.

The demographic profile of many reservation communities parallels that of developing countries, with a high proportion of young people, high birth rates, and high mortality rates (Joe & Malach, 1998). Over half the population of Native Americans is under age 20. The birth rate for American Indians and Alaska Natives in 1991–93 of 26.6 births per 1,000 people was 67 percent greater than the birth rate for all races in the United States in 1992 and 77 percent greater than the rate for the U.S. white population (IHS, 1996a). Similarly, in Canada, indigenous people have a 70 percent higher birth rate than the general population (Monastyrski, 1998)

Death rates of American Indian and Alaska Natives from 1992 to 1994 were more than double the rate for the United States as a whole in 1992 for ages 1–4 and 15–44; 30 percent of American Indians died before they reached 45. However, the Indian rate of death was lower than the U.S. rate for white age groups over 85 (IHS, 1996b).

Language

More than 250 languages are in use among the Native American population. Of the eight language groupings that are used to classify most of the Indian languages, Iroquoian, Uto-Aztecan, Muskogean, Caddoan, and Athapaskan are examples (Joe & Malach, 1998). English is spoken by more than 1.5 million persons in the American Indian population and is the primary language for the younger generation, many of whom do not speak or understand their tribal languages. Almost half a million individuals speak a language other than English, and more than a third of the Native American population do not speak English "very well" (Joe & Malach, 1998; U.S. Bureau of the Census, 1995).

In the late 1800s, the U.S. Bureau of Indian Affairs (BIA) did little to support the loyalty of Native Americans to their dominant languages. The agency established strict English-only rules, under which students were punished and humiliated for speaking their native languages. John Collier, the commissioner of the BIA during the New Deal, condemned and prohibited the exclusion of native languages in the boarding school system, but the English-only rules and punishments persisted unofficially for another generation (Crawford, 1994).

Efforts to reverse the erosion of native languages are beginning. Navajo, Tohono O'odham, Pasqua, Yaqui, Northern Ute, and Arapaho, among many other tribes have adopted policies to promote their ancestral languages. Bilingual education programs have been instituted in Native American schools to assist young children to maintain or learn these languages (Crawford, 1996). As a result of the Native American Languages Act of 1990 and 1992, which protects indigenous languages and authorized a grant program for language conservation, 18 language-revitalization projects were initiated nationwide (Crawford, 1996).

Evidence of Native American language resources now exists on the Internet, including sources for learning Blackfoot, Cherokee, Cree, Lakota, Mohawk, Mohican, Navajo, Oneida, Potowatami, and Quechua (see "Native American Language Resources," 2000). Resources for learning and maintaining Native American languages are increasing for both children and adults.

Selected Social and Economic Characteristics

Common agendas among Native American tribes are the right to self-government, access to high-quality health care and education, and appreciation and encouragement of tribal languages and cultures (Joe & Malach, 1998). Although the different Native American communities attempt to maintain their own tribal identities and to remain separate and distinct from one another, they still have many problems in common. The following educational and occupational characteristics were found in the U.S. Bureau of the Census 1990 data (U.S. Bureau of the Census, 1995b). The data were derived from the 25 largest Native American tribes in the United States and may not reflect the smaller tribes.

EDUCATION

Of the quarter million Native Americans aged 18–24, 63 percent are high school graduates, but only 2.1 percent have bachelor's or higher degrees. For the approximately 1 million persons aged 25 or older, 66 percent are high school graduates, but only 9 percent have four or more years of college as compared to 17.6 percent of the U.S. population as a whole.

Trends in education are illustrated by data on Native American students in 22 public school districts in New Mexico (New Mexico Department of Education, 1998). The average composite scores on the ACT Assessment to assess high school students' general educational development for Native American students who graduated from New Mexico Public High schools from 1995 to 1997 fell below those of all other racial or ethnic groups in the state. In the 1995–96 school year, the dropout rate for all students enrolled in grades 9–12 was 8.5 percent versus 8.6 percent for Native American students. A trend toward fewer Native American student dropouts was notable from 1,135 in the 1990–91 school year to 873 in 1995–96. Furthermore, about two-thirds of the 98 percent Native American student enrollment in the Zuni School District were living in poverty. Other states with many Native American students may have similar rates for academic achievement, dropouts, and poverty.

OCCUPATIONS AND INCOME

The predominant occupations among Native Americans are farming, forestry, and fishing; administrative support or clerical positions; and precision production and repair occupations. The median family income of Native American families in 1989 was $21,619 compared to $35,225 for the U.S. population as a whole. With regard to poverty rates, the incomes of 27 percent of Native American families versus 31 percent of all individuals in the U.S. workforce were below the poverty level (U.S. Bureau of the Census, 1995b). The per capita income of the American Indian population was below $10,000 versus $14,420 for the U.S. population as a whole.

Related Economic and Social Concerns

Native Americans have the highest rates of alcoholism, suicide, and child abuse in the country, although some progress is being made, particularly with alcoholism (IHS, 1996a; Joe & Malach, 1998). A number of Native American groups are developing programs to combat alcoholism. For example, the Blackfoot tribe has a youth alcoholism-prevention program for girls aged 11–19, and the National Association for Native American Children of Alcoholics (NANACOA) established a national network in 1988 (nanacoa@aol.com; Stevenson, 1998), that conducts annual conferences.

Every U.S. census for more than 100 years after the last treaty in the 1800s between U.S. government and Indian nations has found Indian lands to be islands of poverty, with chronic unemployment and rates of disease and early death the highest in the country. These economic and social conditions contribute to the depressed conditions of many Native American families.

There are two extremes of socioeconomic conditions within the archipelago of 554 Native American nations in the United States, far beyond the popular image of modern tribes—from the poverty of the Pine Ridge Reservation in South Dakota, which includes the poorest county in the United States, to the prosperity of the Mashantucket Pequots of Connecticut, who run the largest gambling casino in the country (Egan, 1998). A new generation of Native American leaders, who arose from the sovereignty movement of the 1970s, is assuming authority at the same time that many tribes are becoming prosperous from the earnings of their tribal casinos. Now the tribes' economic, legal, and political strength meet. For example, the leaders of the Goshute tribe leased part of their reservation as a temporary storage ground for nuclear waste in Skull Valley, Utah. The tribe was reprimanded for not following the tradition to be "keepers of the earth instead of protectors of its poisons," but the Goshutes said that they are asserting themselves as a nation within a nation, free to make its own decisions (Egan, 1998). The Muckleshoots Indian tribe of Washington built a casino in 1996. It has become one of the most successful tribal casinos in the country and is a step toward self-sufficiency coupled with jobs.

Since 1988, when Congress approved gambling operations on tribal lands, one third of all tribes have begun to operate some form of gambling enterprise, and although this windfall is unevenly spread, it generates more than $6 billion a year. This venture into gambling has changed the Americans' view of Native Americans (Egan, 1998), even though some of the tribes have not directly received financial benefits from the gambling. Some tribes hire an outside business to run their casinos. The business takes a percentage of the casino's profits that is not returned to the people. In the state of Arizona, the casinos pay a state tax from their profits for the right to operate the casino.

There are some instances in Arizona of the proceeds benefiting the tribe. According to a local newspaper article entitled, "The O'odham people cash in on casino profit" (Duarte, 2000), almost 24,000 tribal members are eligible to receive $2,000 each for a total payment of $49 million from casino profits. These cash payouts are derived from the casino's net profits of $70 million. The tribe's overall economic plan includes $116.5 million in projects, including construction of a nursing home, clinic, community college, cultural museum, radio station, and third casino. Tribes with gambling casinos have had the means to develop cultural programs, to pursue the revival of their languages, to provide scholarships, and to improve their schools. It was one of three Supreme Court decisions in the early 1830s that established the right of Native American tribes to be free from state control, although the tribes remained subordinate to the U.S. Congress. One hundred and seventy years later in the year 2000, this remains the governing framework.

CAUSES OF VISUAL IMPAIRMENTS AMONG NATIVE AMERICANS

Native Americans are at a higher risk for visual impairment than are other groups in the United States because of genetic factors and limited access to appropriate medical care, health education, and good nutrition. Rearwin, Jubilee, Tang, and Hughes (1997) determined that 15 percent of the decreased vision of Navajos was caused by congenital or hereditary conditions, and the other 85 percent was due to acquired visual impairment. When Gay Nord (personal communication, 1997), an optometrist for the IHS on the Navajo reservation in Tuba City, Arizona, reviewed the most common causes of visual impairment in her clinic over a two-month period in 1997, she found that glaucoma (secondary and open angle), cataracts, diabetic retinopathy, macular degeneration, and corneal opacities headed the list. Nord stated that there is a high rate of astigmatism and monocular/amblyopia in childhood because Native American children do not regularly wear eyeglasses. Wearing the eyeglasses during the early years of life potentially decreased the occurrence of amblyopia. In addition, running water is often not available on some of the reservations, and general environmental conditions make the use of contact lenses unsafe. Dobson, Tyszko, Miller, and Harvey (1998) found that the prevalences of astigmatism among children (aged 8 and older) and adults in the Tohono O'odham Nation located in Sells, Arizona west of Tucson were 61 percent and 89 percent, respectively. One third of the children had high-enough astigmatism that eyeglasses were warranted to treat potentially debilitating amblyopia, or lazy eye (Dobson et al., 1998).

Diabetic Retinopathy

Native Americans aged 45–65 have a rate of diabetes mellitus that is about four times greater than the rate in the general U.S. population in the same age group (Ponchillia, 1993). Diabetic retinopathy, a complication of diabetes that leads to the loss of vision, has become a major focus of eye care providers on the reservations. The prevalence of Type II diabetes among Native Americans is 12.2 percent for those over age 19 ("Diabetes Among Native Americans," 2000) and is expected to rise dramatically. One tribe, the Pima Indians of Arizona, has the highest rate of diabetes in the world—about 50 percent of those aged 30–64 ("Diabetes Among Native Americans," 2000). Although data on the exact number of Native Americans who lose their vision because of diabetic retinopathy is limited, the American Diabetes Association ("Diabetes Among Native Americans," 2000) estimated that diabetic retinopathy occurs in 18 percent of Pima Indians and 24.4 percent of Oklahoma Indians. Health and rehabilitation professionals anticipate a large increase in cases of diabetic retinopathy in the future because cultural beliefs, poverty, isolation, and the lack of education and access to basic health care hamper the early diagnosis and treatment of diabetes and its complications. For example, Nord (personal communication, 1997) stated, "The belief of witching is strong here. If you tell them something might happen to them and it does, then that person is the cause of the eye disease . . . I find it very difficult to find sensitive ways to inform people who have traditional beliefs, 17% of whom do not speak English and have little education." (Traditional beliefs about disease and disability are discussed in more detail in the next section.)

Nord also noted that the age at which she sees diabetic patients at the IHS clinic in Tuba City, Arizona, is decreasing: "We see people in their 30s and 40s with a diabetes diagnosis. The numbers keep growing and growing and the potential for the rate of diabetic retinopathy to go up 10 years from now is great." Rearwin et al. (1997) found diabetes mellitus to be the most prevalent (45 cases) of all preventable causes of legal blindness among Navajos in a study of 455 cases.

An example of how diabetic retinopathy can affect Native Americans is Ruth, a 55–year-old Navajo woman. When interviewed by the author, Ruth described how the traditional methods of healing were combined with more modern medical treatments and spoke with much emotion about how her loss of vision has affected her life.

———————

Ruth was first diagnosed with diabetic retinopathy in 1990, when she lived in Rock Springs, New Mexico, in the Navajo Nation. She has since moved to Ganado, Arizona. Ruth has eight children, three of whom were still living at home (a mobile trailer with running water and electricity).

Ruth worked as a dormitory aide for the Bureau of Indian Affairs boarding school for 20 years. One day in March 1990, Ruth noticed her vision was blurring as she drove home from work, and she accidentally sideswiped an oncoming vehicle. She went to the ophthalmologist, who told her that her reduced vision was due to diabetes. Ruth agreed to surgery, but also completed various traditional ceremonies. She said:

"I tried many medicine men because a medicine woman looked in a crystal and said that 11 medicine men needed to be consulted. Two of the 11 men said I should not have had the surgery. I found out that "a nerve" had accidentally been hurt, so my vision was now even worse. I was given many herbs so that I would regain my ability to see. One of them was called Yaz Puchee, or the Beauty Way. I took it and prayed that I would see again. . . . One day I was almost struck by lightning. There was smoke after the lightning . . . like my vision . . . blurry and unclear. . . .

To this day I have not received rehabilitation training. I used to weave, crochet, draw, and make pictures with felt, macramé and make ceramic pots. I crochet by touch, but have been unable to figure out how to weave with my loom. I can't figure out the yarn on the side. . . . My children do the cooking. I miss looking into my grandchildren's faces and watching them play, especially when they are full of excitement and joy. . . . I am divorced now. . . . I assume that my former husband's pride and ignorance got the best of him. I want others in my tribe to know more about how disability affects people and their families.

> Ruth wished that the healthcare system would provide more public education about the effects of diabetes on vision. She did not want anyone else to experience what she went through.

Other Causes of Decreased Vision

In Rearwin et al.'s (1997) study of blindness among Navajos, trauma was the largest single cause of decreased vision and the largest preventable cause. More than 30 percent of trauma-related eye injuries resulted from fistfights and various types of assaults with weapons, such as firearms, baseball bats, and knives. Eye injuries resulting from work and home accidents were also reported.

Congenital or hereditary causes of decreased vision among Navajos were retinitis pigmentosa and oculocutaneous albinism, which accounted for over 50 percent of the cases. Heckenlively, Friederich, Farson, and Pabalis (1981) noted that both types of retinitis pigmentosa, dominant and recessive, have a childhood onset that is easily identified by age 6. They stated that retinitis pigmentosa has been identified in 1 in every 1,800 Navajo children, but that the true incidence is thought to be higher. Heckenlively (1988) stated that the role of heredity is widely acknowledged as a significant determinant of retinitis pigmentosa. Heckenlively (2000) reported that there are actually several types of retinitis pigmentosa in Navajo individuals. Since there has been great progress in diagnosis, it should be possible to track causative genes if families are willing to participate. Stargardt's disease, congenital toxoplasmosis, optic nerve hypoplasia, and oculocutaneous albinism were some of the other congenital causes of visual impairments found in Navajo children.

A neuropathy characterized by weakness, insensitivity to pain, and corneal ulcerations has also been identified as a cause of visual impairment among Navajos to the extent that it has been called Navajo neuropathy (Singleton, 1987; Singleton, et al. 1990). Corneal ulcerations, progressive deterioration of the central nervous system, multiple impairments, low muscle tone, liver failure, and demyelinization of the nerves are additional symptoms.

Reports of the rise in cases of Type II diabetes in children ("Native Americans and Diabetes," 2000) and the rising rate of accidents and trauma (IHS, 1996b, 2000) that place individuals at risk for eye injury strongly suggest that visual impairments among Native Americans are likely to increase. Regardless of the cause of a visual impairment, eye care professionals must offer creative ways to treat the condition through surgery, medicine, and/or regular follow-up visits to the IHS.

For many Native Americans who hold steadfastly to traditional beliefs, the treatment of visual impairments solely through modern medicine is insufficient because it affects the body but not the spirit. Treating the spiritual as well as the physical component of the individual is crucial to many Native Americans. The spiritual leader or medicine person restores harmony by determining the reason why the visual impairment occurred and then recommending treatment that will restore harmony for both the physical and spiritual being. The ability to combine spiritual with physical healing may affect the success of the IHS's treatment of Native Americans with visual impairments.

It is imperative that providers of early intervention, educational, and rehabilitation services be aware of traditional and cultural beliefs that may affect the identification of vision loss, as well as communication with and services to Native Americans. The following section discusses additional cultural beliefs of Native Americans, especially perspectives on disability. Further implications of Native American values are discussed at the end of this chapter.

NATIVE AMERICAN CULTURAL BELIEFS
Beliefs About Disability
The perception of disability varies significantly among Native American tribes. Most Native American belief systems incorporate ideas of multiple causality of illness and misfortune, some

originating from supernatural or natural causes (Joe & Malach, 1998; Joe & Miller, 1987). The supernatural causes may link etiology to witchcraft, spirit loss, spirit intrusion, spells, and various unnatural forces. Illness may also be attributed to various natural disturbances of "balance" (disharmony) brought on by breaking a cultural taboo, acculturation, or accidents not instigated by witchcraft or the harmful wishes of others. Doug Sixkiller St. Clair (personal communication, 1996), a project director of the client assistance program, Institute for Human Development, Northern Arizona University, Tucson, who is of Cherokee heritage, described the meaning of disability, as he understood it:

> I know of no Native language that has any words that directly translate disabilities as English does. Many Indian names infer a disability (Lame Deer, Broken Nose, Walking Stick, Tall Whiteman, etc.); however, these descriptions do not infer inability. Many American Indian cultures revere individuals that the European see as disabled. Some examples of this would be Kokopeli (hunch backed), Mangus Colorado and his sister Lozen (giantism), and Sequoyah (crippled). . . . [N]o one in the culture would be treated special or better than anyone else . . . unless this individual was gifted to such a degree that they can benefit the people as no one else can. Examples of gifted individuals would be medicine people, spiritual leaders, and visionary leaders. . . . Visual impairment (as defined in English) can mean that the individual with the impairment becomes a visionary and [she or] he would hold a special relationship within the culture. However, if the result is that the individual is not a visionary, this does not mean that [she or] he holds a lessened relationship within the culture. Rehabilitation is a word that does not translate. How do you translate segregation, isolation, and labeling in a culture where every one is included? Rehabilitation means to restore, or to put back in order. Well, you can't do this when everyone has a relationship and a position.

When Native Americans are told that a child was born with a disability as a result of a genetic disorder, the diagnosis will not be disputed because it explains *how* the condition occurred, but the parents may turn to their cultural resources to find out *why* the disability occurred. The explanation may be a breach of a cultural taboo. Hopis, a Pueblo tribe in northern Arizona, often believe that an illness or acquired disability is the consequence of an action or attitude (Locust, 1990). They believe that the original spiritual "being" shared with the Hopi people certain rules of life and placed spiritual helpers, the kachinas, near the tribe to protect and help them maintain a certain way of life. The kachinas help teach and guide the Hopis with their songs, prayers, and ceremonies (Mails, 1997). Tragic consequences are most likely to be manifested when a major transgression has occurred, like marrying within one's clan or breaking a kachina taboo. These consequences, such as a disability, are seen not as punishments, but as the logical outcomes that one must bear, although sometimes the reason for a disability remains unclear. In one case, the reason for a daughter's disability is illustrated by the experience of Sophia, a Hopi woman who is the mother of a blind girl, Andrea, and a teacher of students with visual impairments.

Andrea, age 14, was born prematurely, which resulted in retinopathy of prematurity. She has light perception and no other physical or mental disabilities. Andrea attends school in the Tuba City, Arizona, school system on the Navajo reservation, where Sophia is an itinerant teacher of students with visual impairments. Another teacher of students with visual impairments provides Andrea with academic instruction and orientation and mobility services.

Sophia earned a master's degree in education of visually impaired students from the University of Arizona in 1993. She volunteers much of her time outside work and home responsibilities to assist others in her tribe who have children with disabilities. She organized a Hopi support group for new parents of children newly identified with disabilities, gave talks to the local Lions Club, and facilitated parents anonymous, a group of Native American parents of children with disabilities on the Hopi reservation. Sophia implemented a Summer Youth Employment

Program for youths aged 14–18 with disabilities, in 1997, whose program objectives were to teach the students practical skills, such as cleaning tables, doing laundry, folding clothes, and ironing. In the café on the Hopi reservation, she taught the students to set and bus tables; in an office environment, she taught them to file. She recruited the students by sending surveys to families who she knew from her volunteer work in the community. Sophia recognizes her traditional roots by stating that she is a member of the ghost clan. The women in this clan assume leadership roles in the Hopi culture.

Sophia intends to teach Andrea the traditions of the Hopi tribe and assist her to acculturate to the society at large with the help of Andrea's godmother. Sophia wants Andrea to achieve her potential through an excellent education on the reservation. Sophia and Andrea's godmother will soon prepare Andrea for initiation into the tribe. The preparation requires that Andrea know how to weave baskets and bake traditional foods, which Sophia feels confident that Andrea can learn with adaptations and modifications. Andrea's participation in the tribe's traditional ceremonies and customs keeps her active. She spends time socializing with friends after school and baking cookies (under Sophia's direction). Andrea's activities are similar to other children's on the reservation so that Andrea can form relationships that will be important to her continuing success in school and in the celebrations of the Hopi tribe.

When asked about the Hopi beliefs about disability and visual impairment in particular, Sophia replied:

> If your child is born with a defect, you have deviated from the norm. In my case, Andrea is blind because she was a "medical problem." I followed the Hopi belief system. I'm a religious person and believe in Hopi values and the traditional way. When I was pregnant with Andrea, I was overworking. She was born five months prematurely; it had nothing to do with my deviating from the norm or a consequence of something that I had done wrong. Usually in Hopi society, that is the belief, that if you bear a child with a disability, you didn't believe in the system." . . . I married someone within my clan, but I can't really say that this is the

reason Andrea was born with a disability. Maybe because we were married and were within the same clan, something may have caused Andrea to be born early. That's why Andrea was born the way she was, but I'm not sure about this. But that is the belief—we shouldn't marry our clan brothers or sisters. When I was pregnant with Andrea, when I was working, an accident occurred. I fell off the stairs, and I was rushed to the hospital and Andrea was born early. If Andrea had been born at full term and was blind, then I might believe that I had done something wrong.

For some tribes, disability emerges out of an individual's lack of relationships, rather than a medical diagnosis of a physical difference. If a person is unable to give to and share with others in personal interactions, then he or she may have a disability. Joe and Miller (1987) stated that many Native American families are reluctant to define another family member as disabled unless the disability is severe enough to prevent the person from interacting and participating with or relating to others. Individuals who have been labeled disabled but who sustain and develop meaningful relationships with others are unlikely to be defined as disabled or placed outside the family for "care."

The relationships that a person with a disability has with others will lead to a "wellness," according to many native tribes, a harmony of the body, mind, and spirit (Locust, 1985). Harmony is to be at "oneness'" with life, eternity, the Supreme Creator, and oneself; it is an attitude toward life that creates peace. For a person with a visual impairment, it may include compensating for having a visual loss. It is not "events" that happen to a person, but the person's response to those events that matter. Sixkiller St. Clair (personal communication, 1996) defined harmony this way:

> Human beings are made up of a mind, a body, and a spirit. If the body does not function as the average body does, that does not mean that mind and the spirit are not as pure as they were when they were given by the creator. Harmony can still be found.

In most tribes, there is a belief that a spirit chooses which body it will inhabit (Locust, 1994). If a spirit chooses to inhabit a disabled body, then it is the spirit's choice. Many tribes see the spirit not as being "entrapped in a disabled body" (Locust, 1994) or "having the misfortune to be disabled" (Locust, 1994), but as being wise enough and strong enough to inhabit a disabled body. The physical body may have been disabled, but the spirit was not and the spirit had a choice of whether it would use the body or not.

The belief that acquired disability is a logical outcome of a transgression is held by many Native Americans and may affect the identification or treatment of those with diabetic retinopathy, for instance, because individuals may believe that they are experiencing the inevitable results of a transgression at some point in their lives. Each tribe has its own set of moral, religious, or cultural taboos. For example, being near certain creatures, such as some reptiles, spiders and other insects, birds, or animals, can cause illness if tribal beliefs identify these creatures as carriers of negative energy (Locust, 1985). Members of the Apache tribe may become ill if they are near a place where a bear urinated or ate. Locust (1985) described the case of an Apache father whom the tribe considered responsible for his child's deformed hip because he cut down a tree that had been struck by lightning to use for firewood—a transgression because anything struck by lightning is taboo to the Apaches. If the father had been in complete harmony, he would have known that the tree had been struck by lightning and would not have touched it.

A transgression will occur if personal conduct is not in line with the tribe's belief system. Most tribes have some restrictions about touching the dead, cleansing rituals for those who have prepared a body for burial or cremation, and strict procedures for the disposal of the belongings of the dead. Marrying into one's clan is the same as marrying one's sister or brother and hence is strictly forbidden in almost every tribe (Locust, 1985).

Outcomes may be related to the type of transgression. For instance, visual impairments may be attributed to looking at something considered taboo, which makes it difficult to acknowledge that they are the result of diseases or conditions (Ponchillia, 1993). Ruth, the Navajo woman who acknowledged her reduced visual abilities only after being in car accident, attributed her vision loss to the smoke she saw after lightning struck, which is how she describes what the world presently looks like to her.

To prevent a condition from worsening or to prevent future misfortune, the individual or family may turn to tribal healers or practitioners for assistance while they continue to visit an eye care specialist. For example, when a child is born with a visual impairment that is not immediately life threatening, the family may seek consultation from a tribal healer before they consent to surgery for the child, additional medications, or eye examinations from an eye care specialist. Some families may not volunteer information about their traditional practices, in fear that the service providers will not respect their wishes. In the case of Andrea, described earlier, the family used both medical and traditional practitioners:

Sophia returned with Andrea to her home on the Hopi reservation. After working with the family outreach worker for several months, Sophia decided to schedule another ophthalmological examination for Andrea. Sophia took Andrea to Tucson to seek a second opinion from a pediatric ophthalmologist about the severity of Andrea's retinopathy of prematurity. Sophia and Larry, Andrea's father, had observed Andrea and wondered if she had more ability to see than was originally thought. Andrea appeared to be looking in the direction of light and played with toys on a light box that Larry made for her. The second ophthalmologist confirmed the first ophthalmologist's diagnosis of Andrea's eye condition ("no light perception vision"). They contacted an outreach program for families and children with visual impairments. It was at this point that Sophia asked medicine people to perform healing ceremonies with Andrea. Sophia believed that the tribal healers would help restore Andrea to a state of natural harmony or beauty. The family prayed to the longhaired kachinas while attending a dance ceremony. The ceremony gave the family comfort, peace of mind, and a positive outlook on Andrea's future.

Other Cultural Values and Beliefs
ROLE OF THE EXTENDED FAMILY

Most Native American families include both extended and immediate family members. A recurring theme of life and health in native cultures is the circle: Each person is born into a circle of family and community that supports the person and that the person, in turn, supports. Another way to view this circle is as a large extended family in which events that occur to one person affect the group, and vice versa. Shared responsibilities in Native American families involve more than one individual in decision-making and child-rearing responsibilities (Dufort & Reed, 1995). In the Hopi tribe, the godmother is an important adult figure in the lives of children. Sophia explained how Andrea's godmother was selected:

When Andrea was born, she had a baby-naming ceremony, and at that time, I selected the godparents for her. After the ceremony, the godmother takes the role of disciplining and nurturing Andrea. There's a lot of things the godmother has to do for the godchild. She will prepare Andrea for the initiation ceremony, teach her values of life—what to do and not to do. Andrea's godmother is the leader of the women's basket society, so Andrea has to be there to help [and] will have a major role [in that society] when she grows up; she will assume the responsibilities of her godmother. Andrea doesn't know this yet. When she goes through initiation, the godmother tells her what she'll be and do from here on—our traditional values will get taught. The godmother and I will work together. Our extended family is very involved also. . . . My mother, Andrea's grandmother, still believes that Andrea will be unable to carry on the traditions of her godmother. I feel differently. We will teach Andrea to make baskets. She is really good with her hands. I think that it will be easy to teach her to pick out the Yucca for basket making. I think that she can distinguish it from other types of plants we use to make baskets.

In addition to godparents, other extended family members, such as grandparents, aunts, and uncles, may assume child-rearing responsibilities. Aunts and grandmothers are the most common surrogate mothers in the Navajo tribe (Joe, 1982). Mary Jo Martinez (personal communication, 1997), who teaches adaptive physical education in Chinle, Arizona, observed that it is common for family members other than the biological mother and father to raise a child. For example, Martinez told of a parent who approached her one day to say that the parent's sister had given the parent the student who was in Martinez's class. This woman would now function as the mother and raise the child.

The involvement of extended family members in the lives of individuals with visual impairments can ease the efforts of service providers if these family members are included in implementing educational and rehabilitation programs. Since many Native American women help with the day-to-day needs of young children with visual impairments, service providers can teach them ways to improve the children's ability to do many things that are considered important for their families. On the other end of the life span, since Native American elders are usually respected because of the wisdom and experience that come with age, those with acquired visual impairments will be cared for unless the extended family is also taught techniques to help the elders complete familiar tasks that give them pleasure and a sense of independence. To maximize the involvement of extended family members in the instruction of elders, service providers need to learn to communicate effectively with them, as discussed in the next section.

COMMUNICATION STYLES

Communication styles are the cultural guidelines of interaction that influence or regulate the ways in which individuals talk to each other; use or think about silence, body language, and laughter; ask questions; and provide information and elaborate on important points (Dufort & Reed, 1995). Differences in styles of communication may exist between Native Americans and non-Native Americans.

In general, professionals who are not Native Americans ask specific questions and expect the people with whom they are communicating to maintain eye contact as a sign of listening and respect. In contrast, some Native Americans are brought up to show respect for people of knowledge and authority by not asking direct questions and not making eye contact (Dufort & Reed, 1995; Orlansky & Trap, 1987). In many Indian cultures, it is appropriate in certain situations to communicate an issue to a third person who assists in giving the information to the intended recipient (Joe & Malach, 1998). According to Dufort and Reed (1995), in the Navajo conversational style, each speaker takes a turn to make a point without interruptions and often emphasizes important points through repetition or by indirectly stating the points in the words of someone else. Thus, Navajos may be more comfortable providing information in short vignettes and brief narratives, rather than by answering questions. In addition, loud talking is viewed as rude behavior, and it is acceptable to look toward Navajo elders but not to maintain direct or lengthy eye contact, although one can maintain direct eye contact with children (Dufort & Reed, 1995). A light handshake or touching of hands is an expression of polite greeting and leave taking.

Since some English words have no direct translation in native tribal languages, an interpreter can provide the information to the family in the tribe's native tongue. Dufort and Reed (1995) suggested that the family should be consulted about an interpreter, since some families prefer interpreters from within the family and others do not. If an issue is emotional or jargon is used, it is appropriate in certain situations to communicate it to the interpreter, who then gives the information to the intended recipients.

Humor is considered an essential part of Native American life. In some tribal communities, one is expected to have a "joking" relationship with certain relatives (Joe & Malach, 1998). If an individual providing service to a Navajo family or individuals is teased, it is considered a gesture of acceptance (Reed, personal communication, 1997).

Martinez (personal communication, 1997), the adaptive physical education teacher in the Chinle school district, learned that Native Americans shelter their bodies in many ways that are culturally significant. In this account, she describes her experiences with some of her students before she understood these traditions.

> One incident that stands out in my mind was the time I taught square dancing, and some of the children would not hold hands. I didn't know if it was because of their age or if the children were shy. Finally, one student told me that some of them could not hold hands with each other because they were members of the same clan. Ever since that time, I have been careful to pair kids who were not of the same clan (I had to ask) or give pairs of children a handkerchief or rope to hold onto if they were of the same clan. Maybe I didn't need to do this, but I felt safer doing it this way. Another situation took me by surprise. I cut a student's hair to remove some gum. The parent called me the next day and told me not to do this again. . . . I have been on the reservation for 14 years now and regularly consult the school janitor, cook, and families about their beliefs to make sure that I am not contradicting tradition or overstepping any boundaries.

CULTURAL VALUES

Certain beliefs or behaviors may be based on cultural values that may not be obvious to service providers but are important to understand prior to and during communication exchanges. Examples of such values include the following (Locust, 1994):

- Loyalty is to the tribe, clan, and family, not to the school system, agency, or the government.
- The group's unity is binding. Breaking this bond violates unwritten tribal ethics.
- Avoiding disharmony is desirable because being around disharmony can cause a person to be in disharmony.
- The body is sacred to its owner, including the body space around him or her, personal information, and even the person's given name.
- The breaking of maternal bonds with children of both sexes occurs early (at ages 5–9, not 18). It does not mean the end of teaching or supervision, but the end of absolute parental control. For example, children aged 5 and 6 were dropped off at an eye clinic without parental supervision or requests for information.
- The concept of time is culturally determined and is often not measured by a clock. Native Americans mark time on the basis of the seasons, with daily routines gauged by the position of the sun or moon. Human development may be measured according to various tribal customs, such as the naming ceremony, laughs her first laughs, or takes the first step (Joe & Malach, 1998).
- Concepts of education and work are cultural. The amount of and kind of education and work done are related to cultural beliefs from traditional to contemporary.
- Concepts of right and wrong are cultural (e.g., marrying a person within one's own class, using wood for fire that has been struck by lightning).

PROGRAMS FOR NATIVE AMERICANS WITH VISUAL IMPAIRMENTS

Rehabilitation and educational programs have been developed to serve Native American adults and children in their homes and specialized schools. The success of these programs can be attributed to the consideration for Native American beliefs about including family members in the rehabilitation process and to training visually impaired individuals on reservations with family members present so that new skills can be incorporated into the daily routines. Specialized schools also serve a unique role in the education of Native American children and youths, especially if the children and youths are encouraged by their families to attend them to meet educational goals.

Independent Living Programs

The American Foundation for the Blind (AFB)'s Hopi Visually Impaired Project (VIP) (Cummings, 1993) recognized that independent living skills for Hopi individuals with visual impairments should enable them to continue to participate as fully as possible in their extended families and clans. Toward this end, a series of audiotapes specific to the Hopi nation were made to teach persons with visual impairments and their families to carry out different activities even though vision had temporarily affected the ability to complete many activities (Cummings, 1993). The VIP recognized that Hopis with visual impairments wanted to continue to participate in social networks of exchange of goods and services; ceremonies, such as baby namings, initiation rites, and weddings; home and agricultural activities; and activities of religious societies, villages, schools, and the community at large. In short, the aim was to encourage an individual with a visual impairment to find fulfillment as a person in a distinctly Hopi, closely interdependent way, and the training took into account the close connection of individuals in the Hopi society. The VIP found that the extended family is probably the most significant Hopi social unit to recognize when planning the delivery of on-reservation health services.

VIP also identified concerns expressed by individuals with visual impairments and their extended families about their ability to be active through learned skills. Family issues and barriers to training that were found included frustration, anxiety, embarrassment, anger, and the lack of self-confidence because of the inability to complete visual tasks. However, travel to urban centers for intense instruction that related more to another culture was not considered, especially if the skills learned would not be useful at home. Culture-specific daily living skills were emphasized in the areas of the safe use of wood and coal stoves and techniques to use when electricity and running water are not available. Sample adapted activities included making banana (*kwanni*) bread, setting up a quilt frame, putting fabric on the quilt frame, and tying the quilt. Other adaptations included skills for growing and preparing corn, preparing ceremonial-related items, artisan work, agriculture, and food preparation. The VIP (Cummings, 1993) established a database that can be used by the Hopi tribe to design local programs and support services for the reservation's population. Since the family is involved with the day-to-day activities of the individual with a visual impairment, it is common to find other family members absorbing the roles of those who can no longer perform the tasks. This tradition is not specific to the Hopi tribe. Ruth, the Navajo woman who lost her vision to diabetic retinopathy, relied on her children to cook and clean.

Another project designed to provide education and training to Native Americans in their home communities was the AFB Community Outreach Project, funded by a federal rehabilitation training grant (Orr, 1993). In the project, outreach workers in local communities were trained to teach daily living activities to Native American elders with visual impairments and diabetes. Orr (1993) concluded that the project, in which 250 of 1,400 community health workers, representing 78 tribes in 27 states, participated, enhanced the long-term care of older visually impaired Native Americans by helping them gain the maximum level of independent and interdependent functioning. Given the most recent statistics about the life span of some Native Americans (IHS, 1996b), programs like the Hopi VIP and the Community Outreach Project will need to provide ongoing training to tribal members with visual impairments.

Residential Schools

ROLE OF SPECIALIZED SCHOOLS

Prior to European contact, most Native Americans educated their children informally at home with the help of relatives or formally by means of arranged apprenticeships. For example, a young tribal member who wanted to become a medicine person would seek a teacher or mentor (Joe & Malach, 1998). In other instances, clans or societies would take responsibility for training and preparing children to participate in their activities. Nevertheless, most Native Americans are not against formal education. However, as classroom activities and language become increasingly different from those in the familiar home environment, students may lose confidence and self-esteem. Parents of children with visual impairments may find it difficult to decide to have their children leave home to reside and learn at a special school far away because it would mean that the children would be separated from their families, culture, and traditions. However, specialized schools can provide unique services to children with visual impairments that may be helpful in preserving the children's self-confidence and self-esteem, as this author discovered when she interviewed present and former students of the Arizona State Schools for the Deaf and Blind (ASDB) in Tucson.

ASDB has served Native American students for over 30 years (E. Averitt, personal communication, 1998). In the department serving students with visual impairments, 24 percent of the 106 students enrolled in 1998 (23 percent) were of Native American ancestry (L. Albright, personal communication, 1998), and 60 of the 106 students were of high school age. Topor's (1998) survey of four other specialized schools in the West found that the enrollment of Native American students at ASDB was higher than in these schools. The percentage of Native American students enrolled at the four other schools ranged from .007 percent to 20 percent.

Native American students did not always attend the ASDB. In 1933, 100 students of cultural backgrounds other than Native

American were enrolled in the on-campus program. On January 5, 1935, Robert Morrow, superintendent of the school, was instructed by the state legislature to prepare a clause for an amendment to the law regarding the tuition of Native American students and submit it to the state legislature. In 1936, The ASDB (Board of Directors Minutes) demanded a $600 tuition from Fort Defiance, the student's home and local school district, for a student named Odesbah Thomas. Fifteen years later, a tentative charge of $1,000 per year was set for tuition for each Native American student pending the discussion of this fee with the Navajo Indian Agency. The board of directors (ASDB Board of Directors Minutes, 1951–52; 1956) voted to raise the tuition for Native American students from $660 to $1,000 in 1952 and to increase it to $1,650 in 1956. In the early 1980s, the Navajo nation sued the state of Arizona, claiming that Native American students were residents of Arizona and should be allowed to attend the residential school tuition-free like all other Arizona residents, and won. Since then, Native American students have attended the school tuition-free.

Alex, an 18-year-old senior from Pueblo Bonito, a town in northern Arizona, first enrolled at the ASDB during the 1997 spring term. He spoke to the author about how he decided to come to the residential school and what it has meant to him:

I am a Navajo and have five sisters and four brothers. I am the 3rd oldest in the family, but the first to be born with albinism. . . .

I was held back in the first grade because I couldn't "see the numbers." I went to Black Mesa Community School, 1st–7th grade, and played around instead of learned. I went to Hopi High School for one year and learned a lot there. Then I went to Chinle High School in 9th grade. I was enrolled in the special education class. I was taught the same things over and over again. I got bored. I returned to P. High and was enrolled in 10th-grade regular classes. I couldn't understand some of the teachers, couldn't see the chalkboard, my grades weren't good, and nothing was done for me. I don't recall a vision teacher ever helping me. There was so much teasing, I felt like dropping out. In 1995, I came to

Tucson for testing, and I could have gone to ASDB that year. I decided to return to P. High for the next school year. But I felt uncomfortable, and the kids continued to tease me in P. They called me albino, and no teachers intervened; the teasing happened a lot. I decided to come to ASDB the second half of my sophomore year. Before my grandmother died, she told me that she wanted me to do something better with my life. That's one reason I came to Tucson. I was frustrated, and my grandma wanted me to have a better life.

At ASDB, my vocabulary went way up and I read outside class. When I first came to ASDB, I was reading on a 4th-grade level. I think that I went up to an 8th-grade level. In $1\frac{1}{2}$ years, I went up four grade levels in reading.

Seeing all the canes at ASDB was weird at first, but I got used to it. It was also weird because everyone else had vision problems. I started to respect myself after I started at ASDB. In P., I did not respect myself. At ASDB, I got involved in athletics. I'm on the football team and lift weights. I took 1A and 2A wrestling. I took fourth place in the state wrestling tournament. I didn't do this in P.; I didn't have the opportunity. I was teased too much. Now when friends from home see me, they ask how I got so big and broad. They want me to come back and wrestle for P., but I say no.

I will graduate this year. My brother will also graduate in P. ASDB is allowing me to attend the P. graduation with my brother, and we will receive our diplomas at the same time. My family will have to attend only one graduation this way instead of two.

After I receive my high school diploma, I want to go to Pima Community College and come back to ASDB and work in the dorms. I would like to take accounting classes and become an accountant. I might go to the university to get my bachelor's degree. I told my sister that ASDB is a good school. She also has albinism. My sister was having trouble fighting with kids who teased her. My influence helped to bring her to ASDB. She is going to school here now in the sixth grade. My parents wish that I had come to ASDB earlier. I am glad that this school has given me the opportunity to participate in sports, increase my reading level, think about my future, and respect myself.

There are advantages and disadvantages to Native American children attending a residential school. One advantage is that a residential school provides alternatives to their lifestyles and education. For Alex, the switch to ASDB made a difference in his self-esteem, academic achievement, and thinking about the future. In other cases, parents make the decision to send their children to a specialized school at a young age, as was the case with Melfred.

Melfred, a former ASDB student who was born prematurely and has reduced vision caused by retinopathy of prematurity, entered ASDB at age 7. He is grateful that his parents allowed him to attend ASDB. When asked about leaving his family and culture behind, he stated that he has a connection to his heritage that he keeps with him at all times. Melfred spoke fondly of his teachers at ASDB, stating that they were wonderful and "knew what to do." Before he enrolled in ASDB, he attended a boarding school in a town not far from his home in northern Arizona. No services were available to meet his needs as a student with visual impairments, so he did not stay at that school. For Melfred, the specialized school offered instruction from knowledgeable people and a chance to train for a job in computer-aided drafting with animation. Melfred, now age 30, resides in Tucson and freelances as a draftsperson in computer animation.

The school has a tradition of one-week homegoings every six weeks so that Native American students can return to their families who live on reservations far from the Tucson campus. Nevertheless, some Native American families may not want to send their children away to a specialized school for services even if the children will receive an individualized education. Some clans may teach their children about plants, herbs, animals, seasons, hunting, food preparation, child care, and religion. Evenings are often reserved for storytelling and each story has a valuable lesson to impart (Joe & Malach, 1998). Thus, families may decide to keep children at home because they consider it a disadvantage for children to attend a residential school in a foreign environment, where familiar words, values, and lifestyles are absent. In short, a child's educational placement appears to rely on the family's belief systems, traditions, and values about formal education.

IMPLICATIONS FOR SERVICE PROVIDERS

Values are used to help people define who they are, whom they belong to, and who and what are to be regarded as outside their culture. Various authors (Dufort & Reed, 1995; Joe & Malach, 1998; Locust, 1994; Lowrey, 1987; Orlansky and Trap, 1987; Ponchillia, 1993) have suggested that differences in the values of Native American and nonnative people need to be recognized. The knowledge that one has about another's belief system leads to culturally sensitive behavior. It may also increase the chance that the assistance offered by service providers with expertise in visual impairments will be accepted. Educational or rehabilitative interventions may then reduce the effects of the visual loss on the individual and family. According to Joe and Malach (1998), not all traditional Native American values are held by younger generations of Native Americans, but they are still visible and are upheld by others, especially the elders of the tribes.

Some Native American values that have been discussed throughout this chapter are summarized here, and their implications for practice with students and clients with visual impairments are presented as a guide for service providers. These values and implications have been adapted from the work of Cummings (1993), Dufort and Reed (1995), Joe and Malach (1998), Locust (1994), Lowrey (1987), Orlansky and Trap (1987), Orr, (1993), Ponchillia (1993), Quotskuyva (1997), and Reed (1997), and personal communications from Martinez (1997) and Nord (1997), Reed (1997), and Quotskuyva (1997).

1. The extended family is an important part of the circle of life. Group life is primary.
   - Work with an individual or family and supporters as a team.
   - Live in the community and get involved in it at some level to establish rapport. Go to community events and talk to parents.
   - Discuss the family's wishes with respect to removing a young child from a cradle board or other child-tending device. Families may be operating under different beliefs about the usefulness of service provider's strategies.
   - One optometrist stated that it was difficult to obtain information from parents because they dropped their children off at the clinic for their eye appointments, but did not stay. Because child-rearing and parenting styles allow younger children more freedom and expect them to perform tasks that are typically reserved for older children in many other cultures, strategies for obtaining information before a clinic visit can be coordinated with other service providers who visit the families in their homes.

2. Hospitality is valued.
   - Accept food or drinks that are offered; to refuse without explanation is considered rude. If you have just eaten, you may say so and ask if you can take a little bit of the food with you or if you can have water instead of coffee. It is traditional for a host to offer a drink of water.
   - Attend healing, naming, and seasonal ceremonies if invited. It is a sign of acceptance to be invited to traditional functions.

3. Illness or disability is sometimes thought to be supernatural. Rituals and group support provide relief from disability by creating harmony with nature.
   - Show simple diagrams or concrete models of the body or eye to explain the problem more concretely.
   - Death and dying in the Navajo culture was traditionally

taboo; for example, it wasn't acceptable to mention a dead person's name. Consequently, for traditional people, corneal transplants are out of the question because of the relationship of the cornea to the dead person. Younger people may consider a corneal transplant.

4. The concept of the traditional healer–medicine person reinforces the "cure" of the problem.
   - Service providers may be expected to cure the problem, rather than to teach coping skills.
   - Teaching families the reasons behind teaching a skill and the components of the skill can help them make adaptations on their own.
   - Let parents know that you know how to teach a skill that will be useful to their child. Emphasize what the child is capable of doing and what she or he will need to function to "learn to do."
   - Projects that involve hands-on activities to increase the interdependence of affected tribal members are appreciated.

5. Healers traditionally give tangible objects.
   - Check with the family to determine if their spiritual beliefs will allow them to accept toys and mirrors before introducing these objects to a child. Certain animals and dolls may be considered bad luck or evil in certain tribes. When a child requires toys or pictures, consult the family to see if the images or toys are appropriate.
   - Older individuals may appreciate a NoIR lens, cane, or pocket magnifier.

6. Silence is valued; unnecessary talking may be considered foolish.
   - Listen. Be patient when waiting for answers. Do not interrupt or jump to conclusions quickly.
   - Ask broad open-ended questions to give family members a chance to give brief answers with narratives. Tell why you need to know something before you ask a question.

7. Harmony with nature, extreme modesty, and reluctance to show pain or discomfort are valued.
   ♦ Maintain a heightened awareness of the individual's comfort.
   ♦ Pay attention to nonverbal cues; they may give more information than verbal cues about an individual's level of comfort. (Chen, Brekken, & Chan, 1996)
8. Respect elders, experts, and those with spiritual powers.
   ♦ Always recognize, greet verbally, or lightly touch or shake hands with people, especially elders.
   ♦ Use brief eye contact when greeting an elder, but do not maintain it during a discussion.
   ♦ Explore alternatives to accessing health services. For example, elderly support systems for transportation in one part of the Navajo reservation are limited, so some individuals who need regular eye care cannot get rides to the clinic in Tuba City. Others do not make appointments because of family obligations, such as staying with sheep before the shearing season.
9. Humor is important in most tribes.
   ♦ Be aware that teasing behavior is a form of acceptance.
10. It is often assumed that negative actions, thoughts, or words may make bad things happen.
    ♦ Make statements that relate indirectly to the problem you are describing, for example, "I knew of someone who sought help from an eye doctor for his eye difficulty, and it really worked. The treatment was. . . ."
    ♦ Avoid using simulators or blindfolds with a client or family member because the activity may be viewed as a way to cause future blindness.
    ♦ Frame cautionary statements in a positive manner to encourage the family. For example, make statements like "Let's try out these things that are available." or "We will all work with the child to learn something." The service provider should avoid statements such as, "I'll teach your son braille because he will lose all his vision" or

"You should take your daughter to the eye doctor to make sure there's no more loss of vision."

11. Health and vision problems may be viewed as the result of past behavior.
    ◆ Recognize what the individual's belief system is with respect to modern medical treatments. For example, preventive health care may not be part of the culture; hence, such procedures as testing eye pressure, administering eyedrops may seem unnecessary.
    ◆ Give further explanations if the individual is open to hearing and learning about preventive care.
    ◆ If possible, identify a member of the same clan who had successful preventive health care or treatment. Determine if this person would be willing to share information with the person needing medical treatment.
12. The concept of time is viewed differently; it is measured in seasons and months, rather than in hours and minutes. One's lifestyle, environmental factors, and weather all have an effect on one's schedule. The present is more meaningful than the future.
    ◆ Family events and other special events take precedence over appointments with teachers and caseworkers.
    ◆ Appointment times may need to be flexible.

CONCLUSION

The risk of acquired visual impairment among Native American people is high because of genetic predispositions and limited access to appropriate medical attention, health education, and good nutrition. However, the significance of Native American beliefs and practices cannot be overlooked when designing and implementing education and rehabilitative services that will effectively meet the needs of individuals with visual impairments. If service providers are sensitive to and respect traditional beliefs and perceptions, the chances that treatments and services will be successful can greatly increase.

Modern culture and the effects of society on the younger generation have reshaped traditional explanations and perceptions (Joe & Miller, 1987). Thus, the way services are provided to each individual depends on where each family lies on the continuum between traditional practices and the blending of traditional practices with modern education and rehabilitation.

REFERENCES

Arizona State Schools for the Deaf and the Blind Board of Directors Minutes. (1935–36, 1951–52, 1956). Tucson: Arizona State Schools for the Deaf and the Blind.

Chen, D., Brekken, L., & Chan, S. (1996). Project CRAFT: *Culturally Responsive and Family Focused Training* [Video]. Baltimore, MD: Paul H. Brookes.

Crawford, J. (1994). *Endangered Native American languages: What is to be done, and why?* [On-line]. Available: http://www.ncbe.gwu.edu/miscpubs/crawford/index.htm

Crawford, J. (1996). *Endangered Native American languages: What is to be done and why?* [On-line]. Available:http://www.ncbe.gwu.edu/miscpubs/crawford/endangered.html

Cummings, L. (1993). *Hopi Visually Impaired Project:* Final Report to the National Institute on Disability and Rehabilitation Research. New York: American Foundation for the Blind.

Dobson, V., Tyszko, R. M., Miller, J. M., & Harvey, E. (1998). *Astigmatism, amblyopia, and visual disability among a Native American population.* Tucson: University of Arizona, Department of Ophthalmology.

Duarte, C. (2000, November 13) O'odham cash in on casino profit. *Arizona Daily Star,* pp. 1 & 4.

Dufort, M. & Reed, L. (1995). *Learning the way: A guide for the home visitor working with families on the Navajo reservation.* Watertown, MA: Perkins School for the Blind.

Egan, T. (1998, March 8). New prosperity brings new conflict to Indian country. *New York Times,* pp. 1, 22.

Heckenlively, J. (2000). Personal communication.

Heckenlively, J. R. (1988). *Retinitis Pigmentosa.* Philadelphia: J.B. Lippincott Co.

Heckenlively, J., Friederich, R., Farson, C., & Pabalis, G. (1981). Retinitis pigmentosa in the Navajo. *Metabolic and Pediatric Ophthalmology, 5,* 201–206.

Indian Health Service. (1996a). Part 1: Natality and morbidity rates of American Indians. *Trends in Indian Health Service.* Washington, D.C. : U.S. Public Health Service. [On-line]. Available: www.ihs.gov/PublicInfo/publications/trends96.asp

Indian Health Service. (1996b). Part 4: General mortality statistics. *Trends in Indian Health Service.* Washington, D.C.: U.S. Public Health Service. [On-line]. Available: www.ihs.gov/PublicInfo/publications/trends97/97TR3.pdf

Indian Health Service. (2000, September 8). Indian Health Service fact sheet [On-line]. Available: http://www.ihs.gov/AboutHHS/ThisFacts.asp

Joe, J. (1982). Cultural influences on Navajo mothers with disabled children. *American Indian Quarterly, 6,* 170–190.

Joe, J., & Malach, R. S. (1992). Families with Native American roots. In E. Lynch & M. J. Hanson (Eds.), *Developing cross-cultural competence* (pp. 89–119). Baltimore, MD: Paul H. Brookes.

Joe, J., & Malach, R. S. (1998). Families with Native American roots. In E. Lynch & M. J. Hanson (Eds.), *Developing cross-cultural competence* (2nd ed., pp. 127–164). Baltimore: Paul H. Brookes.

Joe, J., & Miller, D.(1987). *American Indian cultural perspectives on disability.* Tucson: University of Arizona, Native American Research and Training Center.

Locust, C. (1985). *American Indian concepts concerning health and unwellness.* Tucson: University of Arizona, Native American Research Training Center.

Locust, C. (1994). *The piki maker: Disabled American Indians, cultural beliefs, and traditional behaviors.* Tucson: University of Arizona, Native American Research Training Center.

Lowrey, L. (1987). Rehabilitation relevant to culture and disability. *Journal of Visual Impairment & Blindness, 81,* 162–164.

Mails, T. E. (1997). *The Hopi survival kit.* New York: Stewart, Tabori & Chang.

Monastyrski, J. (1998). Exploding native population a growing concern. *Wawatay News* [On-line]. Available http://www.wawatay.on.ca/jan29–98/12998s2.html

National Association for Native American Children of Alcoholics. [On-line]. Available http://www.ael.org/erie/ned/ned019.htm

Native American language resources. (2000, October 1) [On-line]. Available: http//:www.plumsite.com/palace/native.htm

Native Americans and diabetes: A statement from the American Diabetes Association. (2000, September 25) [On-line]. Available: http://diabetes.org/nativeamericans.asp

New Mexico State Department of Education. (1998). *Native American student academic achievement levels, drop out rates and students living in poverty.* Santa Fe: Author.

Orlansky, M., & Trap, J. J. (1987). Working with Native American persons: Issues in facilitating communication and providing culturally relevant services. *Journal of Visual Impairment & Blindness, 81,* 151–161.

Orr, A. L. (1993). Training outreach workers to serve American Indian elders with visual impairment and diabetes. *Journal of Visual Impairment & Blindness, 87,* 336–340.

Ponchillia, S. V. (1993). The effect of cultural beliefs on the treatment of native peoples with diabetes and visual impairment. *Journal of Visual Impairment & Blindness, 87,* 333–335.

Rearwin, D. T., Jubilee, H. E., Tang, O. D., & Hughes, J. W. (1997). Causes of blindness among Navajo Indians: An update. *Journal of the American Optometric Association, 68,* 511–517.

Seekins, T. (1997). Native americans and the ADA. *The Rural Exchange, 10,* 1–17.

Singleton, R. (1987). Neurologic syndromes on the Navajo reservation. *The IHS Primary Care Provider, 12,* 44. Chinle, AZ: Public Health Service Indian Hospital.

Singleton, R., Helgerson, S. D., Snyder, R. D., O'Conner, P. J., Nelson, S., Johnsen, S. D., & Allanson, J. E. (1990). Neuropathy in Navajo children: Clinical and epidemiologic features. *Neurology, 40,* 363–367.

Stevenson, J. (1998). *Alcoholism and Native Americans* [On-line]. Available: http://www.geocities.com/Athens/Forum/9235/Alcohol.html

Thornton, R. (1990). *American Indian. Holocaust and survival. A population history since 1492.* Norman: University of Oklahoma Press.

Topor, I. (1998). *Population of Native American students enrolled in 4 specialized schools.* University of Arizona.

U.S. Bureau of the Census. (1995a). American Indian languages spoken at home by American Indian persons 5 years and older in households [On-line]. Available: http://www.census.gov/population/socdemo/race/indian/ailang3.txt

U.S. Bureau of the Census. (1995b). Selected social and economic characteristics for the 25 largest American Indian tribes. [On-line]. Available: http://www.census.gov/population/socdemo/race/indian/ailang2.txt

U.S. Bureau of the Census. (1999a). Population growth rate remains stable, census bureau reports [On-line]. Available: http://www.census.gov.Press-Release/www/1999/cb99-101.html

U.S. Bureau of the Census. (1999b). Projections of the resident population by race, Hispanic origin, and nativity: Middle series, 1999 and 2000

[On-line]. Available: http://www.census.gov/population/projections/ nation/summary/np-t5-9.txt

U.S. Bureau of the Census. (1999c). Table 12: Resident population—Selected characteristics, 1790–1998 and projections, 2000–2005 [On-line]. Available: http://www.census.gov/prod/99pnbs/99statab/sec01.pdf

PART III

Religious Variations and Visual Impairment

Religions and Their Views of Blindness and Visual Impairment

Sandra Ruconich
and Katherine Standish Schneider

Gayla was born prematurely and lost all of her vision as a result of associated complications. She sees her blindness as an inconvenience rather than a roadblock, and it has never stopped her from pursuing her goals. She has two sisters and one brother, and Gayla has been a member of several Christian denominations. Now in her forties, she is married and has two children. Gayla feels close to God and is sure her blindness is not a punishment for a mistake she or her parents made. When she was 4, she recalls receiving "a little packet of something" from a religious friend who told her that if she waved the packet in front of her eyes several times a day, she would be healed. She used the packet for several days, but she remained totally blind. Eventually she threw the packet away.

The denomination of which she is now a member provides at least some of its materials in braille and on tape, and she teaches a Sunday school class and sings in the church choir. She feels members of her congregation generally treat her well. However, she recently acquired a dog guide and has been surprised that her minister asked if the dog needed to accompany her to church and that choir members were reluctant to have the dog in the choir loft. Although Gayla knows of older church members who are visually impaired, she is the only person with a vision loss in her congregation who attends services regularly. Gayla now rides to and from church with her husband and children but before her marriage found it fairly easy to get rides with other church members. She believes her visual impairment has deepened and strengthened her faith.

Although fictitious, this case study represents a composite of responses given by those interviewed for this chapter regarding their experiences and views on the interaction of visual impairment and religion.

Throughout the ages, people have tried to make sense of why disabilities, such as blindness and visual impairments, happen to some people and how to live with these disabilities in faith. This question has always been considered by the world's religions. Indeed, an entire branch of theology, called theodicy, is devoted to explaining evil and suffering. As educational, rehabilitation, and mental health professionals have increasingly realized, religion is a powerful force in many people's lives. Thus, professionals need to understand and include their clients' religious views in counseling efforts. Only then can clients and professionals work together to achieve educational and rehabilitation goals, using the clients' religious values as strengths instead of viewing them as impediments.

This chapter explores how major world religions and their members view visual impairment and blindness. The implications of religious faith for coping with crises, such as the onset of a visual impairment, are delineated. Then the theology of each religion is examined with respect to visual impairment and blindness. Interviews with at least one member of each religion, conducted to explore the respondents' feelings about the interrelationship of their religion and visual impairment, are summarized and analyzed. Finally, suggestions for working with clients who are blind or visually impaired and religious are offered.

In this chapter the word *blind* is often used to include visual impairment, since most religious texts do not differentiate between the two terms. Because of space and time constraints, only the most distinguishing tenets of the world's major religions are included.

THE ROLE OF RELIGION IN EDUCATION, REHABILITATION, AND MENTAL HEALTH

Religious views of visual impairment and blindness can provide a framework for education, rehabilitation, and mental health goals. Since most Americans claim that their religious faith is important to them (Shafranske, 1996), it is logical to assume that religion can play a critical role in the habilitation and rehabilitation process. That religious beliefs may change during times of crisis is supported by at least one study in the field of visual impairment. Erin, Rudin, and Njoroge (1991) found that parents of visually impaired children reported a transition in religious beliefs following their children's births. Immediately after the diagnosis, 20 percent of the parents viewed visual impairment as a punishment for sin, but that proportion dropped to 4 percent as time passed. Furthermore, 32 percent of the parents who were interviewed thought they had been especially chosen by God to raise their special children, and that percentage rose to 45 percent over time. Religious values were a vital part of the healing process for these families.

Numerous studies have shown a positive relationship between religious coping and adjusting to crises and medical illnesses (Pargament, 1996). This coping can be conservational (for example, maintaining one's significance in the face of losses entailed in the crisis) or transformational (such as finding new sources of self-worth). Kemper (1977, p. 147), a Protestant minister who experienced transformational coping after his vision loss, said: "The final destination of the stages of grief is not to 'get over it' or to 'forget it.' Rather, it is to readjust to the reality of painful change." Acceptance, for him, was knowing that he was a creature of the Creator; this knowledge, rather than the mere ability to do things competently, formed the basis of his self-worth.

Religion can provide many benefits to people who are blind or visually impaired. It offers a philosophy of life that deals with the "why" of visual impairment. It encourages reverence for all life, which includes self-acceptance. It fosters realistic hope and nurtures trust—in the universe, in God, in others, and in oneself. It promotes a sense of belonging to a community of caring (Clinebell, 1996).

RELIGIOUS VIEWS OF VISUAL IMPAIRMENT

The Old Testament and Jewish Views

Jewish people look on the Old Testament of the Bible (particularly the first five books) as holy scripture. However, the Old Testament portrays blindness in different ways, depending on the context in which this topic is mentioned. One notion of blindness holds it as a mark of impurity or a blemish that disqualifies one from temple service. Leviticus (21:18–21) warns that "No one who has had a blemish shall draw near; a blind man . . . or a man with a defect in his sight . . . shall not come near to offer the Lord's offering." 2 Samuel 5:9 says: "The blind and the lame shall not come into the house" of the Lord. Some references portray blind people as groping (Isaiah 59:10; Deuteronomy 28:29). Others point out that God may cause some people to be blind (Exodus 4:11), and still others suggest that God punishes sinners by blinding them or their animals (Zephaniah 1:17; Zachariah 12:4).

A second Old Testament view of blindness depicts God as compassionate toward people who are blind, as in references to opening the eyes of the blind (Isaiah 35:5; 42:7; 42:16; 42:18–19). Compassion toward blind persons is also expected of the upright believer (Leviticus 19:14; Deuteronomy 27:18).

Some of the confusion about these two disparate views of blindness arises because in many places in the Bible physical blindness is also used as a metaphor for the lack of spiritual insight. Thus, since no single attitude toward blindness exists throughout the Old Testament, one can only say that blindness is a defect, sometimes caused by God and sometimes pitied by Him. Jewish religious observance spans a wide range of viewpoints, from Orthodox (ultra-conservative), to Conservative, to Reform (liberal). A Conservative rabbi summarized Jewish views of blindness by saying that any abnormality would have disqualified an Orthodox Jew from temple service. However, a blind Conservative rabbi, who now practices Orthodox Judaism, believes the disqualification occurred because "the blemish would distract the people from the divine service," not because the blemish was demeaning (M. Levy, personal communication, April 24,1998).

Conservative and Reform Jews are more liberal in their views. For example, one of the Jewish morning prayers thanks God for opening the eyes of the blind. A student in a Hebrew class wondered if the blind boy in the class said that prayer, too. His response was: "Yes, I say it to thank God for giving vision to other people." The blind boy believed he had other gifts that would bring goodness to the world (Y. Gordon, personal communication, July 7, 1997). Margaret Moers Wenig (quoted in Elshout, 1995, p. 130) summarized the view of blindness set forth in the Torah (the Jewish book of laws) during her sermon at Hebrew Union College's Jewish Institute of Religion: "The Torah preceded the Americans with Disabilities Act by a couple of thousand years in its statement that you should not put a stumbling block in the path of the blind, but be inclusive of them."

The New Testament and Christian Views

Most Christian denominations place more emphasis on the New Testament of the Bible, since it presents Jesus' teachings and promises. Although the New Testament contains some of the same views of blindness as does the Old Testament, it also introduces some different ideas. Jesus healed a number of blind people. Such healings in Matthew's gospel alone include Matthew 9:27–28, 12:22, 15:30–31, 20:30, and 21:14. Two other gospel stories, blind Bartimaeus (Mark 10:46–52) and the man born blind (John 9), deserve particular attention. Bartimaeus was assertive in seeking the restoration of his sight from Jesus, who told him: "Your faith has made you whole" (Mark 10:52). In John (9:3), Jesus disputed the connection between sin and blindness, saying: "It was not that this man sinned or his parents, but that the works of God might be made manifest in him." Luke (14:14) mentions blind people's poverty and suggests inviting them to a feast "because they cannot repay you" (Luke 14:14). New Testament narrators utilized healings primarily to emphasize the power of Jesus, but the Old Testament idea that blindness means ignorance can still be found (Luke 6:39).

Modern Christian Views

Although Christian denominations may differ in their views of blindness or their interpretations of blindness-related biblical text, a common thread of compassion for and support of persons who are visually impaired typifies Christianity. The Christian church's protectiveness of and charity toward blind people led to a priest providing Louis Braille with early education (Kent, 1996). When the poet John Milton went blind, he had faith that God would give him a greater vision to share with others through his poetry. However, in his sonnet on blindness, he also acknowledged the increased passivity his blindness brought: "They also serve who only stand and wait" (Shawcross, 1971, p. 243). The theme of blindness as a blessing given by God is exemplified by Helen Keller (quoted in Belck, 1967, p. 19), a theosophist: "The reason why God permitted me to lose both sight and hearing seems clear now . . . that through me, He might cleave a rock unbroken before, and let quickening streams flow through other lives as desolate as my own once was. I am content."

Three modern trends in Christian theology are briefly discussed because of their implications for professionals who work with individuals who are blind or visually impaired. They are Christian Science, liberation theology, and Mormonism.

CHRISTIAN SCIENCE

Since its inception over a hundred years ago, Christian Science has been a puzzling religion to outsiders. Christian Scientists, often with the aid of Christian Science practitioners, work to cure every condition using spiritual means (Eddy, 1875/1994). They see blindness and visual impairment not as punishments or tests from God, but as rooted in a material view of existence and therefore subject to God's healing laws. Christian Scientists customarily do not mix Christian Science treatment with conventional medical treatment, since the two methods are based on completely different premises. Christian Science explains true existence, or life, as entirely spiritual; conventional medicine works from the assumption that people are primarily physical.

If healing does not occur right away, the Christian Scientist keeps praying until the illness or abnormal condition is healed. Although Christian Scientists often report being healed completely and quickly, some conditions—such as blindness and visual impairment—have involved continuing treatment over months or at times years. In that case, the Christian Scientist may choose to learn braille and other adaptive techniques until normal sight is restored; after the healing occurs, he or she could use the techniques to help others. One practitioner (S. Hansen, personal communication, July 28, 1997) said that in cases she has observed, in which only one parent of an ill or blind child was a Christian Scientist, the wiser of them did not "make the child a battleground for religion," and the Christian Scientist did not fight the other parent's attempts to seek medical treatment.

LIBERATION THEOLOGY

Liberation theology applies Christian principles to issues faced by those in Third World countries and by other poor or marginalized people; feminist theology extends this philosophy to women's issues. The discrimination and marginalization felt by many with disabilities (including blindness) has led to a liberation theology of disability (Eiseland, 1994; Elshout, 1995). This view emphasizes that Jesus was not only a miracle worker, but a boundary crosser; He chose His friends from among the outcasts of society. Because Jesus took on the limitations of humanity and lived among disabled and disenfranchised persons, people with disabilities can be empowered to accept their physical conditions as "survivable" (Eiseland, 1994) and to struggle for justice and self-determination. Thus, they are liberated from second-class, object-of-charity status to full participation, embodiment in an imperfect but acceptable body, and being part of the church. Professionals should therefore walk beside those with disabilities instead of "leading" them. Liberation theology says that God provides strength to struggle, grace to realize that self-worth is not dependent on physical status or actions, and Christ as an example of one who struggles for justice.

Although a liberation theology of blindness and visual impairment has not been officially articulated, it might include the healing of societal inequalities that lead to poverty, preventable blindness, and unequal treatment of blind people; in this view, societal healing is as important as individual healing. Liberation theology might also emphasize the changing of blind people's internalized negative attitudes toward blindness to attitudes of self-affirmation.

Mormonism

Members of the Church of Jesus Christ of Latter-day Saints (also known as Mormons, Latter-day Saints, or LDS) maintain that just as God spoke to people of ancient times through prophets, He also speaks to people of today through prophets. Latter-day Saints believe that the Bible is the word of God but also believe that additional scriptures (such as the Book of Mormon and the Pearl of Great Price) have been revealed to modern prophets.

One tenet included in these additional scriptures is that every person who has ever lived or ever will live on Earth dwelt first with God (Packer, 1991), mental and physical faculties perfectly intact (Smith, 1979). After this earth life is over and all people are resurrected, LDS doctrine says everyone will once again be without physical or mental disabilities (Packer, 1991; Smith, 1979). Some Mormons believe that during their preexistent life of learning and preparation for earthly living, they made choices about how they would come to Earth (for example, they chose to come with a disability, such as a visual impairment).

Another tenet of LDS doctrine is that church structure is patterned after that of the church Christ established, which included prophets and apostles, so the LDS church has 12 apostles. Thornton (1988) mentioned LDS leaders with visual impairments who have served or are serving at church levels from local to international. These leaders include prophets and apostles who continued to serve even if severe vision loss occurred after their call to church service.

Other Religions

Buddhism

Buddhism has much to say about suffering but does not address blindness. Suffering is seen as caused by attachment to a worldly existence. An eightfold path to enlightenment is prescribed, including right actions that will ultimately detach one from this world. The goal is to reach a final state of happiness called Nirvana. The compassion of Buddha is stressed, arguing against a view of Buddhism as being passive about blind people's needs. In actual practice, however, Buddhism may not be as compassionate as Buddha would have wished. Ching's (1982) autobiography, *One of the Lucky Ones*, details her experiences as a blind Buddhist in her native China. Ching was taught that blindness was a punishment for her sins or those of her parents, and Buddhism seemed unconcerned with improving social conditions for blind people.

HINDUISM

The Hindu religion includes many deities and many forms and rituals. It views life's trials as natural and sometimes positive. The good Hindu strives for detachment from things and situations. If one performs the duties and obligations of one's position in life—whether that position is a beggar or a college professor—then one gains merit and may be reborn in the next life at a higher level. Eventually, one hopes to be released from the cycle of birth and death. If blindness helps to detach the individual from the world, it may be seen as a positive factor. However, sometimes blindness is viewed as the result of not making the right sacrifices to the right gods. Mehta (1957), a noted historian and author, has written extensively of his Hindu mother's attempts to cure him of blindness through sacrifices and pilgrimages to holy men. By Western standards, Hinduism may be considered unconcerned with this world, but Hindus may argue that there are three paths to detachment from the world—knowledge, work, and devotion—each of which requires active involvement with life.

ISLAM

Islam honors Mohammed, who preached the existence of an all-powerful and all-merciful God, as a prophet. Because God is in control of everything, blindness and other disabilities are viewed as aligned with His purposes. Blindness is not assumed to be a punishment, but is seen as a test. As it says in the Koran: "There is no blemish in the blind" (XXIV 60:61). In addition, one of the five pillars (beliefs) of Islam is almsgiving to the less fortunate. However, a person who is blind may respond to this charity with patient acceptance that may be mistaken for passive resignation.

INTERVIEWS REGARDING RELIGION AND VISUAL IMPAIRMENT

Interview Summary

All 11 respondents were deeply committed to the religion they currently practiced. Most had accepted and were at peace with their visual impairment, viewing it as one of their many characteristics but not the sole characteristic that defined who they were. Ten said they had a close relationship with God, and six believed visual impairment was part of God's purpose for their lives. None felt their religion discriminated against them because of their visual impairment; only one said some members of their religion might consider visual impairment a punishment inflicted by God. No accommodations had been made for one person, but the other ten respondents' religions provided at least some materials in accessible formats, and some congregations had made special accommodations, such as space for braille books and wheelchair ramps, for their visually impaired members.

In regard to transportation, four respondents walked to church, while the rest got rides; most felt that finding such rides was not difficult. Four respondents were the only visually impaired members of their congregations; the remaining seven respondents' congregations included visually impaired members, but they were generally older and less involved with their churches. Five respondents believed visual impairment was not a factor in the development of their faith, while six respondents were convinced visual impairment had deepened or strengthened their faith.

Perhaps there are two generalizations to be made about those interviewed. First, they felt secure about who they were. They felt secure as people; Paula, for instance, was no longer concerned about her looks. They felt secure as people who happened to have a visual impairment; Lila's "too busy to pay attention" comment typified their comfort level with their disability. They felt secure as people of faith, as exemplified by Melanie's belief in and reliance on "miracles of happenstance"— God's always sending help when she needed it. Second, they were proactive individuals who took the initiative to ensure that they could participate as fully as possible in their religion. Jenny and Bob were active in every aspect of their faith in which they could be active and felt no animosity toward that faith or its authorities. Billy led a prison ministry despite initial transportation difficulties. Melanie coordinated church transportation for herself and others with disabilities. Margaret ignored objections to her being a lector and, once those objections were quieted, brailled pulpit announcements, as well as special hymns and prayers, so that she could do everything a nondisabled lector did. In short, these 11 respondents are outstanding representatives of the religions they practice, and they would be just as exemplary if their vision were 20/20.

Biographical Sketches of Respondents
JUDAISM

Jenny and Bob are Jewish people who live in a northeastern state and are in their 40s. Jenny, an Orthodox Jew, is married and has an older brother and a twin sister. Her visual impairment was caused by what is now called retinopathy of prematurity, a congenital condition resulting from complications associated with premature birth. Jenny has always been totally blind. Asked how she felt about her blindness, she said: "It's regrettable at times . . . , but . . . you just waste energy being bitter about such things, so you just have to accept what . . . God gives to you." She grew up in a Conservative Jewish family, attending the synagogue occasionally on the Sabbath and for high holidays. As an adult, she became Orthodox after attending classes dealing with Orthodox Judaism.

Bob, a Conservative Jew, has two older sisters, is married, and has no children. His visual impairment was also caused by retinopathy of prematurity; he sees "very little light" with one eye and nothing with the other. Regarding his attitude toward visual impairment, he said: "I don't think about it. It's . . . something I've grown up with. . . . I know what my limitations are and I try to work around those." Bob grew up attending an Orthodox synagogue and said he became more active about the time he was preparing for his Bar Mitzvah (the Jewish ceremony in which 13-year-old boys help conduct a service, read from the

Torah, and become men in the eyes of Judaism) when the Jewish Braille Institute gave him braille prayer books. Now he belongs to a synagogue that adopts what it considers the best of both Orthodox and Conservative practices.

CHRISTIANITY

Interviews were conducted with three Christians who represent mainline Protestant, Catholic, and Pentecostal/charismatic viewpoints. Christians come from many denominations, but according to the University of Virginia's (1999) Religious Movements Homepage, denominations encompass developing gifts of the spirit, including speaking in tongues, prophesying, and healing.

Frances, a mainline Christian, lives in a northeastern state, although she has also lived in the South and the Midwest. She is in her 40s, has an older brother and a younger sister, and is single. Frances was born with retinopathy of prematurity, but had "enough [vision] to be mobile" until she was 6 1/2, when a detached retina caused total blindness. In regard to how she felt about her visual impairment she said: "It's just a way of life. I know it's there, but it's not the thing I use to identify myself." Her family is Southern Baptist, and she was brought up in that church, attending church every Sunday and joining the choir as a teenager. Frances said that her parents had—and taught her to have—deep faith. As an adult, she has been active in various denominations, including mainline Protestant. "Everywhere I've gone," she reflected, "I've just said, 'Lord, where do You want me to be?'"

Margaret is a Catholic who lives in a large city in a northeastern state, is in her 40s, and has one younger brother. She is married and has no children. Born with retinopathy of prematurity, she could see objects, color, and "headline print" until she was 9, when she lost all vision except light perception. Her vision has remained stable ever since. Margaret said that her visual impairment is "an inconvenience, . . . but I don't think I really allow it to stop me from . . . enjoying life and having a variety of experiences." Raised in a Catholic family, she participated in religious instruction from kindergarten through high school, attending a Catholic school for the blind until she completed the eighth grade (at that time, the school did not offer a high school program). During high school at her state school for the blind, she "did participate in the planning of the liturgy and things like that" and lectored (read scriptures at Mass) while attending a Catholic college.

Billy, a Pentecostal/charismatic Christian, lives in a southern state. He is in his 50s, had a brother less than a year younger than he who was killed in an accident at age 21, and has a younger stepsister. At the time of the interview, he was engaged and is now married. Billy has congenital glaucoma and radical nystagmus, with some possible strabismus. His vision is 20/200, and although glaucoma can always cause sight loss, his vision has remained stable since he was 9. "I don't struggle with depression any more," he says of his feelings about visual impairment. "I have to wait occasionally for rides. . . . That's the only independence I guess I really miss." As a child, Billy was raised Catholic and attended Catholic school until he was in the fourth grade when he switched to a public school.

A drummer, Billy went on the road with a band six weeks before high school graduation and never graduated. During the next 23 years, he "made a couple of bad marriages," spent more money than he had, and "did drinking and drugging." In 1989, he decided "there had to be more than this to life" and "cried out to God": "If You will just show me . . . what to do, I want to stop doing what I am doing." About three days later, a pastor came to his door, Billy prayed to receive Christ, and he has been "tremendously blessed ever since then." Since that time, he has been drug- and alcohol-free but has never enrolled in a rehabilitation program or experienced withdrawal symptoms. "I just started going to church and started reading the Bible on tape . . . and God has been really gracious to me," Billy said. Six months later his mother converted from Catholicism to "charismatic, born again Christianity" because she saw such a profound change in his life.

CHRISTIAN SCIENCE

Paula, a Christian Scientist, lives in a western state. She is in her 40s, has an older brother and a younger sister, is married, and has children. She is a Christian Science teacher and practitioner, available full time to work with people who come to her with physical or other problems. Everyone in her family was a Christian Scientist. She and her sister have remained active in their religion; her brother joined and became active in another Protestant church "within the past couple of years." Paula was a finalist in the Miss Teenage America pageant. At 14, she began to wear eyeglasses to see things far away. She described her later, more severe visual impairment as a "deterioration of the retina" (she went to an ophthalmologist because she had failed a driver's license examination but could not remember the precise diagnosis). The visual impairment was diagnosed when she was in her early 30s and lasted for about a year, during which time she could not drive or "read any kind of text." She prayed daily for healing, applying the teachings of Christian Science. Currently, her vision is assumed to be 20/20, since she has been able to read "the tiniest line of print" during all subsequent driver's license examinations. In addition, since her vision returned, the licenses no longer indicate a need for corrective lenses. Paula does not know precisely when her vision came back; she knows only that she left her former home in New Jersey with a visual impairment but could see perfectly when she took her driver's test in the West a week later. She became aware of the change when the driver's test examiner told her that she did not need eyeglasses. She said that her vision has remained stable for the past 12 years, verifiable by her continuing driver's license renewals, the most recent of which was in early 1998.

LIBERATION THEOLOGY

Melanie lives in a northeastern state and practices liberation theology. She is in her 60s, has one child, is divorced, and has one younger sister. She is unsure of the cause of her visual impairment, but she knows it is hereditary, that approximately one third of the women in her family have it, and that it typically occurs at midlife. As her syndrome progressed, she went from having acute vision to having trouble reading small print to being unable to read. Currently, she has light perception, and her vision has been stable for some time. Asked how she felt about her visual impairment, she said that she missed flirting, driving, and being able to connect easily with speakers at a conference. "It hasn't stopped me from doing what God has crafted me to do," she stated, adding that as a child she "wanted to know what the world was like from different angles."

Melanie has a variety of other disabilities. She has neurological problems resulting from childhood meningitis and cannot tell where her extremities are. She also suffers from Ménière's disease, a disease of the inner ear that results in dizziness and a constant ringing in the ears. Surgery following an attack of Ménière's disease caused damage to her balance mechanism. She uses a wheelchair because of spinal injuries and impaired balance. She has normal hearing in her left ear but is profoundly deaf in her right.

Melanie's mother and father were both Methodist ministers. Melanie's father died when she was young, and her mother subsequently married a priest of the Church of England. Melanie attended church as a child because of her mother's ministry but did not feel a part of it. She did not go to church as a teenager or as a college student but always felt drawn to the Catholic church and began attending Mass as she grew older. After her stepfather's death, she felt free to become a Catholic and joined this church in 1980. "I always wanted to be a member of the Mother Church," she said.

MORMONISM

Lila, a Latter-day Saint, lives in a western state, is married, and has children. She is in her 40s and has three brothers and two sisters. Lila and her family have always been Mormons. Her visual impairment is the result of retinitis pigmentosa, which, as she recalled, caused legal blindness by the time she was 5 or 6 years old. Lila was reading braille by the time she was 11, and lost the ability to see color when she was 20. At present she sees "some light occasionally." Asked how she felt about her visual impairment, she responded: "Don't notice it. Too busy to pay attention. . . . The frustrating thing is when you want to read something [in] print or go somewhere."

BUDDISM

Usana, an 18-year-old Buddhist from Thailand, attends a school for the blind in a south-central state. The youngest in her family, she has two brothers and one sister. She came to the United States, where one of her brothers lives, to gain computer skills. Usana's visual impairment is the result of congenital cataracts and glaucoma. Although she was born blind, her vision improved when she was 3 or 4 years old, and she currently reads print; she does not know her visual acuity. In regard to how she feels about her visual impairment, she said that she sometimes wishes she could drive or read "real small print like people do." Usana has always been Buddhist. Buddhism is the religion of her family, except for her oldest brother who came to the United States when he was 9 and is now a Christian.

HINDUISM

Anand, a Hindu who was born in India, has lived in a western state for many years. He is in his 60s, has one younger brother, is married, and has children. His visual impairment was caused by optic atrophy that he first noticed when he was 32. His vision has gradually deteriorated ever since, and he now has "travel vision" in his left eye and no vision in his right. He was born into a Hindu family and practices his religion every day by getting up at 4:00 A.M. and praying for 50 minutes. Since there is no Hindu temple nearby, Anand cannot attend services regularly. However, he has no problem attending services conducted by other religions. "All religions are the same," he says. He believes it is the goal of all religions "to help, love, make [a] better life."

ISLAM

Molly is a Muslim who lives in a northeastern state. She is in her 40s, has one older brother, is married, and has no children. She grew up as a member of the Catholic Church, attending church and religion classes once a week, but became a Muslim when she was a senior in college. Her husband is also a Muslim; the rest of her family has remained Catholic. As far back as she can remember, Molly has always been totally blind as the result of retinopathy of prematurity. With regard to how she feels about her blindness, she said: "It definitely impacts on my life. . . . I can't live way out in the country, which I would like to do, because then I would be totally dependent on somebody to drive me everywhere. . . . However, . . . I accept it. There's nothing I can do about it." So far, it has not stopped her from doing anything she really wants to do.

Summary of Responses

The respondents were asked a variety of questions about their feelings about their religion and their visual impairment.

WHERE IS GOD FOR YOU AS A PERSON WITH A VISUAL IMPAIRMENT?

Most of the respondents said that they had a close relationship with God. Margaret's answer was typical: "I love God, and I know that He loves me." Bob felt "more centered" because of his belief in God. Frances and Paula said that they could not have survived the things that have happened to them without this belief. Paula added that her faith kept her from being afraid of her visual impairment and kept her turning toward God; in doing so, she would find comfort, peace, and even joy, eventually concluding that she was "perfect and complete as God's child." Melanie was convinced that "God is everywhere . . . and constantly surrounding me." God confirms His presence to her in that people are suddenly there to help her when she needs help—what she called "miracles of happenstance." Like Melanie, Anand was sure that God is with a person who is visually impaired. He believed that if he helps others, God will send people to help him. Molly commented that Moslems do not cry over things that they can do nothing about visual impairment. She, too, believed that God is everywhere, but did not characterize her relationship with God as the personal, "one-on-one" relationship she understood that some Christians experience.

Six of the 11 respondents believed that their visual impairment was part of God's plan or purpose for their lives. Of the 5 who discussed visual impairment as a possible punishment from God, only Usana thought that it was. She said that she and many other Buddhists, possibly including her mother, viewed visual impairment as a punishment to parents for "something wrong" the parents did in their last life. In contrast, Lila was one of 4 respondents who were convinced that visual impairment was not a punishment. Indeed, she believed that during her pre-Earth life, she chose to be visually impaired while on the Earth. Since she made that choice, she said, "I can move on . . . from feelings of guilt or depression . . . [or] punishment."

HAVE YOU HAD ANY EXPERIENCE WITH FAITH HEALERS?

Four respondents told of positive experiences with faith healers. Margaret went to Lourdes, a place noted for its healing properties, after she was sexually abused by her first husband. "I never thought I'd be able to forgive him," she said. "I went to Lourdes, and I really got the ability at least to pray to want to forgive. And then I did forgive." Three students Frances taught said a prayer of healing for her at a youth program of a charismatic church. Usana prayed daily for improved vision until she was 12 or 13 and sometimes still included this request in her prayers. She felt that those prayers were, at least in part, why her vision "gets better and better" every year. A Hindu high priest visiting the United States gave Anand a blessing about six years ago that, Anand said, caused his vision to improve dramatically. Before the blessing, Anand could not see colors or faces on a television screen. Now he sees colors and faces on television, although he still has to sit closer to the screen than most people with normal vision do, and his vision continues gradually to improve.

Not all experiences have been so positive. Frances remembered the woman who shook a Bible in her face and told her that if only she had enough faith, she could be healed. Molly was 6 or 7 years old when she heard a radio evangelist make a similar statement. She prayed hard and keenly recalled her disappointment when her vision did not improve. In later years, this experience helped to turn her away from Christianity. Margaret described healing services she attended during which people with visual impairments were virtually propelled into participation by other attendees. Melanie vividly recalled a service at which a father was trying to help his daughter, whose neuromuscular condition was so severe that she could not lift her head from her chest, to stand up; ushers came to help the father pull the child from the wheelchair, but to no avail.

Three respondents felt that if God chose to restore their vision, He could do so at any time. Reflecting this view, Molly commented: "Just because He doesn't do it doesn't mean my faith is incomplete." In her work as a rehabilitation teacher and academic instructor for a Catholic organization, Margaret watched clients lose all their remaining vision because they sought healing through voodoo or telephone prayer lines and did not consult physicians. She has shared with these clients the advice of a blind friend, who said that it is not wrong for people to seek healing in nontraditional ways as long as they simultaneously set and work toward rehabilitation goals. Julie Dawson, a blind rehabilitation teacher, stated in a personal communication (July 30, 1997): "When people often pray for a blind person, they pray for what they either think the blind person should have or what they would want were they blind. . . . I would love to have my sight returned. However, sight, in and of itself, does not guarantee security, happiness, peace of mind." Melanie stated: "The body is not crafted to be perfect," adding that when she has asked people during lectures if they are completely happy with their bodies, no one has said yes. "God doesn't care about the wrapping paper on the soul," she concluded. "He cares about how you're *keeping* your soul."

How Does Your Religion View Visual Impairment?

Billy and Frances said that the denominations and individual congregations in which they have worshiped have not considered visual impairment to be a punishment for sin. No objections have been raised to Frances's dog guide attending church with her. Paula explained that Christian Science maintains that all people with disabilities can "escape from their physical limitations." As God's children, she noted, "we have been given only good by Him." Therefore, according to Christian Science teachings, individuals can gain freedom from physical inadequacies and prove their God-given spiritual perfection. As was mentioned earlier, Lila said that Mormonism views visual impairment as a premortal choice made by individuals, not as a punishment. Usana stressed that Buddhism does not see persons who are visually impaired as inferior; rather, it encourages them to aspire to any goal they want to reach. She mentioned a famous blind Buddhist monk who made a statue called "The Honey Statue." Anand stated that he was treated better than other people because of his disability and concluded, "All religions have respect for the handicapped." Molly said that Islam does not view blindness "in and of itself" as a stigma and cited a passage from the Koran in which God mildly rebuked Mohammed for turning away from a blind man who was interested in learning more about the faith and preaching instead to "wealthy, influential people." In the Middle East, she added, there are famous blind Islamic scholars and memorizers of the Koran. Molly thought that a blind Muslim in a Third World country would be economically disadvantaged, but that this disadvantage would have more to do with economics than with religion.

Bob and Jenny stated that Judaism accepts people with visual impairments well, but that there are some things that Orthodox and Conservative Jews with visual impairments cannot do. Although Bob has read the Haftarah (the part of Jewish scripture containing writings of the prophets) in braille during worship services, he could not read the Torah because he had to be physically able to read from the actual scroll on which it was written. Jenny could not light candles for worship on the Sabbath or on high holidays, something women usually do. According to Levy (personal communication, April 24, 1998), the blind rabbi quoted earlier, Orthodox Jews with visual impairments cannot light candles or participate in any ceremony that requires physical vision (such as seeing the light of the candle or reading from the Torah scroll). As a Conservative rabbi, Levy could not officiate at the ceremony of the moon (a monthly ceremony in which it is necessary to see the light of the moon), but he pointed out, if the moon is hidden by clouds, a sighted rabbi is also unable to recite this service. In addition, he stressed the many areas in which blind and visually impaired Orthodox and Conservative Jews can participate (including Sabbath observance, reciting the "Hear O Israel" prayer twice a day, and saying blessings before partaking of food and drink). Jenny and Bob simply accepted these regulations as part of their religion and did not feel anger or animosity as a result. Referring to not being able to light candles, Jenny said, "I don't put any blame or anything. . . . I just feel sad that I'm not able to do that for myself."

Occasionally, Melanie saw a negative reference to blindness in the literature of her religion. She stated that such references are "a judgment from the past," made by people "still burdened" by former stereotypes that blindness is synonymous with darkness, guilt, and evil, and that she was "seeking to alter" these judgments and stereotypes. The priest with whom Margaret initially talked about becoming a lector in his parish did not want her to do so because her dog guide would be with her on the altar. Even a letter from the head of the office of disabilities in Margaret's diocese stating that Margaret had read for the cardinal of her area did not help. Eventually, another priest gave her a chance to lector at a sparsely attended Mass, and a few weeks later she began reading at the noon Mass. Now she is lector coordinator for the parish and a member of the cardinal's archdiocesan pastoral council.

Despite Islam's positive attitude toward visual impairment, Molly said that in the Arab world, dogs are used "as guards and such" and are never allowed in houses. As a dog guide user, she could not take her dog into the part of the mosque where prayers are said, since the dog's saliva is considered unclean. Before she came to the Northeast, she attended a mosque where her dog could be safely left in the back of the building. Her current mosque has no such safe place to leave the dog, and because she felt uncomfortable traveling in this large city without a dog, she was initially unable to attend religious services.

How Are You Treated by Others in Your Congregation?

All 11 respondents said they were treated well; all were active members of their churches. Paula believed that because her visual impairment was not obvious, most people probably did not notice. Anand thought he was treated better than others because of his disability. Billy leads a weekly ministry to prisoners, and the men's ministry of his congregation pays many of the travel expenses associated with this ministry. Frances attended membership classes in her new church as soon as she arrived, became active immediately, and was elected a deacon in less than a year. Melanie generally felt welcome but added, "that's partly because I won't allow myself not to be welcomed." She said that she tried to reach out to everyone, but found that some people are "terribly afraid of blind people and blindness." Usana said that people helped her do things she found difficult to do because of her visual impairment (like lighting candles). Most well-educated Buddhists in Thailand treat her very well, but those with less education, who often live in rural areas, might say something like "You're blind; you can't do anything." Molly feels she's treated like anyone else in her congregation. She finds that specific ethnic groups (e.g., Arabs, Indians, and Pakistanis) tend to stick together, but she attributed this phenomenon to the commonality of their heritage, not to prejudice against visual impairment. Margaret said that some people treated her well and some did not. She has experienced everything from condescension to genuineness. However, she and her husband, who is also visually impaired and an active church worker, have been invited to parties for those who work in the parish. Lila was convinced that her treatment at church was no different from her treatment in other social settings. She agreed with Margaret that people's behavior toward her ranged from condescension to benign neglect to acceptance as normal. "Just because these people are a religious group doesn't mean they're going to be any different" from any other people, she stated.

What Accommodations Have Been Made for You by Your Religion and/or Place of Worship?

Anand said that no accommodations were made for him. Braille materials about Buddhism are available for those who want them, Usana said, but such materials are usually unnecessary until adulthood because parents teach their children about their religion. Bob and Jenny used braille prayer books and other religious texts, available from the Jewish Braille Institute, which are kept in their synagogues. Bob was especially impressed that his small synagogue found room for his bulky volumes and that those in charge were thinking of building additional shelves to store his books. Billy borrowed religious books on audiotape from his regional library for the blind and from Recording for the Blind and Dyslexic. He said that he would feel comfortable asking church members to record books if he needed them. Paula's sister audiotaped weekly Bible lessons and other church materials for her. The First Church of Christ Scientist makes *Sci-*

ence and Health, the book containing Christian Science teachings (Eddy, 1875/1994), Bible lessons, and other Christian Science literature available in large print, in braille, and on audiotape. Lila's church provides braille and audiotaped versions of the magazines it publishes, as well as manuals for teaching church classes. Lila served as president of the young women's organization of her congregation and was, at the time of the interview, an officer in its women's organization; she said that she used a combination of braille and audiotapes to gain access to the materials she needs. Molly said that an English translation of the Arabic Koran is available in braille, and a different translation is available on audiotape from Recording for the Blind and Dyslexic; the Koran and other materials are also accessible via the Internet. Those who read Arabic braille can purchase the Koran and other religious texts in Arabic from Middle Eastern sources. In addition, the Arabic Koran is commercially available on audiotape, as is a version that follows each Arabic verse with an English translation.

Sometimes more extensive accommodations are necessary. Frances has brailled hymns by reading the words from a print hymnal with the Optacon (a device that changes print letters into vibrating images of those letters read with the index finger). She did not have space for braille materials but had some materials on computer disks, especially those she needed as a deacon. She said that the Presbyterian Church USA intends to make all its materials accessible to people with disabilities. Available braille materials currently include the Presbyterian hymnal, the Book of Confessions (faith statements of the church), and the Book of Order (the rules by which services and meetings are organized and conducted). Margaret also brailled special hymns or prayers she needed as a lector. The church typist faxed pulpit announcements (highlighting coffees, food drives, and so forth) to Margaret's office two days before the Mass at which she was to read, and Margaret gained access to these announcements by using either a scanner or a reader to convert them to braille. Because it is often difficult for scanners to read different typestyles or publishing conventions, the typist did not use underlining or bullets in Margaret's copy. Margaret ordered the Mass Propers (weekly readings for Masses) from Xavier Society for the Blind.

Melanie said she required accommodations to gain access to her environment as well as her materials. Environmental accommodations included a niche in the pews that fit her wheelchair, a ramp for wheelchair entrance to and exit from the church, and a lift so she could get to the downstairs cafeteria where her prayer group met. During worship services, she used the parish's FM-enhanced hearing system, which amplified what is spoken into the pulpit microphone and conducted the amplified sounds to earphones she wears. Melanie also sometimes used a smaller amplification device with a microphone and earphones so that a friend sitting beside her could whisper hymn words to her without disturbing other worshipers. Melanie's office staff read materials for her, and she used audiotapes when they were available. The scanner in her office was not connected to the computer and was therefore inaccessible, but she used the computer for word processing.

How Have You Dealt with Transportation to and from Services?

Jenny, Bob, Frances, and Margaret walked to services, but all except Margaret were sure they could get rides if they needed them. Margaret said that the city paratransit service was not dependable, and people in her urban parish did not use cars because it was difficult to find parking spots. Paula's sister drove her to and from church. Usana rode with her parents because she was too young to go to the temple alone, but she thought she could have gotten a ride if she needed one. Before her marriage, Molly sometimes rode with other members of her mosque but then rode with her husband. Lila also rode with her husband, but thought she could get rides with other members if necessary. She tried to avoid asking any one person for rides too often "because I don't want people to avoid me for fear they're going to get asked."

Two respondents' solutions to the transportation issue were

more involved. Melanie and four other people in her parish who were elderly or disabled got rides each Sunday from eight rotating drivers. Drivers who had questions about the schedule the parish Social Concerns Committee sent out every six months called her; she was the parish advocate for access and was influential in establishing this program. Billy got rides with friends when he played drums at church. Regarding his prison ministry, the local bus company paid for his trip to the prison and, as was mentioned earlier, his congregation's men's ministry underwrote his return trip and other related travel expenses. This arrangement was made because Billy could not find anyone who was willing to take him where he needed to go on a weekly basis. Billy had strong feelings about this issue. He mentioned blind friends who could not get rides to and from church. "People are nice to them," he said, "but they don't get really close to them." Such people might offer Billy's friends a ride once or twice, but they were afraid that they would be asked to provide rides regularly.

ARE THERE OTHER PEOPLE WITH VISUAL IMPAIRMENTS IN YOUR CONGREGATION?

Bob, Paula, Anand, and Molly were the only people with visual impairments in their congregations. The remaining seven respondents said that their congregations included other members who were visually impaired, but most of these members were older people who lost vision later in life and were less involved with their churches.

HAS YOUR FAITH CHANGED AS A RESULT OF YOUR VISUAL IMPAIRMENT?

(For people whose visual impairment was congenital, this question was changed to, "Would your faith have been different if you had not been visually impaired?") Molly, Usana, Lila, Jenny, and Bob said that their loss of vision had nothing to do with the development of their faith. In contrast, Margaret thought that had it not been for her visual impairment, "it's possible I'd have no faith today." Having grown up in a tenement where alcohol, drugs, and sex abounded, she responded: "I think I would have joined the forces out in the streets if I had had the independence to do so." However, as a result of her blindness, she spent much of her time reading the classics and religious books. Paula said that her experience with visual impairment strengthened her faith, especially because her recovery was complete. Anand noted that he prayed longer and had deeper faith than he had before he became visually impaired. Frances has struggled with the balance between self-reliance and dependence on the Lord— a struggle she thought she would not have undergone if she had normal vision. "God wants us to acknowledge that He has gifted us and that we're to use those talents we have," she explained; then she added: "We're not to be doormats" and "just wait for things to fall in our laps without taking some initiative." Frances also said that her visual impairment led to "some vulnerability," so that "there is still a need for the deep faith." Expanding on the idea that vulnerability can result in deeper faith, Melanie re-flected: "Coming to grips with the fragility of the human body, if we're in the right stance in terms of our souls and our Creator, turns us toward greater discernment of the meaning of life. . . . I view the impairments that I've developed as painful gifts . . . [that have] caused me to pause and meditate and consider things I [otherwise] would not have considered."

RECOMMENDATIONS FOR PROFESSIONALS

The following recommendations for educational, rehabilitation, and mental health professionals are offered as a springboard for further reflection and dialog in working with religiously com-mitted persons who are blind or visually impaired:

- ◆ Listen to a client's religious beliefs; do not dispute or ignore them. Ask open-ended questions to learn more about the be-liefs of the individual and his or her family. Try to determine how religious beliefs help the client cope.

- If the client's religious beliefs seem to conflict with educational or rehabilitation goals, ask questions about the apparent conflict. For example, a client who does not want to learn braille because he or she anticipates a religious healing can be asked questions, such as these: "Could you learn braille while you wait for the healing to occur?" or "Could you learn braille now so that after your healing you could teach it to others?"
- Cultivate a knowledge of religious resources available in the community, including both groups and individuals. Look for people who support the educational or rehabilitation goals of your agency and who enjoy counseling.
- If, over time, a client's religious views continue to interfere with education and rehabilitation, consider raising this concern with the client and offering to refer him or her to a pastoral counselor. For example, if a client believes that the lack of faith is the only thing keeping him or her from being healed, a pastoral counselor may discuss various kinds of healing and wholeness to help the client move toward a more life-affirming view while maintaining faith.
- Consider bibliotherapy for clients who are concerned about the relationship between disability and religion. Popular Judeo-Christian books that deal with this relationship include those by Kushner (1985), Tada (1990), and Yancey (1990). Autobiographies of persons who are visually impaired and religious have been written by Ching (1982), Hull (1991), Kemper (1977), and Mehta (1957), among others.

Religion can be a powerful force in the life of a visually impaired person. It can provide trust, hope, and meaning in a time of crisis. Professionals who understand how the world's major religions view blindness and visual impairment and how religious beliefs can influence behavior will be best prepared to help clients use their faith in a positive way. Faith can be one factor that aids persons who are blind or visually impaired to move forward in their lives, confident of their worth and secure in the love of a Supreme Being.

REFERENCES

Belck, J. (1967). *The faith of Helen Keller.* New York: Hallmark Cards.

Ching, L. (1982). *One of the lucky ones.* Garden City, NY: Doubleday.

Clinebell, H. (1994). *Counseling for spiritually empowered wholeness.* New York: Hayworth Pastoral Press.

Eddy, M.B. (1994). *Science and health* (Authorized ed.). Boston: First Church of Christ Scientists.

Eiesland, N. (1994). *The disabled God: Toward a liberatory theology of disability.* Nashville, TN: Abingdon Press.

Elshout, E. (1995). Roundtable discussion: Women with disabilities; a challenge to feminist theology. *Journal of Feminist Studies in Religion, 10,* 99–134.

Erin, J. (1991). Religious beliefs of parents with children with visual impairments. *Journal of Visual Impairment & Blindness, 85,* 157–162.

Erin, J., Rudin, D., & Njoroge, M. (1991). Religious beliefs of parents of children with visual impairments. *Journal of Visual Impairmnet & Blindness, 85,* 157–162.

Hull, J. (1991). *Touching the rock.* New York: Random House.

Kemper, R. G. (1977). *An elephant's ballet.* New York: Seabury Press.

Kent, D. (1996). *Extraordinary people with disabilities.* New York: Children's Press.

Kushner, H. (1985). *When bad things happen to good people.* New York: Schocken Books.

Mehta, V. (1957). *Face to face.* Boston: Little, Brown.

Packer, B. K. (1991). The moving of the water. *The Ensign 21*(5), 7–9.

Pargament, K. (1996). Religious methods of coping. In E. Shafranske (Ed.), *Religion and the clinical practice of psychology* (pp. 215–239). Washington, DC: American Psychological Association.

Shafranske, E. (Ed.). (1996). *Religion and the clinical practice of psychology.* Washington, DC: American Psychological Associaton.

Shawcross, J. T. (Ed.). (1971). *The collected poetry of John Milton.* Garden City, NY: Doubleday.

Smith, J. F. (1979). *Answers to gospel questions* (vol. 3). Salt Lake City, UT: Deseret Book.

Tada, J. E. (1990). *A step further.* Grand Rapids, MI: Zondervan.

Thornton, L. W. (1988). Seeing blindness clearly. *The Ensign, 18*(12), 42–47.

University of Virginia. (1999). *The religious movements homepage* [On-line]. Available: http://cti.itc.virginia.edu/~jkh8x/soc257/profiles/profiles.htm

Yancey, P. (1990). *Where is God when it hurts?* Grand Rapids, MI: Zondervan.

CHAPTER 8

Blindness and Visual Impairment and the Religious Community

Virginia Bishop

Maria, a young blind girl, was waiting in line for confession at her church. When it was her turn to talk to the priest, he excused her by saying that she did not have to confess her sins since she was blind. She hurried home happily to tell her mother, who marched her back to the priest immediately. Her mother informed him that blindness was no excuse, and that her daughter must confess her sins just like everyone else.

The role of vision in religious practices may be more important than is generally recognized. Many religious ties involve symbols or rituals (such as crosses, statues, elaborate processions,

This chapter could not have been completed without the assistance of a number of people whose experience and information were invaluable. Grateful acknowledgment of this help is extended to Lynn Borchelt, Tina Herzberg, Anne Corn, Douglas Hind, John Crandall, B. J. LeJeune, Rodger Dyer, Bernadette Kappen, Janelle Felmet, Joanne Murphy, Sylvia Fitzpatrick, Darcy Quigley, Mindy Fliegelman, Lee Robinson, Anne Franklin, Olivia Schonberger, Lesylee Gautreaux, Gerri Test, Ed Guerra, Jim Warnke, Phil Hatlen, Stuart Wittenstein, and Margery Heaton.

and candlelit ceremonies) that are largely visual. Thus, people who are visually impaired or blind may be at a disadvantage in experiencing the emotional significance that is usually spontaneous for sighted members of a congregation. When visual limitations make participation difficult or reduce the significance of the ceremony, they may also limit the personal or emotional bond generally provided by religion. The blind or visually impaired person may feel alone or left out. Members of the congregation may overlook his or her apparent lack of participation, mistaking it for aloofness or disinterest.

Many people find that religion and spirituality are helpful in adjusting to blindness or visual impairment, and professionals and service providers who work with this group need to be sensitive to the role of religion in their clients' lives. Because of this significance and the dedication of the blindness field to inclusion and full access to every aspect of mainstream society, this chapter provides information on how professionals can help individuals who are blind or visually impaired maintain ties to their religious communities.

The extent of each person's involvement in his or her religion may be a matter of both personal preference and visual abilities. Professionals who want to facilitate the connection between people who are blind or visually impaired and their religion may need to guard against projecting their personal interpretations and feelings; however, if the individuality of the visually impaired or blind person is to be preserved, personal choice needs to be part of the inclusion process. This chapter describes the options for the individual in relation to the intentions of the religious community and its members.

The demographic data cited in this chapter were researched through library resources. Since no data could be found that described the number of visually impaired or blind persons in the various religious denominations, extrapolations were made on the basis of the prevalence of those groups in the general population.

Qualitative data were gathered through personal communication with agencies, organizations, theological seminaries, and individuals. A list of organizations or agencies and theological schools was generated from the *AFB Directory of Services for Blind and Visually Impaired Persons in the United States and Canada* (American Foundation for the Blind, 1997), from the *1996 Yearbook of American Churches* (Bedell, 1996), and from personal files. The list of individuals was generated primarily through professional and personal connections. Of these sources, 14 agencies or organizations and 3 theological seminaries (Catholic, Protestant, and Jewish) were contacted once or more by telephone. Of the 23 people who were interviewed about their personal experiences, 7 were visually impaired and 14 were educators in the field of visual impairment.

Information gathered from these sources provided the structure for the chapter. The recommendations at the end of the chapter come from both personal experience and national-international policy documents. The title of one document, *That All May Worship* (Davie & Thornburgh, 1997), reflects the intent of this chapter. The author encourages readers to work to achieve access for persons with visual impairments in their religious communities and to teach clients and students the skills to advocate for full participation in their chosen religious communities.

DEMOGRAPHICS AND DESCRIPTIONS

As of 1995, 163 million Americans (about 63% of the population) were affiliated with some religious denomination. Of this group, 94 percent were Christian, 3.7 percent were Jewish, 1.8 percent were Moslem, and the remaining .5 percent were Hindu, Buddhist, or other unclassified denominations (see Table 1). Of the Christians, 37 percent were Roman Catholic, 22 percent were Baptist, 9 percent were Methodist, 6 percent were Pentecostal, 5 percent were Lutheran, 3 percent were Mormon, 3 percent were Presbyterian, 2 percent were Churches of Christ, 2 percent were

Table 1
Populations of the Major Religions in the United States

Group	Population	Percentage
Christians	153,220,000	94
Jews	6,031,000	3.7
Moslems	2,934,000	1.8
Hindus, Buddhists, and others	815,000	.5
Totals	163,000,000	100

Source: Based on data from J. Wright, *The Universal Almanac* (Kansas City, MO: Andrews McMeel, 1997).

Episcopalian, 1 percent was Reformed, 1 percent was Eastern Orthodox, and 13 other Christian denominations were each less than 1 percent. One third of all Methodists and 3 of the 7 major Baptist groups were primarily African American (Wright, 1997).

The *1997 Catholic Almanac* (Foy & Avato, 1996) noted that 80 percent of Hispanics in the 1990 census listed their religion as Catholic. Five of the major ethnic groups (Irish, German, Italian, Polish, and Hispanic) make up 80 percent of the Catholic population, and about half the new immigrants entering the United States are Catholic. Hispanic Catholics are found largely in the South and West, and the remaining ethnic groups are concentrated in the cities or suburbs of the Northeast and North Central states (Greeley, 1994).

Four million Eastern Orthodox Christians in the United States have ancestries in Greece, the Middle East, and Slavic countries, and three fourths of them belong to the Greek Orthodox or Orthodox Church in America (Pelikan, 1994). More than half the Jews in the world live in the United States, making up 2.5 percent of the U.S. population; although Jewish people live in all 50 states, nearly half of them reside in the Northeast, with large populations in the South and far western states (Neusner, 1994).

Although Hinduism, Buddhism, and Islam are relatively small groups among the American religious population, they represent over 4 million people in the United States. Islam is the third largest religious group in the United States, and it is projected that it will move to second place by 2010; an estimated 1 million American Moslems (especially men) are African Americans, and the remainder are mostly of Asian ancestry (Esposito, 1994). Hindus are of Indian descent, the fourth largest Asian minority (behind Chinese, Japanese, and Filipinos); there are over 150 Hindu temples in the United States (Larson, in Neusner, 1994). Buddhists are primarily of Japanese ancestry, but also include other Asians (Tibetans, Thais, Chinese, Koreans, and Sri Lankans) (Eckel, 1994).

Native Americans who belong to religious communities are primarily Christian, but the influence of tribal traditions and regional cultures has given Native American Christianity many interpretations. Spirituality, in the sense of related to spirits or spiritual or sacred matters, is a common thread of Native American religions and provides a unifying element. The Native American Church as a denomination is a distinct branch that may combine tribal rituals, elements of Christianity, and the use of peyote during certain meetings. The Native American Church has no European or Asian influences, and it provides a common cultural bond for Native Americans (Gill, 1994).

Knowing the prevalence of severe visual impairments may, in turn, provide an estimate of the number of people with severe visual impairments in the various religious communities. It is difficult to locate accurate data about the prevalence of visual impairment because the data vary by definition, age groups, gender, and geographic location. The best statistics available take all these factors into consideration. Table 2 presents an estimate of the prevalence (rate per 1,000) of persons with severe visual impairments in the 1990 population, by age groups. The prevalence of severe visual impairments in the total population was estimated to be 17.3 per 1,000, or 1.73 percent in that year (Nelson & Dimitrova, 1993).

On the basis of the estimate of 17.3 severely visually impaired persons per 1,000 people, and using the membership figures in Table 1, the author estimated that in 1990 there were over 2.5

million visually impaired Christians, over 100,000 visually impaired Jews, over 50,000 visually impaired Moslems, and about 14,000 visually impaired people among Hindus, Buddhists, and other religions with smaller memberships. Of Christian denominations, over a million visually impaired people were Roman Catholic, over 270,000 were Southern Baptists, and almost 150,000 belonged to the United Methodist Church. Readers can estimate the number of members in any other denomination by multiplying that denomination's national membership by .0173. Lindner (1998) provided data on memberships in Christian denominations. Since religious congregations have a different number of children, young adults, middle-aged people, and elderly people, the national percentages may also help determine the possible number of visually impaired persons in the various age groups in any given congregation.

Although many people who are visually impaired belong to religious communities, they may not be active participants. Any congregation that wants to locate its visually impaired members can start with the estimates just given, identify the distribution

Table 2
Estimated Prevalence of Severe Visual Impairment in United States, 1990

Number and Rate	Age							
	0–17	18–44	45–54	55–64	65–74	75–84	85+	Total
Number of severely visually impaired people	95,410	349,350	340,510	600,000	1,068,290	1,190,520	648,680	4,293,3
Rate per 1,000 people	1.5	3.2	13.5	28.4	59.0	118.4	210.6	17

Source: K. Nelson & E. Dimitrova, in "Severe Visual Impairment in the United Sta and in Each State, 1990," *Journal of Visual Impairment & Blindness, 87* (1993), pp. 80–

of age groups within its membership, and design a strategy to reach out to those members who may be visually impaired.

CHILDREN AND YOUTHS WITH VISUAL IMPAIRMENTS

Visually impaired children and youths who are members of a religious community may attend public schools, special day schools or residential schools for blind and visually impaired children, religiously affiliated schools, or may be home schooled. Those who attend public schools are members of both their families and communities. Their participation in religious activities is a matter of family choice, and most parents of children with visual impairments view the religious community as supportive (Erin, Rudin, & Njoroge, 1991). There may be an additional benefit when visually impaired children attend public schools: Not only are they already members of their communities, but their peers do not view them as outsiders. Perhaps the current generation of youths will grow up to include disabled individuals as a normal and accepted part of their social group, and religious communities will not have to seek them out.

Children and youths who attend special day schools usually live at home and are transported daily to and from school; they also remain a part of their families and religious communities. Blind or visually impaired students who receive special educational services in residential schools may be in a different situation, however. The administrators of four residential schools in the United States who were interviewed by telephone reported two possible approaches to religious education at the schools. At the time of enrollment, parents may be asked to indicate both their religious preferences and the extent of their desire for religious training for their children. The schools then contact local religious institutions, matching the religious preferences of the families, and those local institutions take the responsibility for providing any religious training. In these cases, the residential schools usually provide transportation to the local churches or synagogues, but each denomination arranges for the inclusion of students in its religious education program. Another practice that is increasingly common is for residential schools to send students home on weekends. This practice allows for stronger family connections for the students and permits families to attend religious services together. Although this information is based on feedback from only four administrators, these respondents believed that their approach to students' religious preferences reflected those of other specialized schools.

There are no reliable data on how many visually impaired students attend private or religiously affiliated schools. Federal guidelines for students at private and religiously affiliated schools are careful to state that special services provided on the private or parochial school grounds must be "to the extent consistent with the law" (that is, observing the legal separation of church and state). Home-schooled children, whose parents often choose this method for religious reasons, are considered to be attending "private school," and special education services provided to these children observe legal guidelines that apply to private and parochial schools.

Parents who choose to enroll their children with visual impairments in private religiously affiliated schools or to educate them at home do so with the understanding that this choice may affect their children's special education services. Federally mandated Child Find procedures require states and local school districts to "identify, locate, and evaluate" all children with disabilities who reside in their states or districts, including those who attend private or parochial schools (P.L. 105–17, 1997). Following these evaluations and on the basis of those findings, each local school district must develop an individualized plan for providing appropriate special education services (the Individualized Education Program, or IEP) in a free, appropriate public educational program. Parents may still choose to place their children in private or religiously affiliated schools or to home-school them, but in doing so, they give up their right to special services. This does not mean that services cannot be provided if the parents request them, but the funding source for them is not clear. The federal law states that the quality of any offered services must be equal to that available in the public educational setting, but the extent (for example, number of hours) may be different. The local school district is not required to fund services but these alternative services may be provided by public school personnel if they made a free, appropriate educational program available, but most school districts make reasonable efforts to find sources of funding.

Ways of providing services to students who attend religious schools vary from district to district and state to state. Texas's approach to the problem is to allow dual enrollment (that is, a student who is visually impaired is enrolled in a local public school but attends a parochial school), so that the local school district provides materials and services as if the student is attending a public school. Maine uses the Catholic Charities' four regional offices to provide adequate services for visually impaired students in Catholic schools. At least two Catholic schools (St. Joseph's in Jersey City, New Jersey, and St. Lucy's Day School in Upper Darby, Pennsylvania) specialize in services to students who are visually impaired, on either a day or residential basis. It appears that there are a variety of solutions to providing adequate and appropriate educational services to visually impaired students in religiously affiliated schools, but there may still be future clarifying court cases or further explanatory federal guidelines to sort out the problem of who pays for what.

An informal telephone poll of six teachers of students with visual impairments indicated that special education services, materials, and equipment do find their way to visually impaired students in private and religiously affiliated schools and to those who are educated at home. Local school districts purchase and provide modified textbooks that are also used in public schools, but parents are usually required to pay for any modified religious materials needed. If these respondents' experiences reflect general practice, it appears that educators are finding ways to meet the needs of visually impaired students, regardless of where they attend school. However, attendance at a private or parochial school places the responsibility for requesting special services and materials on the parents who chose an alternative school placement.

There is an increasing number of home-schooled children, and many of them are receiving religious education along with their academic instruction. The National Home Education Research Institute (Ray, 1997) estimated that in the fall of 1996 there were 1,226,000 home-schooled children in the United States; using the estimate of 1.5 visually impaired children aged 17 or younger per 1,000 from Table 2 (Nelson & Dimitrova, 1993), one can see that as many as 1,839 visually impaired students are being home schooled. Although these children are considered to be attending "private" school, special education services and materials are usually delivered on the same basis as to those who attend religiously affiliated schools. One teacher of visually impaired students described a unique experience with a home-schooled student who is visually impaired. It seems that the parents originally enrolled the child in a public school in another state and were offended by objectives on the IEP that related to self-care and social skills that they thought were intrusive because they believed those areas are rightfully parental responsibilities. When the parents decided to provide home schooling for religious reasons, the new teacher of visually impaired students was sensitive to their beliefs; she asked the parents how she could help them carry out their wishes. The resulting IEP reflected instructional goals in developing "fine motor skills," thus enabling the parents to provide instruction in dressing, grooming, and other self-care skills. The teacher was able to offer appropriate support while respecting the wishes of the parents in the education of their home-schooled child with a visual impairment. There are also blind parents who want to home school their sighted children, and there seems to be an increasing number of Internet resources for these special situations (B.J. LeJeune, Christian counselor at CARE Ministries, Starkville, MS, personal communication, August 22, 1997). Many special materials are available in braille and large type and on audiotape.

PARTICIPATION IN RELIGIOUS COMMUNITIES BY ADULTS WITH VISUAL IMPAIRMENTS

There are comparatively more visually impaired adults than children and youths, but they may not be as visible. Because many of them are unemployed, underemployed, or retired, they may not have daily contact with other members of their communities. They are a heterogeneous group, with a large variety of visual impairments and a wide range of visual losses. They are found in all cultures, ethnic groups, and neighborhoods. There is as much diversity among people with visual impairments as among the general population, and this diversity may make it more difficult for religious communities that want to promote inclusion to locate them. There is no directory of blind and visually impaired persons and no blind community. Each person has to be contacted, one at a time. The single characteristic that most visually impaired adults have in common is their inability to see well enough to drive, and it may be this factor that tends to keep them from attending religious services.

As people age, the prevalence of visual impairment rises. Elderly blind people tend to isolate themselves, either because they have fewer friends and other social contacts or because they lack transportation. Many families in a religious congregation have at least one extended family member who "doesn't see well anymore." These people may need support to continue to participate in their religious community. Because they are relatives, they may be the easiest to locate, but they may also be the hardest to convince that the religious community will welcome them as active members. They may not know that there are such things as large-print Bibles or recorded devotionals. Father Thomas Carroll emphasized, however, that blindness is no excuse not to attend and participate in religious services. In fact, he said "there is nothing in the nature of blindness . . . which should take the ordinary spiritual care of blind persons out of the regular parish" (Carroll, 1961, p. 371). If religious institutions can provide an environment that is safe, well lighted, and visually user friendly, it may be easier to include older visually impaired people in their weekly religious activities.

Although there have been instances in the past where people have been prevented from full participaton in religious communities, due to a disability, individuals who were interviewed for this chapter were generally positive about their inclusion and cited individualized adaptations that had been made to assist them. There may be many answers to these questions, as they ultimately depend on uniquely individual preferences and abilities and the attitudes of a religious denomination or its specific congregation. For example, a young Jewish woman who was planning to visit a synagogue in a distant town called the rabbi for directions, and during their conversation, he asked if she had any special needs. She replied matter-of-factly that she was a braille reader. When the young woman arrived for the service, the rabbi presented her with a prayer book in braille. He had contacted the local school for blind children and, within the week, had arranged for one of the staff to braille the prayer book for the visitor to his congregation.

Although there is no policy against a blind person participating in communion in either a Catholic or a Protestant church, the manner in which it is done may cause the person to hesitate to participate. Although the emphasis should be on the spiritual meaning of the event, participation sometimes depends more on whether the individual is assertive enough to use a sighted guide, cane, or dog guide to get to the front of the church independently. Will the blind person gain the same spiritual value from kneeling to pray in the pew as kneeling at an altar to which he or she has been guided by an usher? A young blind man in Pennsylvania is accompanied by his sighted wife when he approaches the altar for communion; this solution works for him, but it may not be the preferred approach for every visually impaired person. Each decision about participation must be balanced between the demands of the specific ritual and the abilities and desires of the individual visually impaired person. No single solution will work for everyone, and every situation should be viewed in the context of individual preferences.

VISUAL IMPAIRMENT AND RELIGIOUS LEADERSHIP

The author also investigated opportunities for religious leadership for people with visual impairments. The three theological seminaries she contacted—Catholic University of America, Harvard Divinity School, and Hebrew Union College–Jewish Institute of Religion—did not have any written policy prohibiting a blind or visually impaired person from entering them. All three seminaries reported that at least one student who was blind was currently enrolled. Although the blind students in a religious seminary may have contact with faculty who know little about accommodations for visually impaired persons, seminary students have been able to use a variety of modifications and equipment in fulfilling their academic responsibilities. A young Jewish man reported that he had used an Optacon to read assignments in Hebrew while studying to be a rabbi. Jim Warnke, now an Episcopalian priest (personal communication, August, 1997), devised a system that paired an optical scanner with his computer, enabling him to study at hours convenient to him, sometimes late at night when live readers were not available. The more positive political climate toward disability may have opened the doors of some seminaries and encouraged blind or visually impaired persons to pursue careers in religious leadership, but the students themselves may still take most of the responsibility for accommodations. Although modified study materials are available from a number of sources, seminary students may still have to devise their own ways of gaining access to what is either not available in modified form or difficult to locate.

The seminaries were also asked whether a visually impaired student who completed seminary training could be ordained as a priest, rabbi, pastor, or congregational leader; the responses to this question were less positive. There may be a discrepancy between successful completion of theological studies and the ordainment or hiring of that person as a priest, pastor, or rabbi. In the Catholic faith, a qualified academically trained person with a disability must obtain special dispensation to be ordained as a priest. One of the first blind priests in the United States to be so ordained is in New Jersey. Protestant and Jewish faiths have less stringent rules. One source whom the author interviewed knew of over 50 ordained blind or visually impaired religious leaders who were Jewish, Baptist, Methodist, Mormon, Episcopalian, or Lutheran or members of the Churches of Christ, Assemblies of God, or various independent and related denominations; these religious leaders with visual impairments were from over 20 different states (B.J. LeJeune, personal communication, August, 1997). If this information is representative, visual impairment does not seem to be a major barrier to becoming a religious leader in most denominations, at least for those who were determined and dedicated.

Once ordained, do churches or synagogues actually employ these visually impaired leaders? If employed, how do the leaders perform their duties? One determining factor seems to be whether the religious leader was visually impaired when hired or lost his or her vision afterward. A few whose vision deteriorated while serving as congregational leaders were reportedly dismissed if the church was too small to provide adequate accommodations, but at least one congregation was supportive of its pastor when he began to lose his vision, organizing a corps of drivers and readers to help him continue his leadership role (Weller, 1978).

Religious leaders with visual impairments who actually serve or who have served in the capacity for which they were trained include those in a variety of denominations. A Baptist minister in Texas, a cantor and a rabbi in New York, a Mormon bishop in Wyoming, a Church of Christ minister in West Virginia, an Episcopalian priest in New Jersey, and a Lutheran pastor in Michigan are examples of religious leaders who were described to the author when she was gathering information for this chapter. Clearly, visually impaired religious leaders are employed by many denominations, and visual impairment does not seem to be a limiting factor.

Once employed, do visually impaired religious leaders make any modifications in the services or ceremonies to accommodate their visual impairments? Some leaders have made creative and unique arrangements. Reverend Weller (1978), for example, described his drivers as "assistant ministers" who help to visit sick members of the congregation, administering communion and reading Scriptures. Father Warnke (personal communication, August 1997) memorizes the routine portions of his services and prerecords the changing portions; he then wears an earphone during the service, listening to the tapes as cues for his role in the ceremonies. He is also called on, from time to time, to act as a guest priest at other Episcopal churches. He arrives at least a half hour before the services, uses his white cane to orient himself to the unfamiliar surroundings, and may request a designated acolyte to assist with necessary movement during the service. Father Warnke has been able to devise workable accommodations that allow him to fulfill his role as a religious leader. Leadership-by-example enables him to reach the visually impaired members of his congregation more comfortably and to encourage them to focus on the message instead of the messenger.

INCLUDING PEOPLE WITH VISUAL IMPAIRMENTS IN THE RELIGIOUS COMMUNITY

There seem to be three major outreach issues in uniting individuals who are visually impaired with their preferred religious congregations: finding out who and where these individuals are, assisting with travel to the site of worship, and providing access to the worship environment. Locating each congregation's blind and visually impaired members is not as simple as it sounds. Members of the congregation may be uncomfortable with blind or visually impaired people and focus on defects, disabilities, and differences and hence pity, patronize, or avoid. It is not a matter of bringing "them" into "our" place of worship, but in believing that a place of worship is where all are equal. Until that sense of family defines the congregation, inclusion may be ineffective. A welcoming congregation is the first step toward creating a religious family in which there is "advocacy not avoidance, empowerment not pity, and support not stigma" (Rife & Thornburgh, 1996, p. 36).

Once a congregation has developed a sense of inclusion, it becomes easier to see the people who have been ignored: the elderly family member who is visually impaired who does not want to be a bother; the young adult who cannot see well enough to drive and stays home, rather than ask for a ride; the blind child who has special teachers, books, and equipment in school on weekdays but none on the Sabbath. The congregation may start by identifying the visually impaired or blind people in the congregation. Professionals in the community who work in the field of visual impairment may be able to help in this process.

The greatest single barrier to full participation by blind or visually impaired people in the society is the lack of transportation. In the religious community, it may discourage visually impaired or blind people from even attempting to attend religious services. It could also force attendance at a worship site that is within walking distance or located on a bus route, although that site would not have been the individual's first choice. The single greatest contribution a congregation can make to including people who are blind or visually impaired is to make rides available. Each visually impaired or blind person in the congregation could have a "faith family" or "circle of support," a group of congregational members who are willing to provide rides to religious services and functions. If the group is large enough, it should not be a burden on just a few people, and opportunities to build friendships will be greater. When possible, a visually impaired individual should receive a list of drivers who are willing to drive, so he or she can make arrangements for transportation. The option is an empowering act, not a patronizing one. Because the visually impaired person has participated in the planning process, he or she can have an increased sense of confidence, self-esteem, and equality.

An often-overlooked aspect of transportation is what happens when the car or van arrives at the place of worship. Is the visually impaired person then on his or her own? Or, is someone waiting to assist in orienting the person to steps, entryways, aisles, hallways, or rooms? Not all people with visual impairments are easily oriented, and some cannot move independently and confidently. Most will learn often-used routes in time, but that extra "Can I help?" may go a long way toward creating a warm welcome. However, it should always be extended as an offer, so the visually impaired person does not feel obligated to accompany the person who has brought him or her to the service.

Congregational guides should have some training in how to assist visually impaired people who need orientation or mobility (O&M) assistance, and in the sighted guide technique. Either an O&M instructor or a special teacher of students with visual impairments can also help orient designated congregational guides in a brief training session. This bridge between the car or van and the pew can make attending religious services both friendlier and more comfortable for members of a congregation who are blind or visually impaired.

The visual environment is important to consider in ensuring access. For people who have low vision (that is, can see well enough to read large print, or who use some kind of enlarging device such as a magnifier) lighting is often critical, as is high contrast. A modification as small as increasing the wattage of lightbulbs in hallways, stairways, and rest rooms can help.

Putting high-contrast strips of tape on the edges of steps can also help a person with low vision navigate stairs with more confidence. Braille labels on elevator buttons and on the doors of classrooms or rest rooms can help a blind person find the right location more easily. Including visually impaired individuals in determining modifications will make them feel more at home in their congregations. There are a number of small adaptations that can make a difference between hesitancy and confidence, and professionals in the field of visual impairment can serve as advisers or consultants in implementing them.

Printed materials used in worship services and church activities would seem to require the most modifications, since reading is significantly affected by visual impairment. The kind of modifications will depend on the individual's need. Sometimes materials can be sufficiently enlarged by using a photocopier, a large computer font, or magnification. One woman with low vision described using a hand magnifier to read the Hebrew Torah during her Bas Mitzvah (the Jewish ceremony in which a 13-year-old girl assumes religious responsibilities). If the person reads braille, printed materials may need to be transcribed or specially ordered; recorded materials may also be an option. Each visually impaired person may have a preference about how printed materials should be modified, and this preference should be accommodated when possible. Many resources are already available through organizations of all faiths that produce religious materials of all kinds: Bibles (in many languages, including Hebrew), prayer books, devotionals, Bible studies, special services, classic Christian and Yiddish literature, magazines, calendars, hymnals, and religious education materials. These materials are often available in braille or large print or on audiotape, and most of them are free to visually impaired persons and congregations. Some hymnals may need to be purchased in special media, and consideration should be given to whether a person who is blind wants only the words to the hymns in braille or prefers both words and music in braille.

There is some disagreement about whether braille, large-print, or audiotaped material should be available "in case" a visually impaired person should attend a worship service or should be ordered to fit the individual needs of a person who is visually impaired after he or she begins attending worship services. One church routinely keeps a liturgy in braille, in a three-ring binder, changing the hymns or responsive readings each week. Another church routinely provides the weekly church bulletin in braille for a church member who is blind. If a professional in visual impairment is a member of the congregation, he or she may be willing to braille the weekly bulletin or to enlarge it. One superintendent of a residential school for blind students suggested that if churches would provide materials routinely, people who are visually impaired or blind would feel more comfortable attending. There is no simple solution to this issue, and there may be a little of both sides of the issue in every situation; all congregations must make choices on the basis of their individual situations.

One church congregation, Trinity United Methodist Church in Phoenix, Arizona, has solved the problem of special materials on its own. About 24 volunteers make sure that Sunday school materials, music, worship bulletins, and educational materials are transcribed into braille for about 75 blind United Methodists across the country. One young woman who is blind, who has been attending the Trinity Church for about 12 years, teaches the 2–3 year olds at the Sunday school, using materials prepared in braille by the volunteers. She also uses the braille hymnal because she enjoys singing; she said that the special materials help her make church "a real experience" because she can "participate like everyone else does" (Thompson, 1997). This example emphasizes how the provision of special materials can allow people who are visually impaired or blind to be fully included in and contribute to the religious community and congregational families.

Worship services are only one part of the religious life of a congregation. Most religious communities have a number of in-house functions and extended activities that enrich their members' religious experiences. At the Episcopal Church of the Good Shepherd, in Watertown, Massachusetts, a blind person carries the chalice, another blind person is chair of the Liturgy Committee, and a third blind person is chair of the Board of Directors. Because of its proximity to the Perkins School for the Blind, this church has historically built relationships with the staff and students at the school; it also has many years of experience including blind people in its community and has developed some exemplary and unique ways of modifying materials and/or procedures.

There are a number of other ways in which visually impaired members can make contributions. They can serve as elders, deacons, lay leaders, choir members, teachers, and members of a variety of committees; telephone congregants; and perform office tasks. They can also participate in extended activities, such as retreats, Scouting, church dinners, bake sales, fairs and festivals, and dramatic productions or musicals. There is almost no role or function, from leadership to support, in which people who are blind or visually impaired cannot participate, given transportation, and it is only when they do that they are truly members of their chosen religious families.

Congregations that have already instituted outreach efforts and made it possible for blind or visually impaired people to participate in their religious life have found the benefits of adding these new members. A young blind woman in Pennsylvania reported, "I love singing and feel like I'm part of my church when I sing in the choir." Another woman, who has low vision, said, "I'm a good organizer, and I keep people notified of meetings by phone." A former Lutheran Sunday school teacher told of a blind student in her class who enjoyed it so much that he brought his friends. The sense of belonging is one of the most important achievements any outreach program can foster, and a major goal of all efforts should be to include people who are blind or visually impaired in religious communities.

A PLAN FOR INCLUSION

The United Nations Resolution 48/96, passed in 1993, outlined an endorsed international policy on disability. Rule 12 (United Nations, 1994, p. 30) is quoted here, since it has direct bearing on plans to include visually impaired persons in religious communities.

Rule 12. Religion
States will encourage measures for equal participation by persons with disabilities in the religious life of their communities.

1. States should encourage, in consultation with religious authorities, measures to eliminate discrimination and make religious activities accessible to persons with disabilities.
2. States should encourage the distribution of information on disability matters to religious institutions and organizations. States should also encourage religious authorities to include information on disability policies in the training for religious professions, as well as in religious education programs.
3. [States] should also encourage the accessibility of religious literature to persons with sensory impairments.
4. States and/or religious organizations should consult with organizations of persons with disabilities when developing measures for equal participation in religious activities.

The United Nations' recommendations for accessibility in all aspects of religious life have identified inclusion as an issue of international concern. The plan proposed here describes how to disseminate information as recommended by the resolution. (Among the primary written sources consulted in developing this plan were Bishop 1987; Carroll, 1961; Davie & Thornburgh, 1997; Kelman & Levy, 1976; Kerr, 1973; Martin & Travis, 1968; Rife and Thornburgh, 1997. Personal communications, through telephone calls or letters, were acknowledged at the beginning of the chapter.)

The inclusion of visually impaired people in a religious community does not usually happen by accident; it is more often the result of planned efforts. Although each congregation is different, there are some general guidelines that may help in designing a plan. If there are professionals in visual impairments among the congregation, they can initiate, facilitate, act as advisers or consultants, and make suggestions that will make the religious environment more accessible or more visually comfortable. If enduring change is to take place, some kind of cooperative effort should occur, and this joint effort should include professionals, people with visual impairments, and general members of the congregation. The creation of a task force, committee, or mission statement may be an initial step, followed by a congregational seminar or training session.

During the initial planning stage, there may be some public affirmation of welcome. Examples of such affirmations may be an extra line in the church or synagogue's telephone book or an annoucement in newspapers. Examples may be a statement in a bulletin that "All are welcome. Please let us know what we can do to make this service meaningful for you" or a sign posted in the lobby of the site of worship stating that accommodations are available. Congregational newsletters could carry the message that printed materials are available in enlarged print, braille, or recorded form. If possible, a list of suggestions or guidelines for the congregation can be distributed in advance. An insert in a church or synagogue program could include the following wording:

> Several of our members have visual impairments. Here are some guidelines to help you make them feel comfortable in our religious community.
>
> 1. It is appropriate to use the words *see* and *look* when talking to visually impaired persons. They will know what you mean, and it is not offensive.
> 2. Use the person's name when addressing him or her, and, as a courtesy, state your own name if you are not a close friend (for example, "Hi, Mrs. James. It's Sandy Smith.").
> 3. You don't have to speak louder to a visually impaired person; most do not have hearing impairments.

4. Do not pat a guide dog in harness. The dog is working while in harness and needs to concentrate on safe travel for its owner.
5. It is OK to give verbal cues (such as "We're coming to a flight of stairs") if you are using the sighted guide technique.
6. Do not walk away from a visually impaired person without telling her or him that you are leaving; it is embarrassing to try to talk to someone who has disappeared.
7. If in doubt, do not be afraid to ask the visually impaired person if he or she would like some help; allow the person to accept or reject your help, depending on the task or route or situation. It is friendly to ask, but do not assume that all visually impaired people need help with everything.

Offer a brief training session in the sighted guide technique, conducted by a professional in the field of visual impairment. Although any member of the congregation can learn the basics of sighted guide assistance, ushers for religious services may find the technique especially useful in welcoming a visually impaired person to the worship service.

The accessibility of the worship environment may need to be evaluated for individuals who are visually impaired. Three specific areas for modification may need to be explored, and a professional can be of assistance in performing this evaluation.

Printed materials. Making programs, scriptures, hymnals, study outlines, prayer lists, announcements, devotionals, prayer books, and so forth available in braille or large type or in recorded form will allow persons with visual impairments to express their preference, depending on their primary reading medium.

Rituals or ceremonies. When a ritual or ceremony involves movement from one location to another, some adaptation may be needed. One option may be to arrange for assistance from a friend, family member, usher, or other individual, although the visually impaired person should always have the choice of moving independently. Another option may be to bring the ceremonial elements to the pew, so that a visually impaired person can participate fully with minimal assistance. People with visual impairments should be encouraged to let others know their preference if they need assistance so that arrangements can be made.

Lighting. Many visually impaired persons use vision to travel, and many are able to read print, sometimes with enlargement or optimal lighting. Check the lighting in hallways and stairs because these areas may be darker than others. If there are steps or stairs, the edges of the steps may be highlighted with contrasting paint or tape to make them more visible. If there are elevators, place braille labels on the control buttons.

The next step in implementing a plan for inclusion is to identify visually impaired people in the congregation. Members can be surveyed to see if anyone has a family member, friend, or neighbor who is visually impaired. Elderly members of the congregation are particularly likely to be visually impaired.

When individuals are identified, transportation needs can be determined. Groups of people who can provide rides can be organized; even four people taking turns can share the responsibility, and each will be on call only once a month. When possible, the person with a visual impairment should have the opportunity to be oriented in advance of the first visit to the worship service. This orientation is best done by one person, so the blind or visually impaired individual can concentrate on remembering where there are steps, doorways, pews, hallways, rest rooms, and other landmarks.

The visually impaired person should be invited to become involved in congregational activities, such as singing in the choir, teaching Sunday school, helping on telephone teams, writing articles for a newsletter, or using computer skills. Getting people involved in activities can help them develop a sense of belonging and can help others recognize their abilities.

A final consideration in the plan for inclusion is the evaluation of how well the plan is working. This type of planning is ongoing, and it may change as the congregation changes. The most obvious way to measure progress is to ask the blind or visually impaired members of the congregation for comments and suggestions. During their routine visits to all members of the congregation, religious leaders can ask the members who are blind or visually impaired about how support services (drivers, readers, and guides) are working out and whether adapted materials are adequate. These visits should not be only evaluation sessions; they can also provide opportunities for private discussions. Members may identify other blind or visually impaired individuals who may be interested in joining the religious group.

CONCLUSION

"Religion offers community to our lonely human souls" (Rabbi Harold Kushner, quoted in Rife & Thornburgh, 1996, p. 5). When the religious community seeks to include all who are interested, it fulfills that mission. The process of involving an individual with a visual impairment in a religious community requires attention to the person's abilities and need for information, but it is not difficult to do. Even a few people can make changes. In the words of the noted anthropologist, Margaret Mead (quoted in Rife & Thornburgh, 1996, inside front cover), "Never doubt that a small group of thoughtful, committed citizens can change the world. Indeed, it is the only thing that ever has." Every congregation can begin to make that change.

REFERENCES

American Foundation for the Blind. (1997). *AFB directory of services for blind and visually impaired persons in the United States and Canada* (25th ed.). New York: AFB Press.

Bedell, K. (Ed.). (1996). *1996 yearbook of American churches*. Nashville, TN: Abingdon Press.

Bishop, V. (1987). Religion and blindness: From inheritance to opportunity. *Journal of Visual Impairment & Blindness, 81,* 256–259.

Carroll, T. (1961). *Blindness: What it is, what it does, and how to live with it.* Boston: Little, Brown.

Davie, A., & Thornburgh, G. (1997). *That all may worship: An interfaith welcome to people with disabilities.* Washington, DC: National Organization on Disability.

Eckel, M. (1994). Buddhism in the world and in America. In J. Neusner (Ed.), *World religions in America* (pp. 203–218). Louisville, KY: Westminster/John Knox Press.

Erin, J., Rudin, D., & Njoroge, M. (1991). Religious beliefs of parents of children with visual impairment. *Journal of Visual Impairment & Blindness, 85,* 157–162.

Esposito, J. (1994). Islam in the world and in America. In J. Neusner (Ed.), *World religions in America* (pp. 243–258). Louisville, KY: Westminster/John Knox Press.

Foy, F., & Avato, R. (Eds.). (1996). *1997 Catholic almanac.* Huntington, IN: Our Sunday Visitor, Publishing Division.

Gill, S. (1994). Native Americans and their religions. In J. Neusner, (Ed.), *World religions in America* (pp. 11–32). Louisville, KY: Westminster/John Knox Press.

Greeley, A. (1994). The Catholics in the world and in America. In J. Neusner (Ed.), *World religions in America* (pp. 93–110). Louisville, KY: Westminster/John Knox Press.

Kelman, N., & Levy, M. (1976). The Jewish blind. In S. Strassfield & M. Strassfield. (Eds.), *The second Jewish catalogue* (pp. 167–173). Philadelphia: Jewish Publication Society of America.

Kerr, J. (1973). Our blind spot. *Spectrum, 49* (1), 25–28.

Larson, G. (1994). Hinduism in India and in America. In J. Neusner (Ed.), *World religions in America* (pp. 177–202). Louisville, KY: Westminster/John Knox Press.

Lindner, E. (Ed.). (1998). *Yearbook of American and Canadian churches, National Council of Churches of Christ in America.* Nashville, TN: Abingdon Press.

Martin, C., & Travis, J. (1968). *Exceptional children: A special ministry.* Valley Forge, PA: Judson Press.

Nelson, K., & Dimitrova, E. (1993). Severe visual impairment in the United States and in each state, 1990. *Journal of Visual Impairment & Blindness, 87,* 80–85.

Neusner, J. (1994). Judaism in the world and in America. In J. Neusner (Ed.), *World religions in America* (pp. 151–176). Louisville, KY: Westminster/John Knox Press.

Pelikan, J. (1994). Orthodox Christianity in the world and in America. In J. Neusner (Ed.), *World religions in America* (pp. 131–150). Louisville, KY: Westminster/John Knox Press.

P.L. 105–17 (1997). Individuals with Disabilities Act (IDEA) Amendments of 1997. 20 U.S.C. 1412(a)(3)(A) and (B).

Ray, B. (1997). *Home education across the United States.* Purcellville, VA: Home School Legal Defense Association.

Rife, J., & Thornburgh, G. (1996). *From barriers to bridges: A community action guide for congregations and people with disabilities.* Washington, DC: National Organization on Disability.

Thompson, G. (1997, July 19). Church helps blind to sing and serve. *Arizona Republic*, p. R2.

United Nations. (1994). *The standard rules on the equalization of opportunities for persons with disabilities.* (Resolution 48/96). New York: United Nations.

Weller, R. (1978). *Blind—and I see!* St. Louis: Concordia.

Wright, J. (Ed.). (1997). *The universal almanac.* Kansas City, MO: Andrews McMeel.

PART IV

Gender, Sexual Orientation, and Visual Impairment

Women with Visual Impairments

L. Penny Rosenblum

"I think it is really hard to separate out what is gender originated and what is disability related. I think sometimes in people's eyes disability is the bigger factor. . . . Women's issues are very important, but I don't know how we can separate [the two]" [Beth]

When women who are blind or visually impaired examine their identities and roles in society, they often find it difficult to separate the influences of gender and visual impairment. Despite their individuality, however, they share some common issues. This chapter explores how women who are blind or visually impaired view themselves in society, particularly in relation to self-concept, sexuality, relationships, child rearing, independence, education, and careers, using interviews to highlight the women's varied experiences. The chapter ends with recommendations for professionals who work with these women.

DEFINING THE POPULATION

In the United States, an estimated 34.2 million people (17.5 percent of the population) over age 15 have a disability that is evident in a functional limitation (such as not being able to climb a flight of stairs, read a page of print, or hear a conversation). Of these 34.2 million people, 9.7 million have difficulty reading a page of print (Kraus, Lewis, Stoddard, & Gilmartin, 1996). McNeil (1993) reported that 5,679,000 women over age 15 (5.6 percent of all women in the United States) have a functional limitation in seeing (for instance, difficulty seeing words and letters in regular print). In addition, an estimated 929,000 women (0.9 percent of all women) report not being able to see words at all.

Women with disabilities, including visual impairments, earn less money than do their male counterparts. Although the gap in earned salaries is closing, it is still substantial. Szymanski and Parker (1996) noted that 37 percent of all employed men versus 75 percent of employed women earn less than $20,000 a year.

One must recognize that there are tremendous variations in the functional vision and life experiences of these women. Furthermore, as age increases, the percentage of women with visual impairments also increases, resulting in some distinctive issues for older women (McNeil, 1993). Jackie, Paula, and Tammy illustrate the variations in the population of women with visual impairments. Their experiences provide a framework for looking at the issues that women with visual impairments face.

Jackie

Jackie, a 45-year-old Caucasian woman with congenital low vision (significantly reduced visual acuity of 20/2000), is married and the mother of two daughters, one who is a high school senior and the other who is in her early 20s. Jackie, her husband, and two daughters have lived in their suburban home for over 20 years. Jackie is a print reader, although as her vision has decreased, she has come to rely more frequently on readers and books on audiotape. She has learned to read and write the letters of the alphabet in braille, but does not choose to use braille.

Jackie grew up with an older brother and younger sister and remembers that her parents often worried about her, paying more attention to her than to her siblings, partly because of the need to help her extensively with schoolwork. Jackie attended college, where she used readers and books on audiotape to gain access to materials. After college she worked part time for a year as a teacher before she and her husband started a family.

Jackie's family is the center of her life. She dated little before she met her husband. Although her husband is sighted, they met at a program for individuals with visual impairments, where they were both working for the summer. Her husband has been a teacher of children with visual impairments for 30 years. Jackie feels that her husband is sensitive to her visual impairment and is willing to alter his schedule and assist her when needed. Raising children and managing a household often present Jackie with challenges. When her children were young, she thought that she had to "stay on top of them" to monitor their safety. She found that transporting the children by walking to various activities required her to have good travel skills. Now that Jackie's children are grown, she said, "I sometimes wish I had the independence of all the other people around here who can jump in their car and go."

Jackie believes that her visual impairment has influenced her interactions with others. For example, because many people in her community do not realize how limited her vision is, when they wave to her from across the street and she does not wave back, they think she is not friendly. Even her children's friends who spend time at the house often do not comprehend Jackie's visual impairment. "The kids think I have eyes in the back of my head. [In reality] I can listen from the other room and figure out what they are doing."

Jackie feels independent in her own home, but is quick to acknowledge that she is not independent outside it. When shopping or traveling outside her neighborhood, she goes with a family member or friend. She does not use a cane and must rely on a sighted companion in unfamiliar areas.

Paula

Paula is a 42-year-old congenitally blind African American woman who lives in a large city and is employed as a program manager. Paula was the fourth of six children (the youngest of the girls in the family) and does not know if she got treated as a "baby" more out of birth order than because of her blindness. When she and her siblings went out to play, her brothers and sisters were held accountable if she got hurt. As an adult, she is the only sibling who has lived outside the city in which she and her siblings were born. She finds that her siblings come to her for advice regularly, though they still continue to worry about her being safe and independent. Personal safety is a concern for Paula: "I tend to be more open about my whereabouts. I want many people to know where I am and what I am doing. I want people to check up on me. I recognize that I have a greater level of vulnerability in the community. I'm sensitive to that vulnerability and I'm not ashamed to get assistance if safety is an issue. . . . My sighted girlfriends jump in their cars at 10 o'clock at night to get a pizza. I wouldn't even go in a cab at that time of night."

Although she does not have any children, Paula has her nieces and nephews. She is surprised at the sensitivity of these young people and believes they are proud to have an aunt who is blind. Many of her nieces and nephews bring friends by her house to "show me off, have me read braille or cook for them; . . . they think it is cool to have a blind aunt when they become teenagers."

Paula missed going through the same rites of passage as sighted teenagers, specifically getting a driver's license, and remembers resenting the lack of freedom. Her close friends were all sighted, and she felt accepted by them. She did not meet other visually impaired people until she was in her late 20s and became involved in consumer organizations for people with visual impairments. Now she has both sighted friends and visually impaired friends.

Educated in public schools, Paula found that she has always had to prove herself academically to teachers and later professors. Being a woman, blind, and African American, Paula thought, has opened educational opportunities for her because of affirmative action. She commented, "I was a three for one as far as scholarship committees were concerned. Talk about minority representation when you give me funding!" Paula said that her blindness has had a significant impact on her employment opportunities. She lamented, "I don't want to sound pessimistic, but I wonder who, what, and where I would be without my blindness. I'm probably not where a sighted woman would be if we were equal. Maybe it has more to do with the practical things. If where the better jobs are isn't accessible by public transportation, then I'm not going to [get them]."

Paula believes that it is important for her to educate others about visual impairment. She noted, "I have to remind people that I am here and competent. I feel obligated to educate people for when they meet the next blind person. I advocate for what someone else [who is visually impaired] might need. We're not all the same." Another avenue for advocacy is participation in consumer organizations, something Paula does with a vengeance. She wants people to be comfortable with their visual impairments and to recognize that they can lead full lives. As for her own life, she stated, "I really can't complain [about being blind]. I can't think of what I missed. Driving a car? I haven't missed getting to the places I want to go. I've had a wonderful life, frankly."

Tammy

Tammy, aged 39, is Caucasian and the mother of five adopted children ranging in age from 10 to 18. She and her husband, Joel, have been married for 23 years. Tammy began to experience problems with her vision in her mid-20s, lost much of her sight over a six-month period, and lost her remaining sight gradually over several years. Tammy recently went through training and received a dog guide. Her children were resistant to the idea of her getting a dog guide because they thought people would stare. Once their friends acknowledged that the dog guide was "cool," the children quickly adjusted to the dog.

Tammy has experienced many challenges as a woman with a visual impairment. When her vision began to deteriorate, the eye specialist recommended that she not drive until the cause was determined. For six months she did not drive, but then the eye specialist recommended that she obtain a state identification card. When she applied for the card, her driver's license was taken from her, and this event forced her to face the permanency of her vision loss. She felt isolated and alone. One of her greatest concerns was that she would not be able to see her daughters in their wedding dresses or the faces of her grandchildren.

Tammy attended a rehabilitation program, where she felt she did not belong. She remembered, "I thought everyone was mean. I was uncooperative. Really I was just scared." Learning orientation and mobility (O&M) skills, how to cook with limited sight, and how to write checks gave Tammy a sense of independence. However, she thought that she often does not get to exert her independence. Joel or the children are quick to do things for her, even when she says, "I can do this for myself. I don't need your help."

Tammy finds that she continually must educate the public. Often, a waitress or salesperson will talk to her companion, rather than to her. For example, in a store, the salesperson will ask her son, "Would she like this in a bag?" Tammy believes that people have preconceived notions about what blind people can and cannot do on the basis of their prior experiences. Often their experiences are with older family members, so when they meet a woman in her late 30s who can write her own checks, they do not know how to respond.

Other Women Who Were Interviewed

In addition to Jackie, Paula, and Tammy, a number of women with visual impairments volunteered important information that illustrates the main topics of this chapter. Carol is a 35-year-old Caucasian woman with low vision who does not work and has no interest in working. She uses public transportation and taxis for travel and believes that the greatest impact her visual impairment has on her life is limited transportation. Liz, a 32-year-old African American social worker who is married and has no children, lost her vision at age 8 and is a braille reader and dog guide user. Diane is a 75-year-old Caucasian woman who began to lose her vision at age 62 because of macular degeneration. It took her time to adjust and reestablish her independence both with her family and in the community. She is actively involved in a center-based program for adults with visual impairments in her community. Kelly, a 37-year-old Caucasian woman who is functionally blind, is employed in a hospital where she is the only person who is visually impaired. She finds that she must work hard to prove that she is a capable employee, not simply the token disabled person on staff. Beth is a 31-year-old congenitally blind, Caucasian graduate student who reads braille and uses a variety of technological devices (including a portable note taker, computer, and audiotapes) to meet her needs.

Although women with visual impairments have vastly different experiences, they have some things in common. The most important may be their desire to be independent. When asked what issues are important for women with visual impairments, many cited independence—both in doing for oneself and in traveling. Tammy expresseed a common feeling, "If I could boil everything down in a nut shell, it would be my independence. I want to do everything by and for myself. For example, going to the grocery store. I want to go pick out my own groceries, not have my husband pick them out for me."

WOMEN, VISUAL IMPAIRMENT, AND SOCIETY

Women with visual impairments are a heterogeneous group. Their roles within society are influenced and shaped by both their gender and their disability. All individuals with disabilities face many challenges in this society. For those whose disabilities are more obvious (such as wheelchair or cane users), people instantly recognize their disabilities and often make judgments based on their perceptions of the disabilities. For those with less obvious disabilities (like low vision and asthma) their actions are often misinterpreted by people who are unaware of the disabilities. For example, a woman who does not see a man who is attracted to her wink at her from across the room will not respond with a wink or a smile. The man may interpret her lack of a response as a lack of interest, when she simply did not see his overture.

Society's Views of Women with Disabilities

Although there is a dearth of information on women with visual impairments in the literature on visual impairment, information in the literature on women with disabilities, primarily physical disabilities, is helpful in laying the foundation for understanding the issues that visually impaired women face. The feminist literature is also of value in examining the roles of women in Western society, but that literature contains little information on elderly women and women with disabilities (Morris, 1991)—an indication that these populations are frequently overlooked.

Although the number of disabled women in the United States is growing, scientists and policy makers have traditionally studied the affects of disability on men (Hanna & Rogovsky, 1991; Thurer, 1991). For example, the medical community has explored sexual issues and options for men who are paralyzed, but has conducted little research on these issues for women who are paralyzed. The emphasis on men is also seen in the media. When a disabled character is included in a television show or movie, the character is more often a man than a woman (Morris, 1991). As a result of the emphasis on men in this society, there are often subtle differences in the availability of services (such as job training programs, medical treatments) to disabled women compared to disabled men. This practice reinforces the societal perception that women are less capable or worthy than men (Lonsdale, 1990; Thomson, 1997; Thurer, 1991). In this society, many find it more acceptable for a woman to become disabled than for a man to become disabled because passivity, docility and dependence are viewed as characteristics that are more common in women than in men (Hillyer, 1993; Lonsdale, 1990; Morris, 1991; Vash, 1981; Wendell, 1996). Thus, expectations for women with disabilities are often lower than for men with disabilities.

In feminist theory, women are considered by society to be "the other" class, that is, a less fortunate or less able group (Thomson, 1997). Individuals with disabilities and chronic illness are also considered to fall in this category (Thomson, 1997; Wendell, 1996). The consequences of being in "the other" group are great for those with disabilities. For example, because of the society's rigid definition of independence, those who cannot care for their own physical needs or find employment because of their physical limitations are not considered independent (Wendell, 1996). Independence is also defined as productivity (Hillyer, 1993), so when a disability interferes with a woman's productivity in caring for children or holding down a job, the woman is viewed negatively by society. Disabled people do not have a place in this society and are not included in much of everyday life; for example, they rarely are depicted in television programs and films or have adequate transportation options in their communities. Disabled individuals and women must often work to become part of the mainstream society, which revolves around heterosexual, employed, white men. When an individual is both disabled and a woman, it can be a challenge to gain full acceptance into society (Thomson, 1997).

In this society, women with disabilities are stereotyped in one of two ways: either as happy and mentally healthy, accepting their disabilities and willingly seeking and accepting assistance from others, or angry and bitter about the fate they have been dealt. Women in either category may appear invisible to others (Browne, Connors, & Stern, 1985; Wendell, 1996). Both types of women may be perceived as needing help, the first one asking for and accepting help graciously, although running the risk of appearing dependent, and the second one demanding assistance in such a way as to cause society to feel sorry for her.

A woman with a disability who does not want to be perceived as dependent, passive, angry, or bitter faces societal barriers. For a woman with an adventitious visual impairment, fighting the stereotypes can be a challenge, for she has not only to understand and accept her own feelings in adjusting to her disability, but acknowledge the feelings and attitudes of others (Kolb, 1985). The attitudes of others are deeply ingrained. For example, Western societies often have rigid perceptions of what is sexually attractive and what is not (Lonsdale, 1990). Since disability is not considered sexually attractive, women with disabilities are often viewed as being asexual and not sexually desirable (Thomson, 1997; Thurer, 1991; Wendell, 1996). A typical assumption is that these women do not have sexual feelings or relationships that include sex, do not get married, and hence do not bear and raise children (Fine & Asch, 1985; Hanna & Rogovsky, 1991; Lonsdale, 1990; Thomson, 1997). When women with disabilities do marry, their rate of divorce is higher than among women without disabilities and men with disabilities (Hanna & Rogovsky, 1991).

In this society, a woman's perceptions of physical attractiveness, including sexual attractiveness, affect her self-image and psychological well-being (Lonsdale, 1990). These perceptions are influenced by society, especially the value men place on women with "beautiful" bodies that conform to the male stereotype of sexuality (Wendell, 1996). Thus, women are not reinforced (led to believe) in the concepts that bodies come in many shapes and sizes, that bodies with physical deformities are beautiful, and that the physical limitations of a body do not lead to a weak or inferior person within the body (Wendell, 1996). For women with congenital disabilities, the disabilities are part of their self-image, and they must struggle against society's negative perception of them. They are more likely than men with disabilities to internalize society's rejection of them, and they more often identify themselves as disabled than do their male counterparts (Fine & Asch, 1985). These tendencies may result, in part, from the desire to fit in or to please others. If no one has ever spoken with a disabled woman about her potential to marry and raise children, she may assume that marriage and children are not within her reach because of her disability. An adventitiously disabled woman will have to "rework" her self-image to reflect both her own and society's views of the disability (Lonsdale, 1990). This is not an easy task, and many adventitiously disabled women struggle with doing so.

In addition to issues of self-image and psychological well-being, women with disabilities often have more limited role choices and role models than do men with disabilities (Fine & Asch, 1985). The traditional roles for women (homemaker, teacher, and human service worker) may not be as attainable for women with disabilities as for women without disabilities. Entry into fields that are traditionally male (such as business and engineering) are also more difficult for these women. Thus, there are a higher unemployment rate and fewer training programs for disabled women than for disabled men (Fine & Asch, 1985).

Although women with disabilities have gained more recognition and acceptance over time, they still face many challenges. Breaking down the negative stereotypes and stigmas imposed by society is still important for many women with disabilities.

Society's Views of Visual Impairment

Visual impairment is often viewed negatively and is feared. Terms such as *blind, visually handicapped,* and *visually disabled* are perceived as negative (Rosenblum & Erin, 1998). Furthermore, having a visual impairment is believed not to be "normal," and the negative ramifications of this lack of normalcy can affect all aspects of an individual's life (Harsh, 1993). Moreover, whether a visual impairment is congenital or adventitious affects a woman's perception of her disability. Women who are adventitiously blind or visually impaired have to examine their own negative feelings about their impairments and how these feelings affect who they are as visually impaired persons (Tuttle & Tuttle, 1996). Women who are congenitally blind or visually impaired grow up with their disabilities, but often question how their lives would have been different if they were sighted. Whether a woman is congenitally or adventitiously visually impaired, she inevitably faces challenges imposed by society's attitudes toward visual impairment.

Double Barrier

Disabled women are often "doubly disadvantaged" economically, socially, and psychologically compared to women without disabilities and men with disabilities (Fine & Asch, 1985). They have two barriers to overcome: those related to the stereotypical behaviors (docility, passivity, and dependence) that women are expected to exhibit and those related to the behaviors that are believed to be representative of individuals with visual impairments. Thus, a woman with a visual impairment must struggle with both society's perceptions of women and with perceptions of people who are disabled (Wendell, 1996). For example, blind or visually impaired women have difficulty entering careers that are traditionally male and are for sighted people, such as science and medicine (Hutto & Hare, 1997).

When women who are blind or visually impaired are successful and independent, they often are subject to unwarranted admiration. This admiration can make them feel as if they are being idolized simply because they have done something (for example, obtained an advanced degree or been hired by a business) that women without disabilities do every day (Lonsdale, 1990). If they are not successful, they are perceived as failures because of their disability (Lonsdale, 1990). The challenges that being a woman and being visually impaired impose can be exhausting, both emotionally and physically.

GROWING UP AS A GIRL WITH A VISUAL IMPAIRMENT

Women who are congenitally blind or visually impaired or lost their vision in childhood are influenced by their experiences growing up as visually impaired girls in their families, schools, and larger communities. It is during childhood that one develops the necessary skills for later social interaction. Even in infancy, parents engage in different types of play with girls than they do with boys (Feldman, 1998). Play with boys involves more rough and tumble, while play with girls involves more face-to-face interaction. Infants with visual impairment are not as responsive as sighted infants to their parents; they often do not exhibit the expected responses when parents smile and make exaggerated facial expressions (Warren 1984, 1994). Since parents may be unsure of how to interact with their infant girls who are blind or visually impaired, these babies may not have the opportunities to practice and learn about social interaction to the degree that sighted babies do.

Preschoolers learn about the world through play and interaction with objects and others (Feldman, 1998). By the end of the preschool years, girls prefer to play with other girls and boys prefer to play with other boys (Feldman, 1998; Patzer, 1985). Thus, they have learned from the larger society that there are gender differences and it is preferable to associate with one's own gender. Because preschool-age children also prefer to play with peers who are physically attractive and similar to them (Patzer, 1985), they may choose not to play with a child with a visual impairment because the child is perceived to be "different" or "not normal." Furthermore, since children who are blind or visually impaired are often behind sighted children in their play skills, they spend much of their play time alone (Skellenger, Rosenblum, & Jager, 1997; Warren, 1984, 1994) and thus have limited opportunities to learn from their peers.

During the elementary and adolescent years, friendships become essential. Girls have more intimate friendships and a greater number of best friends than do boys (Ritz, 1992; Sharabany, 1974). Children who are perceived to be physically attractive find it easier to establish friendships (Clark & Ayers, 1991; Patzer, 1985). Children and adolescents with visual impairments have fewer friendships than do their sighted peers (MacCuspie, 1992; Rosenblum, 1997), are often perceived as being less socially competent (MacCuspie, 1992), and spend more time alone (Wolffe & Sacks, 1997). For example, Carol found that since her parents restricted her participation in activities, such as roller skating, bike riding, and team sports, it was difficult to develop friendships with other girls. If she could not do the same activities as the sighted girls, they were not interested in spending time with her. Thus, Carol remembered spending a lot of time with her family and little time with children in the neighborhood. Since it is through friendships that one gets to practice social interactions; learn about dating and relationships; and experience trust, loyalty, and intimacy; not having friends can have negative ramifications for visually impaired adolescent girls as they move into adulthood. For instance, Beth remembered that she was socially on the fringe in high school because the other girls were not comfortable interacting with her. She often would not be invited places, such as the movies, because people would assume she could not enjoy movies. As adolescent girls move into womanhood, they bring with them their prior experiences with family, friends, and peers. When they are visually impaired, their potential for having had fewer or unsatisfactory social experiences is great.

WHO AM I?

This section examines women's perceptions of who they are as both blind or impaired persons and women. Many of the issues that women with visual impairments face are also faced by men with visual impairments. Similarly, some issues experienced by women with visual impairments are experienced by other women as well. Thus, it is important to look at women's issues globally and then to highlight the often subtle differences for women with visual impairments. Most women with visual impairments acknowledge that being visually impaired is an important characteristic of who they are and one they do not wish to alter.

Self-Concept

One's self-concept is influenced by interactions with family, friends, and society. Like their male counterparts, women who are blind or visually impaired often question who they are and how they are perceived by society. When they meet others, they often feel the need to prove themselves by, for example, choosing outfits that match, eating in restaurants, traveling in unfamiliar cities. The emotional energy in always having to be "on" can exhaust a woman with a visual impairment. Some believe that it is necessary for them to educate the public, whereas others find that always being "watched" is overwhelming and prefer to spend time alone or with their families or friends.

It is not uncommon for women with disabilities to attempt to portray themselves as not having disabilities and to try and pass as normal (Hillyer, 1993; Morris, 1991). Women who have low vision may try to "hide" their visual impairments, especially in unfamiliar social situations. For example, Kelly admitted that she sometimes "fibs" and tells someone that she can see something when she cannot. She noted, "You don't want to be different, so there is an actor in you which surfaces at times. Also, you learn to do things unobtrusively and to plan ahead." Similarly, Carol telephones a restaurant ahead of time to learn what the specials are, so she does not have to ask her date or friend to read them to her. She does not want to feel dependent on others; instead, she wants to show that as a woman with a visual impairment, she is capable of independence.

Other women do not find their visual impairments to be obstacles; rather their visual impairments help them build self-confidence and widen their experiences. Sometimes, their visual impairments may be the reason they meet someone who later becomes an important person in their lives. For example, Natalie, a 57-year-old woman who is adventitiously visually impaired, met her second husband because of her visual impairment; they fell in love when they were taking classes at a rehabilitation center because of their recent decrease in usable vision. In some instances, a visual impairment may give a woman opportunities that might otherwise not be available, such as a scholarship to attend college or access to a job training program. As was noted earlier, Paula found that the combination of being a woman, blind, and African American gave her access to financial resources not available to other African American women or other women who were blind. For still others, a visual impairment may serve as a catalyst to a career path that opens many doors and allows them to meet a variety of sighted and visually impaired people. These enriching experiences stemming from being women with visual impairments play defining roles as the women strive to understand who they are and their roles in society.

A woman who is visually impaired may have both positive and negative experiences related to her disability and gender, which, in turn, have an impact on her self-concept. These influences are individual and vary throughout a woman's lifetime. Feeling impelled to behave in such ways as "fibbing or "planning ahead" or believing that she is being judged or evaluated because of a visual impairment is likely to lower a woman's self-concept because the amount of energy that she has to put into planning how to handle these issues can be taxing.

Role Models

Many women have role models whom they look to as examples or mentors, whether these role models are actresses, singers, religious figures, teachers, family members, or friends. Hutto and Hare (1997) found that a factor that contributed to successful employment for visually impaired women was the presence of role models in their lives. Paula's first role model of a successful blind woman was Helen Keller, to whom she was introduced in *The Miracle Worker* (Gibson, 1957). Later, Paula had a blind resource room teacher who showed her how one can adapt and live in a sighted world. The one disadvantage, she thought, of having this teacher as a role model was that for years she believed that the only profession available to her was teaching.

Many women with visual impairments do not know successful women with visual impairments to whom they can look for guidance, models, or inspiration. Peanstiehl (1983) noted that most women who did not report a visually impaired role model in their lives thought that having one would be a positive experience. Kelly thought that it is important for visually impaired women to find successful professionals who can serve as positive role models and that they can do so through blindness organizations (such as the American Council of the Blind and the National Federation of the Blind). A role model who is also visually impaired can be inspirational and supportive, especially for a woman with an adventitious visual impairment. For example, when Tammy attended a rehabilitation program after she lost her vision, she met an older woman who had diabetic retinopathy. Tammy observed how gracious and patient this woman was with others, especially the public, and strove to act as this woman did. Meeting other women with visual impairments can help a woman adjust as she examines how the visual impairment affects her self; her role in society; and the adaptations necessary to continue to be an independent, productive person.

Sexuality and Physical Appearance

Images of women who are physically and sexually attractive—and do not have visual impairments—dominate the mass media. Much of a person's understanding of physical attractiveness is learned through vision and is acquired early in childhood. For women, more so than men, their perceptions of their body image and physical attractiveness are closely related to their self-image (Hillyer, 1993).

Some visually impaired women think that the appearance of their eyes (for example, prosthetic eyes, irregularly shaped pupils, or nystagmus) or the need to use optical aids (like prescription lenses and magnifying glasses) detracts from their perceived attractiveness. Liz remembered that in college, she was not allowed to pledge a sorority because of the appearance of her eyes. Even now, she said, "I think the appearance of my eyes can be a deterrent to people approaching [me socially]. Not so much with kids but more so with adults." Tammy also thought that the appearance of her eyes interfered with her interactions with others. Since she is constantly asked, "Are you tired? Do you have a headache? Did something happen to your eyes?" when she does not wear dark glasses, she tries always to wear dark glasses in public, rather than explain her visual impairment.

Many blind or visually impaired women believe that their attire, makeup, and hairstyles are more closely scrutinized than those of sighted women. For example, Paula noted, "If a sighted woman comes into work with her hair a mess, people say, 'Oh, she's having a bad hair day.' If I come into work that way, they say, 'Oh, she's blind and can't take care of herself.'" To succeed in the world of work, women with visual impairments often feel they must be aware of the latest fashions and have an up-to-date wardrobe to be equal with their coworkers. Some choose not to wear makeup because they are concerned that they cannot apply it appropriately, whereas others, such as Tammy, work hard to learn how to use modifications to apply makeup successfully. Other concerns are the additional time required to organize clothes to ensure that items match and the need to take a family member or friend along to ask a salesperson to assist while shopping for clothes. As Tammy said, "There are few people I trust to help me pick out clothes or makeup. There is one woman I know who I take shopping with me. I don't trust the salesperson or my husband. My daughter does a pretty good job, but she wants me to dress the way she does. Green nail polish is not for me!"

For women, physical appearance and attractiveness are closely tied to intimacy and sexuality. Sighted women often get more information about sexual topics from friends, television, and written materials than do women with visual impairments (Welbourne, Lifschitz, Selvin, & Green, 1983). The lack of accurate information and societal perceptions inhibit the sexual activity of many women with visual impairments. Welbourne et al. (1983) found that the mean age of first intercourse for blind women was 21 compared to 17 for sighted women. The blind women in the study attributed this difference to difficulty meeting men, not recognizing and responding to flirting, negative societal attitudes toward blindness, and not feeling physically attractive. Since women with visual impairments often find it difficult to establish relationships that lead to intimacy, Kirchner, McBroom, Nelson, and Graves (1992) found that women who were legally blind were less frequently married than women who were sighted or men who were legally blind. Women with visual impairments may not believe they are capable or worthy of intimate relationships or desirable to potential partners.

For women with visual impairments, concerns about sexuality and physical appearance are individual. Some women believe that their visual impairments have little impact on sexuality and physical appearance, while others believe that their visual impairments greatly affect these two areas.

Safety

There are several levels of safety. One level involves protecting one's body from physical injury caused by hazards in the environment, such as cutting a finger with a knife, banging a knee by walking into the edge of a table, or breaking a bone from falling down a flight of stairs. Women who are visually impaired or blind must monitor their own safety and teach others to help keep the environment clear of potential hazards. Tammy's youngest child learned as a toddler to move toys from the center of the room and to pull her by the hand if there was an obstacle in her path. Tammy taught her coworkers to leave doors either completely open or completely closed and not to move furniture without telling her. Because family members, friends, and coworkers tend to want to protect a woman with a visual impairment from potential harm, it is imperative for her to assert her independence in a positive way so as to be autonomous and self-sufficient.

Another level of safety involves threats to the individual by other people. In this society, women are more vulnerable than men to such threats to their safety and women with disabilities, including visual impairment, are more vulnerable to assault than their sighted counterparts (Andrews & Veronen, 1993; Pava, 1994; Sobsey, 1994). As Beth commented, "I've been very lucky, but I know I'm more vulnerable than most women. I like to walk around by myself, and I don't like to ask people for rides when I'm three blocks from my house."

Pava's (1994) survey of 105 women with visual impairments found that 29.7 percent had been targets of unsuccessful, attempted assaults, including both physical assaults (like beatings and muggings) and sexual assaults (rape), and 16.2 percent had been actual targets of assault. Similarly, over 50 percent of congenitally blind women in Welbourne et al.'s (1983) study reported having one or more forced sexual experiences. To combat vulnerability, women with visual impairments take precautions, such as using drivers or taxis at night, not traveling alone in unfamiliar areas, or stopping only women to ask for assistance. Many have considered getting a dog guide not only for independence, but for an added measure of safety. Moreover, many choose where they want to live with safety in mind.

Although they work on feeling safe and not allowing concerns about their safety to interfere with their lives, most women who are blind or visually impaired believe that they take their increased vulnerability into consideration when making decisions. Pava (1994) advocated the need for women with visual impairments to participate in training programs to learn self-protection techniques. Given that an estimated 2 in 3 women with disabilities experience some form of sexual assault (Sobsey, 1994), this recommendation is warranted for women who are blind or visually impaired.

Independence

Being an independent adult is expected in our society, though no one is truly independent of everyone and everything (Morris, 1991). To be perceived as independent, one has to care for one's own needs, including travel, housing, and finances. Women are acculturated to be interdependent, or to put others' needs before their own, to care for others, and to accept others caring for them (Hillyer, 1993). Women with visual impairments are even more susceptible to being interdependent than independent because of the nature of their disabilities. For example, having to enlist others to assist with transportation, to read mail, or to identify the color of an article of clothing can cause a woman who is blind or visually impaired to feel that her independence is significantly compromised. As Beth explained, "it has been a struggle not to let my blindness affect my independence."

Like Beth, other women who were interviewed for this chapter reported that they often felt frustrated in regard to their level of interdependence with significant others in their lives. They identified two levels of independence: internal, when one is in control of life choices and is not dependent on others to make decisions, and external, when one is able to gain access to the environment and travel through it successfully. Although nondisabled men and women also strive for independence, women with disabilities, such as blindness or visual impairments, frequently have to work doubly hard to exercise their independence (Hillyer, 1993; Morris, 1991). They often believe that they place more emphasis on both types of independence than do nondisabled women, partly because they are overly conscious of not wanting to depend on others. They must demonstrate to their family members, friends, and the society at large that they can be self-sufficient by traveling in their communities, obtaining employment, and managing a home. In this regard, it is critical to have a "tool box" of choices to meet the daily demands of every situation. For example, when a woman with low vision needs to read mail, she can employ a sighted reader, use a computer scanner, or use a closed-circuit television system. Internal independence allows one to examine the options that are within one's resources and to make the choice that is best for a situation.

For most people who are blind or visually impaired, the greatest barrier to external independence is transportation. Decisions about employment, housing, and lifestyle center on access to transportation (Corn & Sacks, 1994). The need to plan for transportation dramatically decreases one's spontaneity and choices and increases one's frustration and feelings of isolation. For example, Diane believes that giving up her driver's license initially caused her to lose much of her independence. After several years of having to rely on others for transportation, she received O&M training. Now she is able to walk safely using a cane and to travel using city buses. She lives in a part of the city where she can take advantage of many services without having to rely on others for assistance. When she needs assistance, she has learned to arrange for it and to reciprocate appropriately, thus exerting her internal independence.

Diane is similar to many of the respondents in Corn and Sacks's (1994) study of the transportation experiences of 110 adult nondrivers who were visually impaired. The respondents were asked to rate 25 potential obstacles to transportation using a 5-point Likert-type scale (from 1 = no frustration to 5 = a high amount of frustration). Women reported a significantly higher level of frustration than did men. The obstacles that caused greater frustration for women than for men included planning means of transportation ahead of time, walking in dangerous areas alone, requesting rides from others, and ensuring security while traveling. Similarly, the respondents with low vision reported significantly higher levels of frustration than did those who were blind. The women also perceived that their inability to drive affected their lifestyles to a greater extent than it did their male counterparts with regard to their social lives, ability to live independently, and employment opportunities. Kelly said that she often does not attend plays or lectures in the community because she cannot get to these events by public transportation and lacks the financial resources to hire a driver or taxi for recreational activities. Thus, she sometimes feels "left out of the loop because I don't have a car to get me to the fun places."

For many women with visual impairments, the lack of independence they experience is frustrating. Women with visual impairments who report that they generally feel independent tend to be good travelers who have developed effective advocacy and problem-solving skills in addition to their ability to use a variety of transportation options.

INTIMATE RELATIONSHIPS: FAMILY, ROMANCE, AND CHILDREN

Relationships with family members and romantic partners are two types of relationships that are important in women's lives. This section examines the impact of blindness or visual impairment on these two types of relationships and on raising children.

Family

The family is responsible for children's initial socialization, values, and experiences. Women who are blind or visually impaired who report being successful in their careers have indicated that their families provided an atmosphere in which they could ask for assistance when needed. In addition, their families were willing to make accommodations and expected them to participate in all aspects of family life (Hutto & Hare, 1997).

Although many blind or visually impaired women who shared their experiences for this chapter reported a nurturing family environment, others said that their parents and siblings were overprotective. Kelly noted that she developed independence at a residential school for blind students and that her family "babied" her tremendously and still does. Family members sometimes think that they need to "take care" of a woman who is visually impaired—a need that often strengthens a woman's need to seek both internal and external independence. Diane said that her two adult sons are anxious about her and try to take care of all her needs. She has had to gain her independence from them in much the same way that they gained their independence from her when they were teenagers.

Dating and Marriage

Many people in the United States believe that women with disabilities, including blindness or visual impairment, are asexual and do not have romantic relationships or marry and have families (Fine & Asch, 1985; Kroll & Klein, 1995; Thurer, 1991). Women with visual impairments are less likely to marry and raise children than are women who are sighted or men who are visually impaired (Kirchner, 1995). Since marriage is a contributing factor to self-sufficiency and economic success in the United States, many women who are blind or viually impaired are not viewed as independent (Kirchner, 1995) because they are not married. However, many women with visual impairments do have romantic relationships and marry, and their partners are often sighted. Peanstiehl (1983) found that visually impaired single women did not want to marry men who were visually impaired because they thought that doing so would compound their problems and impede their privacy in reading mail and deaing with financial matters.

Women with visual impairments often find that the hardest part of dating is to meet men who are comfortable with women who do not fit the "norm." Beth has had many boyfriends in her 31 years, a fact that she attributed to being blonde, petite, and outgoing. "Guys who wanted to date me were guys that were on the edge," she said, indicating that she meant socially on the fringe. "They were interested in me. They were always relaxed about the blindness stuff. When I was 24 or 25, I dated 4 or 5 people: one I met on the bus, one I met through work, one [who] was the son of a colleague. With one, it started out with, 'I really admire you and the things you can do being blind.' We kept talking and had things in common like biking and restaurants. Initially, that was the only way he knew to start, even though he was attracted to me as a woman." Beth recognized the need to make potential partners relaxed when it comes to her blindness and to help them realize who she is as a complete woman.

Liz said that her family expects her husband to take care of her (that is, to go shopping with her, provide transportation, and read mail), but she does not agree with this philosophy. Yet she admitted that her husband sometimes takes on this role. She noted that then he "feels resentful when it comes to transportation. On a weekend, he wants to kick back, and I need some help getting to the store." Liz described her relationship with her husband as first an acquaintanceship, then a friendship, and finally a romantic relationship and said that the slow start stemmed from his need to see beyond her blindness. This belief was echoed by other women, who acknowledged that on the first few dates, men are often overly concerned about the visual impairment and must be "taught" such things as when to provide clarification of the environment. For example, in public, the man must remember to identify verbally people whom the woman may not recognize by voice alone. Some men "learn" so well that they take on a caregiving role—a role that most women with visual impairments, who are looking for "equal" partners, not brothers, do not think is appropriate. When Tammy and her husband Joel married, she was fully sighted and believed they had an "equal" partnership. As her vision decreased, Joel took on more responsibilities, such as driving the children to activities, vacuuming, grocery shopping, and paying bills. At times, Tammy feels as if he treats her as another child in the family. When she lost her sight, she questioned whether he was staying with her out of a sense of duty, rather than love. With time, she has come to realize that he still loves her, regardless of her disability. She believes that it is important to communicate with her husband so that both of them can share their feelings openly about the visual impairment. She does not think that her husband views her as less of a woman. Their sexual relationship has never been affected by her visual impairment.

Each relationship has its unique issues, just as do relationships between men and women who are sighted. Paula, for example, reported dating both blind and sighted men. She explained that when she dates a blind man, she does not have to spend as much time explaining her blindness, although there are still communication and control issues as in all relationships. She also said that when she dated a sighted man who did not want her to carry a cane, she did not know whether he was embarrassed to be seen with a woman using a cane or wanted to make her totally dependent on him.

It is possible for women with visual impairments to have romantic relationships. Breaking societal stereotypes and forging relationships with partners who are accepting takes time and patience. As with other aspects of life, women with visual impairments must often be their own advocates to succeed in romantic relationships.

Raising Children

Women with visual impairments are less likely to bear and raise children than are women who are sighted (Kirchner, 1995) because fewer of them marry or believe that visually impaired women can be "good" mothers who can meet all their children's needs and monitor their children's safety. Yet many women with visual impairments successfully raise children by planning and making adaptations. To monitor their infants' and toddlers' movements, they may put bells on the children's shoes, use harnesses in public, or give the children sound-making toys. Once the children learn to speak, these mothers teach them always to answer verbally when called. Using their other senses, especially hearing, is critical to these mothers' effective parenting.

The mothers who were interviewed for this chapter reported that when their children became toddlers they understood that to show things (such as toys and pictures), they had to place them in their mothers' hands. When children enter school, they may resent having mothers who are unable to drive. Joan, a 40-year-old totally blind single mother, said that from the age of 8, her daughter resented when they had to use public transportation and would often not talk to her at the bus stop or sit with her on the bus. These behaviors caused Joan great anxiety because she was unable to monitor her daughter's safety. As a teenager, her daughter has come to rely on friends for transportation, but often comments to Joan about the unfairness of having a mother who is "not normal." Tammy has found that her children's reactions to her loss of vision have varied. Initially, her son who was in elementary school did not want her to come to school because he was embarrassed to have friends see her using a cane. She recognized that her children can lie to her more easily than they could if she was sighted. For example, her teenage daughter may tell her the kitchen is clean, but Tammy later discovers that her daughter "cleaned up" by stacking all the dirty dishes behind the bread maker. Tammy has come to understand that these behaviors are typical of children and that her children are not necessarily picking on her when they take advantage of her limited vision. There are times when child rearing can test the patience of any woman, and women with visual impairments are no exception.

Of course, some children accept their mothers' visual impairments and do not feel angry or embarrassed. For example, Diane's two grown sons, daughters-in-law, and five grandchildren all accept her visual impairment. They have been willing to learn methods, such as the sighted guide technique, to assist her and to make adaptations in their homes (like reducing glare and increasing contrast) to accommodate her vision loss. Diane believes that the support of her family enabled her to accept her loss of vision more easily. Children can benefit from having mothers with visual impairments. For one thing, they learn empathy for individuals with disabilities. Tammy noted that her children are independent and good decision makers because they have had many opportunities to "fend for themselves." If they want to be involved in an activity, they know that they must take responsibility for arranging transportation. When she is helping a child with homework, the child must read the directions to her and accurately describe the material. These types of experiences, she thought, have helped her children to grow and mature.

Children's reactions to their mothers' visual impairments vary. In the case of a woman with an adventitious visual impairment, the age of the child when the mother became visually impaired and the reactions of the mother and other family members influence the child's acceptance of the visual impairment. If a mother has been visually impaired from the time of the child's birth, the child will always know the mother as visually impaired.

EDUCATIONAL AND CAREER OPPORTUNITIES

This section examines two areas that are closely related: the educational and career experiences of women with visual impairments. One's attitudes toward and values regarding education and careers are shaped during childhood and are influenced by one's family and available opportunities. The educational and career experiences of congenitally visually impaired women often differ from those of adventitiously visually impaired women, who went through part or all of the educational system as sighted persons and thus could make use of educational opportunities without difficulty and were not confronted with negative attitudes, limited materials, and restrictions in transportation.

Educational Experiences

The childhood educational experiences of many women with congenital visual impairments did not maximize their potential. Carol struggled to see the chalkboard and other written materials in elementary school. She recalled that since the teachers did not take the time to assist her in gaining access to materials, she quickly lost interest in school. Carol graduated from high school, but was not encouraged to go to a trade school or college. Although she has sold hot dogs at an arcade and worked at a license plate factory, she now collects a small pension resulting from her father's death. She stated, "I don't want to go to school or work. I don't have it in me." To Carol, being legally blind, not being a woman, has been a negative factor in her educational and vocational experiences.

Like Carol, other women often perceive that their visual impairments restrict their educational opportunities. Common issues include the lack of access to printed materials, others' assumptions that the content is too difficult, and the increased amount of time it can take to complete assignments. Proving one's capabilities to teachers, parents, and counselors is critical for women who want equal educational opportunities. A woman who lacks self-confidence may not believe she is capable of succeeding academically. Tammy said that she was not accepted to the private college in her town because of her visual impairment. Her application was simply ignored by the administrators in spite of multiple visits and telephone calls. The administrators of the public college in her town were reluctant to accept her, but recognized that under the Americans with Disabilities Act (ADA) they had to make accommodations for her. She believes that her educational opportunities have been greatly restricted because of her visual impairment.

Other women with visual impairments successfully navigate the educational system and earn bachelor's, master's, and doctoral degrees. They are able to demonstrate their capabilities in spite of the limitations imposed by their loss of vision. The use of technology (such as portable note takers, scanners, and laptop computers) has greatly enhanced access to written materials for people with visual impairments. Women who are visually impaired can gain access to educational opportunities because of the requirements of affirmative action.

However, even as they successfully move through the educational system, women who are blind or visually impaired often have limited knowledge of appropriate careers for which they can prepare. Kelly recalled that since she did not have any blind role models when she was in college, she majored in special education because she did not know of any other careers at which blind women had succeeded. Kelly typifies many blind and visually impaired women who often chose college majors in the service professions because they did not know that other choices were available to them.

Women who are adventitiously blind or visually impaired typically completed high school or college before their vision decreased. For these women, educational opportunities focus on rehabilitation services received through rehabilitation teachers, private agencies, or residential facilities. For women who have been sighted and now must learn adaptive techniques to shop, cook, clean, sew, and organize their clothing, additional training is essential to success. Diane believes that the instruction in home management and O&M training she received through a private agency enabled her to live independently again. Tammy also acknowledged the benefits of participating in a rehabilitation program and later a dog guide training program. It is through such programs that women are able to regain control of their lives following their loss of vision.

In this society, most people view education as a door to career opportunities, economic advancement, and independence. To maximize their potential to succeed, women with visual impairments must have access to education and receive necessary supports (such as live readers and computer technology). The benefit of providing rehabilitation services as a form of reeducating women with adventitious vision losses must also be recognized.

Career and Employment

The careers that women who are blind or visually impaired have traditionally entered (for example, teaching, psychology, social work, and secretarial work) are low paying and often emphasize caring or helping others (Hutto & Hare, 1997). As with educational opportunities, they have entered these occupations because of their limited role models and societal expectations of what are appropriate careers for women with visual impairments.

Another concern is the availability of actual employment opportunities for women with visual impairments. Both women and men with visual impairments have reported being unemployed or underemployed (McNeil, 1993), although since the passage of the ADA in 1990, a greater number of blind and visually impaired people have found jobs (Kirchner, Johnson, & Harkins, 1997). Women with visual impairments still face barriers to employment. Corn, Muscella, Cannon, and Shepler's (1985) survey of 41 visually impaired women, 39 percent of whom were adventitiously visually impaired and 61 percent of whom were congenitally visually impaired, found that the women thought they faced greater barriers to employment than did sighted women, including rehabilitation counselors' attitudes, their own lack of confidence in their skills, employers' attitudes toward their advancement, and a greater need for safety precautions. Corn et al. concluded that both the self-perceptions of women with visual impairments and employers' attitudes toward employing them are the key barriers. For example, Liz thought that she was not hired as an itinerant social worker because the employer did not believe she could use public transportation and drivers to fulfill the job responsibilities. She said that employers often scrutinize her work more than that of her coworkers because of her blindness. However, she noted that once she is hired, employers are generally willing to make accommodations (such as tape recording her phone messages and purchasing a speech synthesizer for her computer).

Women with visual impairments often want to work, but the barriers they face, both real and perceived, can inhibit their success. Kirchner et al. (1997) found that 44 percent of the 264 adults with visual impairments they surveyed were interested in working but were not employed, and 12 percent were not interested in employment. The latter group gave reasons based on perceived barriers (such as transportation), rather than a distaste for work.

In spite of the barriers to employment, many blind and visually impaired women are employed in competitive jobs with sighted people. Successfully employed women share characteristics that enable them to advance in their careers. These characteristics include intelligence, self-discipline, a strong personal self-concept, self-esteem, drive, motivation, risk taking, creative thinking, assertiveness, strong written and oral skills, self-reliance, determination, and perseverance (Hutto & Hare, 1997). The foundation for success in employment is based, in part, on one's positive self-esteem, educational experiences, and support systems.

Many people believe that those who have college degrees obtain better jobs and are more satisfied with their jobs. However, Kirchner, McBroom, Nelson, and Graves (1992) found that a college education was not as great an economic advantage for legally blind adults as for sighted adults. Although individuals with college degrees were three times more likely to hold professional, managerial, or technical jobs than those without them, the level of satisfaction experienced by legally blind adults was less. This difference may relate to many visually impaired individuals' need to prove themselves on the job and the subsequent emotional strain this creates. Kelly said that on a new job, it takes about a year for her to prove that she is a capable, competent employee, not simply the token disabled woman on staff.

Clearly, women who are visually impaired or blind can obtain satisfying jobs in a variety of fields. Yet, their unemployment rate remains high (60 percent to 70 percent), and their salaries are low (Kirchner et al., 1992). The need for equality is most evident when the employment of these women is examined.

RECOMMENDATIONS FOR PROFESSIONALS

Each woman who is blind or visually impaired is a unique individual and has had her own experiences gained through her interactions with family, friends, and society. The age at which she experienced her decreased vision, her attitudes toward blindness or visual impairment, and the attitudes of others around her influence her perceptions of who she is. Similarly, the professionals with whom she comes in contact also bring their experiences and beliefs to their interaction with her. Thus, it is necessary for professionals to be sensitive to the belief system of a woman who is blind or visually impaired and to their own beliefs about the role of these women in society.

Professionals have many responsibilities to women who are visually impaired or blind. First, they must help those women who lack self-confidence to recognize their strengths and assist them in developing the self-assurance they need to be successful. Provisions for individual and group counseling should be part of any program serving these women. In this regard, it is crucial to develop a network of successful women who can serve as role models and mentors for other visually impaired women. Key avenues for finding such women are consumer organizations (like the American Council of the Blind and the National Federation of the Blind) and electronic discussion groups, such as Lowvis and Aernet, both of which can help women with visual impairments recognize that other women are facing similar issues and can help them meet or otherwise gain contact with others who understand issues that sighted family members or friends can not comprehend.

Second, professionals need to recognize the importance of independence, both internal and external, and strive to promote independence as an achievable goal for women who are blind or visually impaired. Through education and guidance, blind and visually impaired women can come to understand that independence is not equated with a driver's license; rather, it is the ability to make choices and determine the direction in which their lives are headed. To have the greatest number of choices, these women must have access to educational opportunities, both those related to their visual impairments (such as O&M training) and postsecondary education. In addition, since these women have easier access to educational and career opportunities if they are competent travelers, professionals need to promote their development of O&M skills, help them obtain any necessary training, and advise them of all potential transportation options. Professionals can also help blind and visually impaired women understand the frustrations they may experience as nondrivers and how they can reduce these frustrations.

Third, professionals need to work with women who are visually impaired or blind to determine the reasons they are unemployed and to reduce the number of barriers to gainful employment. These women must be encouraged to look at the entire spectrum of careers, not just those in the human service professions. Professionals must not only assist them, but must promote understanding among educators and employers to ensure that society recognizes the potential of women who are blind or visually impaired.

Another consideration is the role of professionals in assisting adolescents who are blind or visually impaired. Giving young women information about educational opportunities, the range of careers available, and assurance that they can be wives and mothers, is important. In addition, since young women with disabilities are potential targets for sexual assault, it is imperative that professionals help them to recognize their vulnerability and teach them the skills to monitor any unwanted sexual advances. Young women who are blind or visually impaired must recognize that they have opportunities in spite of their vision loss and gender. They are the future, and it is imperative for professionals to assist them to achieve equality and autonomy.

CONCLUSION

This chapter has examined the issues that many women who are blind or visually impaired face. All woman are individuals, and thus, their experiences vary dramatically. A woman's visual status and gender are key components of her personality. A woman's attitudes, influenced by society, affect how she faces the challenges set before her. Professionals can aid women with visual impairments in maximizing their potential and independence and becoming active members of their communities. As Kelly noted, "Having a visual impairment and being a woman has driven me to be more independent. I have been told at times I am too independent. I don't want to be a burden to others. I simply want to be my own person and do the same things other women do."

REFERENCES

Browne, S., Connors, D. & Stern, N. (1985). *With the power of each breath.* San Francisco: Cleis Press.

Clark, M. L., & Ayers, M. (1991). Friendship similarity during early adolescence: Gender and racial patterns. *Journal of Psychology, 126,* 393–405.

Corn, A. L., Muscella, D. B., Cannon, G. S., & Shepler, R. C. (1985). Perceived barriers to employment for visually impaired women: A preliminary study. *Journal of Visual Impairment & Blindness, 79,* 458–461.

Corn, A. L. & Sacks, S. Z. (1994). The impact of non-driving on adults with visual impairments. *Journal of Visual Impairment & Blindness, 88,* 53–68.

Feldman, R. S. (1998). *Child development.* Upper Saddle River, NJ: Prentice Hall.

Fine, M., & Asch, A. (1985). Disabled women: Sexism without the pedestal. In M. J. Deegan & N. A. Brooks (Eds.), *Women and disability: The double handicap* (pp. 1–5). New Brunswick, NJ: Transaction Books.

Gibson, W. (1957). *The miracle worker: A play for television.* New York: Alfred A. Knopf.

Hanna, W. J. & Rogovsky, B. (1991). Women with disabilities: Two handicaps plus. *Disabilty and Society, 6,* 1, 49–63.

Harsh, M. (1993). Women who are visually impaired or blind as psychotherapy clients: A personal and professional perspective. In M. E. Wilmuth & L. Holcomb (Eds.), *Women with disabilities: Found voices* (pp. 55–64). New York: Haworth Press.

Hillyer, B. (1993). *Feminism and disability.* Norman: University of Oklahoma Press.

Hutto, M. D., & Hare, D. (1997). Career advancement for young women with visual impairments. *Journal of Visual Impairment & Blindness, 91,* 280–295.

Kirchner, C., Johnson, G., & Harkins, D. (1997). Research to improve vocational rehabilitation: Employment barriers and strategies for clients who are blind or visually impaired. *Journal of Visual Impairment & Blindness, 91,* 377–392.

Kirchner, C., McBroom, L., Nelson, K., & Graves, W. (1992). *Lifestyles of employed legally blind people: A study of expenditures and time use.* Mississippi State: Mississippi State University Rehabilitation Research and Training Center on Blindness and Low Vision.

Kolb, A. (1985). Assertiveness training for women with visual impairments. In M. J. Deegan & N. A. Brooks (Eds.), *Women and disability: The double handicap* (pp. 87–94). New Brunswick, NJ: Transaction Books.

Kraus, E., Lewis, E., Stoddard, S., & Gilmartin, D. (1996). *Chartbook on disability in the United States, 1996: An info use report.* Washington, DC: National Institute on Disability and Rehabilitation Research.

Kroll, K. & Klein, E. L. (1995). *Enabling romance: A guide to love, sex, and relationships for the disabled (and the people who care about them).* Bethesda, MD: Woodbine House.

Lonsdale, S. (1990). *Women and disability: The experience of physical disability among women.* Nooundmills, England: Macmillan Educational.

MacCuspie, P. A. (1992). The social acceptance and interaction of visually impaired children in integrated settings. In S. Z. Sacks, L. S. Kekelis, & R. J. Gaylord-Ross (Eds.), *The development of social skills by blind and visually impaired students* (pp. 83–102). New York: American Foundation for the Blind.

McNeil, J. (1993). *Americans with disabilities: 1991–1992: Current Population Reports (Series P-70, No. 32).* Washington, DC: U.S. Bureau of the Census.

Morris, J. (1994). *Pride against prejudice.* Philadelphia: New Society.

Patzer, G. L. (1985). *The physical attractiveness phenomena.* New York: Plenum Press.

Pava, W. S. (1994). Visually impaired persons' vulnerability to sexual and physical assault. *Journal of Visual Impairment & Blindness, 88,* 103–112.

Peanstiehl, M. R. (1983). Role models for high-achieving visually impaired women. *Journal of Visual Impairment & Blindness, 77,* 259–261.

Ritz, S. (1992). Intimate friendship and social competency through early adolescence (Doctoral dissertation, Virginia Commonwealth University, 1992). *University Microfilms International,* 9310463.

Rosenblum, L. P. (1997). Adolescents with visual impairments who have best friends: A pilot study. *Journal of Visual Impairment & Blindness, 91,* 224–235.

Rosenblum, L. P., & Erin, J. N. (1998). Perceptions of terms used to describe individuals with visual impairment. *RE:view, 30,* 15–26.

Sharabany, R. (1974). Intimate friendship among kibbutz and city children and its measurement (Doctoral dissertation, Cornell University, 1974). *University Microfilms International,* 1613066.

Skellenger, A. C., Rosenblum, L. P., & Jager, B. K. (1997). Behaviors of preschoolers with visual impairment in indoor play settings. *Journal of Visual Impairment & Blindness, 91,* 6, 519–530.

Sobsey, D. (1994). *Violence and abuse in the lives of people with disabilities: The end of silent acceptance?* Baltimore, MD: Paul H. Brookes.

Szymanski, E. M., & Parker, R. M. (1996). *Work and disability: Issues and strategies in career development and job placement.* Austin, TX: Pro-Ed.

Thomson, R. G. (1997). *Extraordinary bodies: Figuring physical disability in American culture and literature.* New York: Columbia University Press.

Thurer, S. (1991). Women and rehabilitation. In R. P. Marinelli & A. E. D. Orto (Eds.), *The psychological and social impact of disability* (pp. 32–46). New York: Springer.

Tuttle, D. W., & Tuttle, N. R. (1996). *Self-esteem and adjusting with blindness: The process of responding to life's demands* (2nd ed.). Springfield, IL: Charles C Thomas.

Vash, C. L. (1981). *Psychology of disability.* New York: Springer.

Warren, D. W. (1984). *Blindness and early childhood development* (2nd ed.). New York: American Foundation for the Blind.

Warren, D. W. (1994). *Blindness and children: An individual differences approach.* New York: Cambridge University Press.

Welbourne, A., Lifschitz, S., Selvin, H., & Green, R. (1983). A comparison of the sexual learning experiences of visually impaired and sighted women. *Journal of Visual Impairment & Blindness, 77,* 256–259.

Wendell, S. (1996). *The rejected body: Feminist philosophical reflections on disability.* New York: Routledge.

Wolffe, K., & Sacks, S. (1997). The lifestyles of blind, low vision, and sighted youths: A quantitative comparison. *Journal of Visual Impairment & Blindness 91,* 245–257.

CHAPTER 10

Men with Visual Impairments

James Warnke
and Eugene Bender

It is still painful to remember my age-mates excitedly going off to sign up for Little League baseball or the Cub Scouts and being told that I could not play or participate because of my "eyesight problem." I can still recall hiding in the wooded area behind the Little League practice field listening to my father coach all my friends on a Saturday morning and wondering, usually tearfully, how I would ever be a "real boy" [a phrase from the movie *Pinocchio* that was popular at that time] like them. [Sid, aged 52]

The expectations placed upon boys and men in today's mainstream culture can have a pervasive effect on the self-image and self-identity of boys and men who are blind or visually impaired throughout their life span. In the era of generic service delivery and a one-size-fits-all philosophy in human services, it seems particularly important to the authors to be specific in addressing the issues of men who are blind or visually impaired. Furthermore, the interest in women's issues in the arenas of sociology, psychology, and anthropology has sparked an interest in similar specific issues related to men.

This chapter examines, from a developmental point of view, the life-cycle issues that men who are blind and visually impaired confront in this society. It explores how congenital and adventitious visual impairment and blindness affect men's sense of themselves as men as understood in the broader American culture of today. Since other chapters in this book deal with issues of men who belong to diverse racial and ethnic groups or have different sexual orientations, the population discussed here is essentially heterosexual white men who live in North America and speak English as their first language.

After discussing pertinent statistical data, the authors present a brief reflection on boyhood and adolescence and then address the phases of young manhood, middle age, and elder men. In each case, they outline the primary issues of phase-specific adjustment and developmental issues and describe the experiences of both congenitally and adventitiously visually impaired males.

STATISTICS

The U.S. Bureau of the Census reported that in 1994, 48.9 million persons in the United States were disabled (McNeil, 1997). Almost 23 million were men, 9.9 million with disabilities described as severe. Over 8 million said that they had difficulty seeing words or letters in ordinary newsprint even when they wore corrective lenses, and 1.5 million reported that even when they wore corrective lenses, they could not see the words or letters in newsprint.

The majority of disabled Americans are unemployed, and of those who are employed, it is estimated that the majority are underemployed. For example, McNeil (1993) reported that only 26 percent of 563,000 adults aged 21–64 with severe functional limitation in seeing print were employed. The rest were either unemployed and looking for a job or out of the workforce. Although the Americans with Disabilities Act (ADA) has engendered much hope for competitive employment for disabled men, particularly men who are blind or visually impaired, there is clearly much to be done. Common barriers to employment for individuals with visual impairments include

- transportation
- the lack of skills and education
- employers' attitudes
- government-sponsored work disincentives (meaning that income from employment can result in the reduction or elimination of benefits, such as Social Security disability payments and Medicaid)
- vocational rehabilitation counselors' heavy caseloads
- problems in providing adaptations (McBroom, Crudden, Skinner, & Moore, 1998)

Since much of a man's identity and sense of self are tied to his ability to work and earn a living for himself and his family, these statistics are sobering, to say the least.

BOYHOOD AND ADOLESCENCE

"The Child is Father of the man," or so the poet William Wordsworth wrote. To understand men's responses to visual impairment and blindness and the consequences of these impairments for men in this culture, one must look back at boyhood and adolescence. The authors use the term *boyhood*, rather than *childhood*, here deliberately to highlight the characteristics of this phase of development as it is experienced specifically by boys. Since there is no equivalent male term for adolescence, that term will be used in this chapter.

In the mainstream culture, young boys are expected to strive in sports and games and to do well in academic subjects. They are also expected to master the world of the peer group from a young age by learning the skills of cooperation and assertiveness and their sometimes delicate interconnectedness. The authors suggest that it is no accident of language that before a boy becomes a "mister," he is, in the more antiquated usage of English, referred to as "master." In this culture, men have traditionally had to establish their claim to respect (and fear) early on. They do so on the playground, in the street, on the basketball court, and on baseball and football fields long before adolescence begins. Frequently, the normal athletic contests of childhood that foster bonding and the creation of social hierarchies are either severely compromised or impossible—and, in any case, truly frightening—for boys with visual impairments. Many of the events described in Kuusisto's (1998) autobiography, *Planet of the Blind*, reflect these realities in vivid and terrifyingly accurate images. The fear and humiliation when a classmate stole Kuusisto's eyeglasses and called him "Blindo"; the enormous energy it required to pass for sighted; and the physical pain experienced in the neck, shoulders, and lower back from holding books an inch from the eyes to try to keep up with schoolwork are experiences that many children with visual impairments have probably had.

Many boys with visual impairments deny their disability, either out of their own needs or the perceived needs and expectations of their families. Many of these boys go onto the baseball field, trip over the bases, run head-on into their teammates, and endure a hundred beatings of one kind or another just to be part of the gang. More typically, some boys re-create the world and write the hero's role for themselves, either eradicating the blindness or visual impairment altogether or transforming it into a positive or at least a mysterious trait. One boy may retreat into books or art, radio or television, while another may adopt an overtly aggressive or haughty demeanor to scare away all who would question his "manhood." Others may just retreat into themselves, avoiding contact with their peers altogether.

Engaging in heroic fantasies fueled by history or popular art and culture allows some blind or visually impaired boys to endure what feels like the indignities of the disability, such as frequently having to ask for help, not being able to participate in certain athletic activities, and wearing thick eyeglasses. Sometimes these fantasies draw others to them, if only for a short while, to hear their stories or play out their daydreams. As the architect of these imaginings, the boy who is blind or visually impaired is in a positive position of control, a position that persons with disabilities are rarely allowed to have.

Denial of the disability, while unrealistic, is also a mechanism of defense that some boys who are blind or visually impaired use to assuage their pain and maintain a sufficient sense of themselves to face the world each day. Denial can range from more reality based and adaptive to less reality based and pathological. People without disabilities, including supposedly responsible care providers like parents and teachers, are often quick to remind a boy who is blind or visually impaired of his limitations. Indeed, some boys hear the following messages much too frequently: "Visually impaired boys can't play sports. Boys who are blind cannot use tools, ride bikes, or ever, ever drive cars." Hearing statements such as these enough times suggests to many blind or visually impaired boys that all they can do is be passive, be grateful to those who are unselfish enough to help them, and be quiet—in other words, at least in their minds, adopt the attributes that are often ascribed to girls.

In adolescence, the developmental emphasis on mastery continues, but its targets expand to include the areas of same-sex friendships, opposite-sex friendships, romantic and sexual relationships, and the self-mastery required to make and implement vocational and career choices. Self-mastery also includes the development of the personal identity and self-regulated self-esteem necessary to choose peer groups and to be individuated enough by the beginning of manhood to be in, but not always of, these same peer groups.

For some visually impaired boys and adolescents, these multilevel, multidimensional, interconnected strivings for intrapersonal, interpersonal, and situational mastery are challenges, indeed. Although their successful achievement is far from impossible, it is interesting to note that the boyhood challenge, "OK, now do it with your eyes closed!" to a fellow who has just exhibited a high level of prowess in some activity is one of the few such challenges that can be declined with honor on the street, in the school yard, or on the playing field. For many visually impaired boys and adolescents, the mastery of these challenges is frequently frustrated or deferred, achieved only with adaptation or such extreme requirements of time and energy as significantly to negate their positive effects, or is attainable only with the assistance of a sighted person, thus depriving a youngster of the coveted feeling, "I did it all by myself," that is so important for the development and maintenance of high self-esteem.

Daryl, a middle-aged man explains:

I remember how the elation and pride I experienced at being the last one chosen for the junior varsity basketball team in my freshman year of high school was somehow polluted by the neurotic fear that the coach had chosen me only because the team stunk anyway and he felt sorry for me and the very realistic self-evaluation on my part that I would be truly unable to keep up with my teammates in the fast-paced visually challenging environment of a real game.

Men frequently report in psychotherapy or rehabilitation that they learned early to keep experiences like these to themselves. The retraumatization that can occur when well-meaning listeners minimize the emotional impact of these experiences by labeling them overstated or hysterical is akin to that reported by adult survivors of childhood physical and sexual abuse.

Doubts about one's ability to be a "real boy" frequently translate into doubts about one's ability to be a "real man." In a culture that frames manhood in terms of the competence to produce, perform, and keep up independently and unaided in the highly competitive areas of work and career, social and intimate relationships, and recreation, "real men" walk alone, move quickly, exhibit competence, and get the job done. In a culture where real men do not make excuses, the reasonable accommodations necessary for boys or adolescents who are visually impaired even to begin to keep up, no less excel, can begin to sound, to the boys and adolescents themselves, like unreasonable excuses for incompetence and performance that sometimes seems to be chronically "a day late and a dollar short."

An example is John, an 18-year-old unmarried white male who was totally blind and entered a four-year college after a successful academic career in a small high school, where he had been accommodated with a full-time classroom aide and adaptive technology under the watchful eyes of his parents and teachers. He found the jump to dormitory living and self-management so stressful that after a successful first term, he was unable to cope with the situation and required intensive counseling and an extended period of orientation and mobility training before he could again take on the greater demands for autonomy and independence required of him in the college setting.

For many, the symbol of masculinity in early 21st-century America is the ability to drive an automobile. To obtain the coveted driver's license at age 16 or 17 is, for the adolescent male, to wrest control of his life from the oppressive adults who have always decided where he would go and when he would go there and with whom he would go. Now, literally "in the driver's seat," the adolescent male crows, "I'm going now." "I'm going later." "If you want to come along, get ready now!" The adolescent male who is visually impaired or blind at this crucial juncture remains dependent on his parents, siblings (often younger siblings, which really stings), and friends. He can "go" at their convenience. Still a child in the passenger seat, he is denied this crucial rite of passage into adulthood, usually forever, and avenues for attaining age-appropriate developmental milestones are frustrated and made infinitely more difficult in his eyes, as well as in the eyes of the society at large. Not having the opportunity to participate in activities that are typical for adolescents can result in costly personal consequences, such as isolation from the peer group, nonparticipation in social activities that are needed to develop friendships with young men and young women, and unfamiliarity with job and career training opportunities in the community that will later facilitate entrance into the workforce.

For men who become visually impaired in early, middle, or late adulthood, the result is frequently a sense of being thrust back into the earlier phases of developing mastery and competence at a time when they should be in possession of these characteristics. They may experience a sense of being boys or adolescents again or even perpetually, struggling to remaster the skills of life but now having to master the requisite adaptive skills as well. What, then, are the effects of and responses to visual impairment for men of different phase of life as they work, play, and love their way through life in this culture?

YOUNG MEN AND THE TRANSITION TO "MANHOOD"

Young men are launching themselves into the worlds of work and career, romance and love, and recreational experiences. Having acquired the embryonic identity requisite to begin to live as an adult man in the real world of the present time and culture during the crucible of adolescence, they begin in earnest to seek employment, cultivate relationships and engage in courtship, and cultivate themselves through hobbies and community service.

For the young man who is congenitally visually impaired, this phase means the emergence from the accommodations and supports not only of his family of origin but of the special education system as well. Even if he has spent all or most of his time in the educational mainstream with only minimal support, the step into competitive employment is often a quantum leap. The accommodations promised and provided by the ADA, even at their best and most appropriate, can never be as fine tuned and incremental as those provided in the educational setting. Furthermore, the burden of responsibility now shifts from the educational institution to the individual and his family. The practical and psychological effects of this shift cannot be minimized. Much like the burden of proof in law, which, in the U.S. system, leaves the responsibility for proof on the prosecution and the presumption of innocence on the defense, this shift presumes that individuals will become, in effect, their own case managers and advocates and that it is their responsibility to negotiate whatever reasonable accommodations they require.

Employment

As national surveys (see, for example, Crudden, McBroom, Skinner, & Moore, 1998) indicate, young visually impaired men are not as successful as their sighted counterparts in obtaining employment. Practical difficulties in transportation and acquiring print materials in accessible formats and the anxieties of those in gatekeeper positions in meeting and interviewing a visually impaired man, perhaps for the first time, complicate an already complicated and highly competitive situation. Some visually impaired young men whom the first author interviewed for this chapter suggested that being a good or even a superior candidate for a job or career position is not good enough for a visually impaired man. Like Tony, they thought that they must be "supercompetent" even to have a chance:

Tony, a visually impaired social worker, believed he was granted only a *pro forma* interview at a major community mental health facility serving children because the executive director and medical director had decided before they even met him that a visually impaired man could not possibly be an adequate therapist for children. This young social worker held two master's degrees with honors and had excelled in graduate field placement.

Although these obstacles to employment are not enough to knock most young visually impaired men out of the competitive workforce, they are frequently experienced as psychologically burdensome at best and can delay entry into a chosen job or career path. Young men who are visually impaired often find themselves, like actors or musicians, needing to work a succession of less than lucrative day jobs or to be dependent longer than they would like on their families of origin while they struggle to break into the "mainstream" or the "big time" of their vocational choices.

An important point in this regard is the need for a helping network in searching for meaningful work. If networking is important for all young men in this arena, it is essential for young men who are visually impaired. The authors have heard for some 20 years, and know from their own experience, that one is most likely to be seriously considered and given a chance to prove oneself in employment if the way has been paved by a friend, mentor, or associate in the potential employer's or gatekeeper's network. These anecdotal observations were confirmed in Crudden et al.'s (1998) study in which the participants attributed their employment to successful networking with coworkers, customers, and others, rather than to a service delivery system. "Michael is legally blind, but you'll see that it's no problem" or "Max is visually impaired, but he is the most competent person you will find," said by a trusted colleague to a potential employer, can be the best guarantee of an interview that is not just a *pro forma* exercise.

Typically, young adulthood is characterized by activity, mobility, and relationships. A young man who is congenitally blind or visually impaired, is competent in orientation and mobility (O&M) skills, and is interested and socially able to keep on and keep up is likely to be successful and, therefore, to feel successful, as the following case of Sam illustrates:

Sam, a 20-year-old totally blind computer professional, is successfully employed in his chosen profession and is living with a sighted woman who is a successful professional in her own right. He has designed his life to include residing in an area where public transportation to and from work is quick and easy by local standards and enjoys, with her, the recreational opportunities of the region. Sam describes his life as "as good as it gets" and himself as well on the way to being all that he would wish himself to be.

In contrast, a man, such as Louis, whose adjustment to his disability has been less than adequate is likely to feel the crunch of being left out and left behind:

Louis, aged 25, with a degenerative visual impairment that will most probably lead to total blindness, was raised in a family where the rule was to deny his disability and pretend it did not exist. His size and strength allowed him to accrue false hopes of an athletic career because he was able to play high school football for his small rural team. The academic accommodations given to the school's athletes encouraged his grossly overinflated evaluation of his academic abilities and allowed them to go substantially unchallenged until his graduation. Louis then found himself unable to compete either academically or athletically in college and soon flunked out. He was left with a deep sense of personal failure and poor self-esteem that led to clinical depression and intense anxiety.

Relationships

In addition to the quantum leap into the world of work in young adulthood, there is a quantum leap into the world of relationships. Young men develop working relationships with colleagues; lasting friendships, both same and opposite sex; and romantic, loving, and sexual attachments. Men who are blind or visually impaired must master the relational minefield with no or a limited ability to read the nonverbal components of communication that make up a substantial part of social situations. Many sighted persons are unaware of the magnitude of coincidental learning or learning by visual observation that takes place each day while they are otherwise cognitively engaged. Everything from appropriateness in dress and demeanor to knowing whether a quip is intended as a joke or an insult is mediated or validated visually.

Although it is not impossible to negotiate social relationships without access to nonverbal cues, the inherent difficulties should not be minimized. In young adulthood, men move from a learning mode based infinitely less on direct verbal instruction, as was customary in childhood and adolescence, to one that is based infinitely more on visual observation and imitation. A young man who needs to be told how to dress, how to interact socially in a wide variety of social situations, or to interact skillfully in the myriad rituals of social relatedness is, by the very fact of having to be told, judged to be less than adequate. Unless he is skillful enough to ask tactfully, he probably will not be told but, rather, will be silently (and therefore to him, invisibly) judged and found wanting.

The subtle interactions of flirting, dating, courtship, and sexual intimacy are of particular concern in this regard. Difficult for many young men in this culture, they are especially challenging for those who are visually impaired or blind, since they rely intensely on the interaction of nonverbal and verbal cues and responses and because the penalties for not "playing the game" well can be immediate and painful and bode poorly for the development and maintenance of an appropriate sense of self and self-esteem.

Imagine the social dilemma of the totally blind man in his 20s who mistakes the kindness of a female coworker for a romantic interest. Or, conversely, consider the young man at his 10th high school reunion who was asked by a female classmate why he had never asked her out. When he answered that he had no idea that she would have responded positively to such an invitation, she told him that she was crazy about him and had given him the eye all the time. To his chagrin, he discovered that he had completely missed or misunderstood her nonverbal flirting behaviors in a way that had deprived him of a potentially delightful romantic relationship.

Recreation

Since much of what young men in this culture think of as recreation involves some form of "going" and "doing," as well as the capacities for interpersonal communication and social interaction, this area, too, presents special challenges for visually impaired young men. Young visually impaired men who developed recreational areas of special interest and expertise in childhood and adolescence—such as competence in an athletic activity, music, or a unique hobby like Civil War reenactment or karate—frequently receive positive social rewards because they are both visually impaired and recreationally competent (thus being viewed by peers as being able not only to "do it," but to do it with their eyes closed). However, those who have not developed such interests often find themselves adrift and bored.

Losing Vision

Those who experience significant vision loss or blindness for the first time during young adulthood frequently feel as though they have hit a brick wall. Having just begun to traverse the geography of young adulthood as sighted persons, they now feel like strangers in a strange land, unable to function visually as before but not as yet equipped with the basic "blindness skills" that would allow them to function adequately as visually impaired persons. These blindness skills include O&M skills for getting around—in and around one's home, workplace, recreational spots, and the like—using such adaptations as sighted guide assistance, a white cane and/or a dog guide; the skills necessary for reading in adaptive formats, such as braille and large print, reading with recordings, and computer literacy; and the practical daily living skills related to cooking, personal care and hygiene, and other ordinary activities that allow a man who is blind or visually impaired to function independently in his world and in the world at large.

One of the most important points made by Tuttle and Tuttle (1996) is that one can adjust to one's larger life with blindness or visual impairment only if one has adjusted to the blindness or visual impairment in the first place. That is, before a man can truly be comfortable learning and using these kinds of blindness skills, he needs to accept psychologically and emotionally the reality of his vision loss. Moreover, the use of adaptive aids, procedures, or devices or persons as assistants is acceptable for a man who is blind or visually impaired only if he and others around him experience these adaptations as objects that he uses, not things that he needs or depends on or cannot really cope without.

The visually impaired young man is faced with a mainstream culture that expects him to move in, move up, and make a place for himself. He is expected to get a job, go after a career, make friends, find a partner, make commitments to all these and, generally, to make a life for himself. He is expected to be proactive, not reactive.

As simple as this point seems, its importance cannot be overestimated. The young man is expected to do these things himself. He is not expected, if he is to think of himself as a man, to wait for someone else to make his place or his friends or his relationships for him. In this 21st-century culture, men do these things for themselves.

MEETING MIDDLE AGE

The middle years are, for many men in this culture, a time of consolidation, revision, and reassessment. Economically, career men often think of themselves as being at the peak of their earning curve and "topped off" in or on a particular career path. Socially, men look around and place themselves. In their intimate lives, men are well beyond the beginnings and are either consolidating marital and familial situations or working on their alteration in the service of starting over. Fathering is established in its patterns, and a man now has enough personal history that he can profitably reflect on it. Not yet old, a man cannot reasonably expect to pass for young any longer and, if he is wise, the reality that these are what will become the "good old days" has begun to dawn on him. Realizing that he has worked hard for a long time to get where he is, it occurs to him that he will be working hard for a long time still. Too old to depend on parents or family of origin any longer, he is still far too young to depend on his own children or those mechanisms of support (such as social security or a pension) that the society has prepared for elders. In this culture, this is the age of self-sufficiency and independence at its most rigorous.

The man who is blind or visually impaired moves through this period of life with his sighted confreres. He is 5 to 10 times more likely to be unemployed or underemployed. His income is likely to be less than, and his vocational and recreational options are likely to be inferior to, his age-mates'.

If he is working, it may have taken him longer to find a job and/or to find a suitable position in a desired career path. He may feel that he is playing catchup while all the time he is trying just to keep up. Those who have mastered well the "skills" of visual impairment (O&M, accessible formats for reading and writing, transportation, and the like) are frequently sailing, or at least paddling, along in the mainstream of American life.

One frequently sees human-interest stories in newspapers or on television about the ever-growing number of visually impaired or blind men who are leading successful and interesting lives. They own computer companies, teach karate, attend Ski for Light, have become partners in their law firms, and have graduated from medical schools. Those who are less fortunate or less accomplished frequently feel that they are either up the creek without a paddle or are valiantly rowing against the current of the current events of their lives and the life of the society. Although education and technology promise the opening of many doors once closed to men who are visually impaired or blind in the worlds of work and social life, the authors believe that blue-collar men who are blind or visually impaired may have *fewer* options and opportunities than they did even a decade ago. Illustrative of this point is Leonard, D'Allura, and Fried's (1998) study, which confirmed that a higher proportion of people with visual impairments who are employed have higher levels of education and reported having computer skills.

Men who become visually impaired in this phase of life are often hit hard, both emotionally and practically. Those who are faced with the gradual or imminent loss of vision, from a variety of medical conditions, frequently experience great anxiety and dread while they attempt to conduct their daily lives in good style and good spirits. Even in this age of the ADA, they often struggle to conceal their emerging visual impairments from friends and employers, fearing, sometimes accurately, that the consequences of prematurely revealing their loss of vision will be dire socially and economically. For them, the prospect of no longer being able to drive and to conduct their personal and professional affairs as before and the physical and psychological consequences of vision loss itself can form a matrix of intersecting traumas that is infinitely greater than the sum of its parts.

Those who incur sudden visual impairment or blindness through illness or a traumatic injury face a reorganization of their emotional, interpersonal, and practical lives that rivals that of any other traumatic disablement. Over 20 years of clinical and rehabilitation experience have taught the authors that full and adequate adjustment to blindness or significant vision loss in this phase of life can take from 2 to 5 years.

Personal relationships change dramatically with the onset of a disability. In the initial period of adjustment, one experiences a greatly heightened dependance on spouses, children, friends, and colleagues. In a phase of life when roles and accommodations in interpersonal relationships are fairly well established and operational, the tidal wave of adjustment required to manage life with a visual impairment or blindness frequently upsets the usually delicately balanced mobile of interpersonal and social relatedness.

Having to depend can be difficult or even humiliating for a man with a firmly established sense of independence. The wife and children can be at a loss as to how to deal with their own feelings about the man in their lives as he struggles to adjust and cope. They can also have difficulty in adjusting to their own new roles as sighted guides, driver assistants, and readers. These and other concomitant shifts in interpersonal roles and power can take more than a little getting used to for everyone concerned, as they did in George's family:

George, a 46-year-old airplane mechanic who was totally blinded in an industrial accident, struggled for five years to regroup and reorient. After a long and difficult recovery from the physical traumas of his injuries, he began to battle the depression, anger, anxiety, and confusion associated with the psychological adjustment to blindness, complicated by a posttraumatic stress disorder precipitated by the accident itself. His wife became the breadwinner of the family, a role she would never have chosen on her own, as he became Mr. Mom for the three children of the family. The children struggled to work through their own adjustments to their father's disability and the new and unexpected structure of their family. All in their own ways mourned the life they might have had if the accident never happened and accepted the life they had not had individually and with one another. Although all survived and actually adjusted well, George commented at the close of the five-year period of reorganization: "It's like someone tossed a hand grenade into my life. I'm not even the same man I was before I got to be blind. I'm OK now, but I am not the same."

It can be particularly disconcerting for men and their families at the upper ranges of middle age to experience and adjust to blindness or visual impairment because they are not ready, emotionally, financially, or socially, to retire and are so established in their patterns of living and financial and social commitments that they find change and adaptation difficult, as was the case with Philip:

A successful 59-year-old engineer, Philip began to lose vision rapidly. He and his wife had planned to retire within six years to play golf, their shared passion, and to travel, a pleasure they had long deferred to raise and educate their two children. Philip's adjustment to his visual impairment was complicated by the fact that it had made the couple's carefully laid plans for their later years go tilt. He was frustrated and angry much of the time for a period of months because he hated having to adjust to new ways and new things and new adaptations and was enraged at the loss of the future he had hoped to provide for his wife and himself and for which they had both worked and sacrificed for so long. Relief came when the couple discovered a travel agency that specialized in customers who were disabled and found that they could still travel in a way that they could enjoy and that was within their means. To this day, they mourn the loss of the golfing they had hoped for. Even several serious attempts to play the game in an adaptive format frequently enjoyed by other blind or visually impaired players would not, in this case, bridge the gap between what they had been able to enjoy before the vision loss and the less satisfying adaptive experience.

ELDER MEN

It is estimated that 60 to 70 percent of men who are blind and visually impaired in the United States are over age 65 (J. Casabianca-Hilton, personal communication, 1999). Vision loss from a wide variety of causes is seen as almost inevitable as a man grows older and must be understood in the larger context of the natural aging process.

Once again, the inability to drive is a paramount concern in the adjustment of many men. Particularly if the man has been the primary driver in his family, the shift in who sits in the driver's seat and who is in the passenger seat may be a significant factor in a couple seeking professional counseling in relation to vision loss in this phase of life. However, the fact that retired men frequently leave the driving to bus drivers on trips with local senior centers or other senior-oriented social groups goes a long way to soften this blow, as does the fact that older parents are frequently driven by their adult chilren.

When blindness or visual impairment interfere with the ability of older men to read, watch and enjoy television, sightsee, or interact with the grandchildren, the result is frequently depression, anxiety, and a deep sense of hopelessness. That most emotionally healthy men come to expect at least some diminishment of their physical abilities as they grow older counteracts the fact that older persons often do not feel comfortable learning and adapting in new ways.

The older a man gets, the more likely he is to have friends and family members who are also visually impaired. Knowing others who have the same problem may soften the sense of aloneness in the disability that sometimes plagues younger men, as the following example shows:

Several senior men found camaraderie in a self-help group for blind and visually impaired persons at their local senior citizens' center. They encouraged each other to use the sighted guide and white cane techniques that they had individually resisted using before they joined the group. The time their wives spent together while the group met also helped them to feel that they were all in this situation together and to recover from the sense of isolation they had all previously experienced.

RESPONDING TO MEN WHO ARE BLIND OR VISUALLY IMPAIRED

What makes the difference in life is not just what happens to a person, but how the person and others react and respond to what has happened. This can also be the case with living with blindness or visual impairment, regardless of its onset. There is a continuum of reactions and responses to visual impairment and blindness that ranges from the adaptive and healthy to the maladaptive and pathological—both for the individual man involved and for all those who are significant to him, whether they are intimately or socially involved in his life. Healthy and adaptive reactions and responses are based on the realistic, incremental acceptance of the vision loss and the adjustment and adaptation required to continue life optimistically and with joy. This process involves riding the rapids of the mourning-like process of emotional adjustments; acquiring, through education and rehabilitation, the skills necessary to continue in the worlds of work, play, and loving relationships; and accepting and taking responsibility for one's reactions and responses to being a blind or visually impaired man.

Unhealthy and maladaptive reactions and responses are rooted in the individual, in the pathological extremes of denial and avoidance. These responses leave a man adrift in the cycles of denial, rage, and depression that are a common reaction to vision loss. In this situation, a man either cannot mobilize himself to believe that there can be a meaningful life for him after vision loss or because of visual impairment or loses himself in the grandiosity of unrealistic goals and expectations, projected rage, and blaming others.

Similarly, those who are related to the man, either by intimate personal relationships or roles that are of societal significance to him, can react along the same continuum of responses. These responses form a complex of interreactions that, to a greater or lesser degree, become predictive of the man's relative success in adjusting to his disability and to living with it. Society's relative success in fostering the adaptive integration of men who are visually impaired or blind into the fabric of the mainstream of American life is determined by the real people in each man's network of family, friends, and colleagues. The more routinely that men who are adjusting to vision loss can find and create places for themselves along the more healthy and adaptive range of this continuum and their families, communities, and the society at large can find and create ways to support and foster such achievements, the better it is for everyone.

Of particular importance in this regard are the various professionals who the blind and visually impaired man and his intimate others encounter in their adjustment to his disability. Men who are visually impaired or blind need consultants and coaches, not caregivers or codependant pseudo-parents. They need professionals who know their jobs and know their clients. They need information and options expressed in clear and useful language by persons who are compassionate and truthful, engaging yet respectful of autonomy, and optimistic yet rooted in the nonnegotiable realities of what is really happening.

To be of real help to men who are blind or visually impaired, those who are intimately involved with them, either personally or professionally, may consider the following suggestions:

- Learn as much as you can about the particular situation of the man involved, including the nature of his visual condition, its history and prognosis. Knowledge paves the way for understanding and empathy.
- Become familiar with the usual adaptations and ways of assisting men who are blind or visually impaired. Local agencies that serve blind and visually impaired persons and national consumer organizations are helpful in this regard. Read their literature and attend their meetings.
- Become aware and sensitive to your own reactions and responses to blindness and visual impairment in general and to the man with whom you are dealing specifically. Understanding, empathy, and respect always start with how you are really feeling and reacting and how you are really thinking.
- Finally, be aware that you cannot be truly helpful all by

yourself. You need to connect with others in the man's social, personal, and professional network to be most effective. Together, you can make a common effort and receive communal support. It is difficult to imagine that this point could be overemphasized, and every reasonable effort to network should be fostered.

In the complex matrix of the medical, educational, rehabilitation, and mental health worlds of the early 21st century, a multidimensional, multidisciplinary approach to services for men who are blind or visually impaired stands the best chance of success for these individuals and the greatest chance of satisfaction for the various professionals who are involved in each case.

The more that blind or visually impaired men can respond with and be responded to with respect, competence, and courage, the more they can live, love, and work with joy and competence and contribute their time and talents that are so dearly needed for this society to thrive and develop.

REFERENCES

Crudden. A., McBroom, L. W., Skinner, A. L., & Moore, J. E. (1998). *Comprehensive examination of barriers to employment among persons who are blind or visually impaired* (Technical report). Mississippi State: Mississippi State University, Rehabilitation Research and Training Center on Blindness and Low Vision.

Kuusisto, S. (1998). *Planet of the blind.* New York. Dial Press.

Leonard, R., D'Allura, T., & Friend, B. (1998). *Factors associated with employment: A follow-up of vocational placement referrals.* Poster presentation, International Conference for Education and Rehabilitation of the Blind and Visually Impaired. Atlanta, GA.

McBroom, L. W., Crudden, A., Skinner, A. L., & Moore, J. E. (1998). *Barriers to employment among persons who are blind or visually impaired: Executive summary.* Mississippi State: Rehabilitation Research and Training Center on Blindness and Low Vision.

McNeil, J. (1993). *Americans with disabilities: 1991–92: Current Population Reports,* (Series P-70, No. 33). Washington, DC: U.S. Government Printing Office.

McNeil, J.(1997). *Americans with disabilities 1994–95: Current Populations Reports (Series P-70. No. 61)*. Washington, DC: U.S. Government Printing Office.

Tuttle, D. W., & Tuttle, N. R. (1996). *Self-esteem and adjusting with blindness: The process of responding to life's demands* (2nd ed.). Springfield, IL: Charles C Thomas.

Gays, Lesbians, and Bisexuals with Visual Impairments

Kay A. Ferrell and Patrika Griego

If we are to achieve a richer culture, rich in contrasting values, we must recognize the whole gamut of human potentialities, and so weave a less arbitrary social fabric, one in which each diverse human gift will find a fitting place.
— Margaret Mead (1963, p. 322)

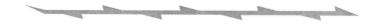

The sexuality of persons who are blind or visually impaired has never been a topic of great concern in education. Little, if any, research has been done, and the number of articles written on the topic is minuscule. The reluctance to acknowledge the sexuality of people with visual impairments stems from society's reluctance to discuss sexuality in general and the myths frequently associated with blindness (see, for example, Lowenfeld's 1981

The authors dedicate this chapter to the memory of Matthew Shepard, the nephew of an esteemed colleague and teacher of students with visual disabilities. Shepard's death makes the risks all too clear and the need for tolerance all too compelling and reminds us that our work is, after all, about families.

discussion of the history of society's treatment of blindness). Educators do not question the need to mediate the environment for children with visual impairments, except when it comes to sex education. Children whose ability to observe dating mores, flirting, or body language and whose understanding of sexuality is often derived from verbal descriptions based on abstract concepts that cannot be easily demonstrated tactilely seem particularly vulnerable to misunderstandings, misperceptions, and abuse.

In this context, it is not surprising that even less information is available about gay, lesbian, and bisexual individuals who are blind or visually impaired, both adults and youngsters. As new treatments for AIDS prolong the lives of people with HIV, it is likely that more and more gays and lesbians who are HIV positive will require educational or rehabilitation services as a result of AIDS-related retinitis. Similarly, with the population growing older and thus subject to age-related sensory impairments, it is equally likely that gay and lesbian partners will require those services as they age.

In working with gay, lesbian, and bisexual individuals with visual impairments, it is important to remember three points:

- ◆ The visual impairment itself can hamper the development of a healthy self-concept, which, in turn, may affect sexuality (Tuttle & Tuttle, 1996).
- ◆ The gay, lesbian, and bisexual community is subject to hostility, ridicule, and intolerance, even to the point of violence, from the heterosexual community (Wolfe, 1998).
- ◆ Although both visual impairment and homosexuality are often invisible characteristics, that fact does not protect their owners from fear, risk, stigmatization, and prejudice.

In this chapter, the terms *homosexual* and *homosexualities* encompass what Honeychurch (1996, p. 340) defined as "diverse experiences subsumed as non-heterosexual. Through the use of the plural form, the wide range of dissident sexualities that constitute homosexual desire, behavior, and identity are recognized and inscribed as non-monolithic." This and other terms used throughout this chapter are defined in Sidebar 11.1. As Capper (1999) pointed out, research on this topic is difficult to conduct, partly because of the way "heterosexuality becomes normalized as natural" (Britzman, 1995, p. 153), in which everything non-heterosexual is viewed as deviant, and partly because individuals who are willing to talk about the subject are generally those who live a more open or activist lifestyle. The reader is cautioned against overgeneralizing the information presented here and urged to "tak[e] into account the multicentered nature of identity, rather than [focus] only on sexual minority identity" (Griffin, 1996, p. 4).

HISTORICAL BACKGROUND AND SOCIAL ISSUES

History of Attitudes toward Blindness and Visual Impairment

The loss of productive, talented individuals from participation in the workforce and society because of negative stigma surrounding blindness and visual impairment affects the ability to participate, contribute, and be a voice in society. World War II marked a significant shift in the attitudes toward and treatment of those with visual impairments. Until blinded veterans returned from the war, demanding to have independence in their lives and in society, there was little investment in promoting the abilities and capabilities of visually impaired or blind persons. The development of orientation and mobility (O&M) services at Valley Forge Hospital and Hines Veterans Administration Hospital (Bledsoe, 1980) helped veterans blinded by the atrocities of war overcome both physical and psychosocial barriers.

As more and more veterans with visual impairments moved back to and functioned successfully in their communities and families, the need to expand O&M services and to provide

≋ *Sidebar* 11.1.
**Definitions of Terms Related to People
Who Are Gay, Lesbian, or Bisexual**

---

bisexuality: A sexual orientation in which a person feels physically and emotionally attracted to people of both genders.

"coming out" (also "coming out of the closet" or "being out"): The process by which a person acknowledges, accepts, and, in many cases, appreciates his or her lesbian, gay, or bisexual identity and often reveals his or her sexual orientation to others. This process occurs for different people in a variety of places and ways.

heterosexism: The assumption that all people are or should be heterosexual.

heterosexuality: The sexual orientation in which a person feels physically and emotionally attracted to people of the opposite gender.

homophobia: The fear, dislike, and hatred of same-sex relationships or those who love and are sexually attracted to others of the same sex. Homophobia includes prejudice, discrimination, harassment, and acts of violence brought on by fear and hatred.

homosexuality: The sexual orientation in which a person feels physically and emotionally attracted to people of the same gender.

internalized homophobia: The fear and hate of one's own homosexuality or bisexuality by many gay and lesbian individuals who have learned negative ideas about homosexuality throughout childhood.

invisibility: The constant assumption of heterosexuality that renders gay and lesbian people invisible and seemingly nonexistent.

sexual orientation: A person's emotional, physical, and sexual attraction and the expression of that attraction.

transgender identity: A gender identity that is different from one's biological sex and the identification with and desire to be of the oposite biological gender.

Source: Adapted from Youth Pride, *Creating Safe Schools for Lesbian and Gay Students: A Resource Guide for School Staff* (1997, April). [Available from Office of Diversity Affairs, Council for Exceptional Children, 1920 Association Drive, Reston, VA 20191].

high-quality training for O&M specialists was recognized. University programs were instituted, professional associations were formed, standards were developed, and the education and rehabilitation of individuals with visual impairments greatly improved (Blasch, Wiener, & Welsh 1997). People who were blind or visually impaired continued to move toward full integration with such developments as

- the professionalization of the field and the development of more college and university training programs (Gallagher, 1988; Spungin & Taylor, 1986);
- the application of the Equal Protection Clause (the 14th Amendment) of the U.S. Constitution to education and employment, resulting in federal laws, such as the Individuals with Disabilities Education Act and its amendments, that guaranteed the right to free appropriate public education in the least restrictive environment;
- the passage of civil rights legislation that prohibited discrimination against persons with disabilities (the Americans with Disabilities Act);
- strong advocacy by consumer groups; and
- the promise of technology that would make print accessible to all persons with visual impairments.

History of Homosexualities

The history of the gay, lesbian, and bisexual culture is difficult to examine because of society's bias against homosexuals and because historians have usually considered the sexual orientation of historical figures to be irrelevant. Nevertheless, both lesbians and gay men have been politicians, philosophers, educators, athletes, writers, artists, and more, and the homosexual community claims many prominent figures in history, including Alexander the Great, Aristotle, Francis Bacon, James Baldwin, Julius Caesar, Willa Cather, Leonardo DaVinci, Elton John, Michaelangelo, Plato, Marcel Proust, Richard the Lion Hearted,

Sappho, Socrates, Gertrude Stein, Andy Warhol, Walt Whitman, Oscar Wilde, Tennessee Williams, and Virginia Wolff (Cown, 1988; Duberman, Vicimus, & Chauncey, 1989; Mathison, 1998). Gay, lesbian, and bisexual individuals have played an essential role in building society, despite the discrimination and persecution they have experienced because of their sexual orientation. Since the emergence of European culture in America, homosexuality has been "tainted . . . with the stigma of sexual perversion" (Lang, 1998, p. 17).

Two major events shaped the culture of homosexualities in the United States. The first was World War II, in which the rallying of all Americans for the war effort increased the mobility and reduced the isolation of gays, lesbians, and bisexuals. The armed forces at that time overlooked many things—including racism and homophobia, as well as some physical disorders—in their ranks because so many troops were needed for the war effort. It was not until after the war that an organized effort to create a hostile and suppressive environment toward homosexuals became pervasive in the United States. (Duberman et al., 1989).

The second major event was the Stonewall riots. In 1969, a routine raid by police on the Stonewall Inn, a gay bar in New York City's Greenwich Village, met with resistance from the bar's patrons, and riots continued for five days. This event marked what most people consider the beginning of the gay rights movement in the United States, although many efforts to eliminate institutionalized discrimination against gay, lesbian, and bisexual individuals occurred before then (Duberman, 1993).

Marcus (1992) noted that much of the institutionalized violence against homosexuals can be traced back to European roots, epitomized by the rise of Nazi Germany and its planned campaign to annihilate homosexuals. The Nazi government eventually eliminated the first organization founded for homosexuals, the Scientific Humanitarian Committee, which had encouraged education about homosexuality and supported the struggle for equal rights. In Nazi Germany, gay men were routinely executed, and lesbians were not even acknowledged because they did not fulfill their childbearing role to promote the Aryan race (Harrison, Thyer, & Wodarski, 1996).

Today, violence toward and prejudice against gays, lesbians, and bisexuals is still widespread, even in communities that are normally tolerant of diversity among their members. As Wolfe (1998, p. 47) noted: "There is no culture war in America, but on the question of gay rights, fairly severe battles are likely to be fought for the foreseeable future." As a result of this oppression and prejudice, gay and lesbian youths are more likely to attempt suicide than are heterosexual youths (Remafedi, French, Story, & Resnick, 1998). Peyser and Lorch's (2000) 1997 study reported that 46 percent of homosexual high school students in Massachusetts had attempted suicide in the previous year. Sidebar 11.2 presents statistics on the disturbing effects of the continuing prejudice against people with homosexualities on gay and lesbian adolescents and young adults.

As Leland (2000, p. 48) noted, "Hate crimes like the murder of Matthew Shepard and Pfc. Barry Winchell, beaten to death in his bunk at Fort Campbell, Ky., . . . shatter" the myth of security some homosexuals might feel at the beginning of the 21st century. Although tremendous advances have been made in society as homosexuals have entered the mainstream of politics and television, there is still "a contradictory mixture of progress and resistance."

Double Whammy

Combine the barriers faced by a person with the social stigmas of both visual impairment and homosexuality and add the person's limited ability to monitor visually and interpret the social situation or climate, and it is not surprising that gay, lesbian, and bisexual individuals who are blind or visually impaired are so difficult to identify in society. Coming out of the closet is difficult enough for people without disabilities; when a person cannot see what is on the other side of the closet door, skepticism and fear predominate.

≈ *Sidebar* 11.2.
Statistics on the Effects of Prejudice on Gay and Lesbian Youths

Suicide

Gay, lesbian, and bisexual youths are at increased risk of attempting suicide (Remafedi, French, Story, Resnick, & Blum, 1998). Suicide is the leading cause of death among adolescents who are homosexual (Kulkin, Chauvin, & Percle, 2000).

School Dropout

In a national study, 28 percent of gay and lesbian high school students dropped out of school because of harassment resulting from their sexual orientation (Remafedi, 1987).

Isolation

Approximately 80 percent of lesbian, gay, and bisexual youths report severe isolation problems (Hetrick & Martin, 1987; Radowsky & Siegel, 1997). Some of this isolation stems from estrangement from their parents and rejection by peers (American Psychological Association, 2000).

Violence

During high school, 45 percent of gay students and 20 percent of lesbians reported experiencing verbal harassment and/or physical violence (National Gay and Lesbian Task Force, 1984). Remafedi (1987) found that 37 percent of gay and bisexual male adolescents had experienced discrimination, 55 percent had experienced verbal abuse, and 30 percent had experienced physical assults from heterosexual adolescents.

Homelessness

Twenty-six percent of gay and lesbian youths are forced to leave home because of conflicts with their families over their sexual identities (Remafedi, 1987).

HIV/AIDS

Approximately 15 percent of all persons with HIV in December 1999 were 13–24 years old. African-American and Hispanic gay

(continued on next page)

and bisexual men are infected with HIV at younger ages than white men, and 23 percent of all people diagnosed with AIDS are women. Only 47 percent of AIDS diagnoses in December 1999 were in gay men (CDC, 2000). The increase in cocaine use among adolescent gay and bisexual men was a significant, independent predictor of the failure to use "safe-sex" strategies (McNall & Remadefi, 1999).

Student Attitudes

Almost 97 percent of students in public high schools reported regularly hearing homophobic remarks from other students (Massachusetts Governor's Commission on Gay and Lesbian Youth, 1993).

Staff Attitudes

Almost 53 percent of students in public high schools reported hearing homophobic comments made by school staff (Philadelphia Lesbian and Gay Task Force, 1992).

Health Issues

About 68 percent of gay adolescents and 83 percent of lesbian adolescents used alcohol, and 44 percent and 56 percent, respectively, used other drugs (Hunter, 1992). Between 1994 and 1997, the use of marijuana, cocaine, and amphetamines increased significantly among gay and bisexual men (McNall & Remafedi, 1999).

Depression

Depression strikes homosexual youths four to five times more severely than it does heterosexual youths (Hammelman, 1993).

Source: Adapted from Youth Pride, *Creating Safe Schools for Lesbian and Gay Students: A Resource Guide for School Staff* (1997, April). [Available from Office of Diversity Affairs, Council for Exceptional Children, 1920 Association Drive, Reston, VA 20191].

DEMOGRAPHICS

Population

The number of individuals who are gay, lesbian, or bisexual and visually impaired in the United States is unknown. However, it has been estimated that approximately 8 to 10 percent of the general U.S. population is gay, lesbian, or bisexual (Hyde, 1990; Kelly, 1990). The prevalence of visual impairments among children has been estimated to be 0.2 percent (Wenger, Kaye, & LaPlante, 1996). Given that the U.S. population was over 275 million in February 2000 (U.S. Bureau of the Census, 2000), there could be as many as 55,000 gay, lesbian, and bisexual individuals with visual impairments, particularly since the incidence rate increases with age. However, this estimate is difficult to verify because (1) it includes people of all ages, some of whom have not reached puberty; (2) persons with homosexualities do not volunteer their sexuality in any census; and (3) a declaration of sexual orientation is not required to be eligible for disability services. Additional factors, such as racism, sexism, fear, and prejudice, may keep people from revealing their homosexuality.

Geographic Distribution

The population of gays, lesbians, and bisexuals with visual impairments is evenly distributed throughout the country. Adults appear to migrate toward urban centers greater than 500,000 in population, such as New York, Los Angeles, Miami, Washington, DC, and Chicago (CDC, 2000), where they may feel more open about their homosexuality and where there are communities of gays and lesbians, but generally, gays, lesbians, and bisexuals are no more or no less blatant about their sexuality than are heterosexuals. Geographic distribution is simply not relevant; gay, lesbian, and bisexual individuals live everywhere in the country.

Predominant Visual Etiologies

Because the exact number of individuals with visual impairments who are also homosexual is not known and their impairments have not been identified, it is difficult to determine the primary visual etiologies. Logically, eye conditions that occur in the general population also affect people who are gay, lesbian, and bisexual, and those that are more predominant among certain ethnic groups would affect individuals in these groups who are homosexual as well. Except for visual disorders associated with the risk of acquiring AIDS, (such as cytomegalovirus) (Kapperman, Matsuoka, & Pawelski, 1993) or age (such as cataracts or macular degeneration), the visual etiologies found among homosexuals with visual impairments is unknown.

Cultural and Community Implications

The cultural implications of being gay, lesbian, or bisexual and visually impaired or blind are complex, since there is great diversity in the social, economic, ethnic, and religious backgrounds of homosexuals, and the only common thread is their sexual orientation and the culture that has emerged through their struggle for civil rights, including the language, symbolism, and music of the gay and lesbian community. Being gay or lesbian does not mean that one understands visual impairments, and being visually impaired does not mean that one understands homosexuality. Being gay or lesbian and visually impaired simply means that one belongs to and may identify with more than one community at a time. It does not guarantee acceptance in either community.

Families

Informal discussions with gays and lesbians led the authors to conclude that most of their families of origin were heterosexual. In the stories these individuals told about coming out to their heterosexual parents, the parents' responses seemed to fall into three categories:

1. The parents were affirming and accepting.
2. The parents expressed love for their homosexual child, but

the child understood that the topic of sexuality was not to be openly discussed or displayed.

3. The parents disapproved of and rejected the homosexual child.

The experiences of children raised by homosexual parents are not significantly different from those of children raised by heterosexual parents' (American Psychological Association, 1998), according to interviews with three teenagers, one of whom is visually impaired, whose mothers are lesbians. The parents of these teenagers gave permission for their children to speak with us and encouraged them to speak openly. These teenagers—Max, Chloe, and Josiah—are doing well in school, in their families, and in their relationships with friends. They attend church, play guitars and video games, and probably spend too much time on the Internet.

Max lives with his lesbian mother and her partner for part of the week and with his heterosexual father and his partner the rest of the week. He appears to have a close relationship with both parents. "Being raised in a minority gay household," he said, "has taught me to love everybody and [to] realize [that] things like being gay don't fall under generalization and stereotypes. We're not that different from my friends' families, but our household is not the same either. Stereotypes just don't describe our household!"

Max stated that he had two kinds of tolerance. One type allows him to disagree with something, but simultaneously show respect for all people and treat them well. He attributes this kind of tolerance largely to his experience of having a lesbian mother. "I am more aware and careful about what I say," he said. "I've been the one on the other end, the one comments are made about." The second type of tolerance is more religiously based. Max stated that while he tolerates others' different beliefs, he still believes that his path was the right one. He saw no contradiction in these two types of tolerance and thought they were mutually inclusive.

Max does not hide the fact that his mother is a lesbian, although he does not tell his friends either. "I don't *not* take friends home because of my mom. I don't hide it, but I don't prepare them before they come over either. My friends have always been good people who wouldn't care about it anyway, so it never comes up. I think they know." Max also said that he did not think he had experienced any type of discrimination or prejudice at school because of his mother's sexuality, but he noted that he attended a "very progressive school." He stated, "Lots of the kids at school are openly gay and lots of the teachers, too, but that wouldn't happen at a public school. . . . The only bad thing about my mom being gay is that she knows most of my teachers, because they're gay, too."

Because Max was 6 years old when his mother became involved in a lesbian relationship, he said that he could not remember a specific time when he realized she was gay. He just gradually learned, as he did about other personal family information, when it was appropriate to speak about it and when it was not.

———————

———————

Chloe, a teenager who is visually impaired, was adopted by a lesbian couple when she was a toddler. She has attended schools for students who are blind throughout most of her educational experience. Chloe described her childhood as a happy one. She likes school, where she is an accomplished athlete. When asked what it was like growing up with lesbian parents, Chloe reported, "It really didn't matter. My home was the same as my friends' who had moms and dads for their parents. . . . I liked to have my friends come over. . . . Everyone we were around was always nice." Chloe, like Max, also thought that she was tolerant of people's differences.

Chloe's mother is currently single, and believes that her lack of a partner minimizes the effect of her sexual orientation on Chloe's life because it is currently a nonissue. Chloe's mother stated that Chloe was sensitive about trying to "fit in," as many teenage girls are. She thought that Chloe's greatest problem at the time of the interview was the impact of her visual impairment on her social life, and she pointed to the inability to read nonverbal cues as a deterrent in Chloe's development.

———

Josiah lives with his grandmother, grandfather, and mother, who is a lesbian. In the interview, he stated that his mother's sexual orientation is no one else's business and he does not discuss it at his public school. "No one knows." He also does not think that his mother's sexual orientation has had any impact on his social or school activities. If his close friends ask about his mother, he makes no attempt to hide her sexual orientation, but replies that she is bisexual. "It's no big deal; it's just not anybody's business." Like Max, Josiah did not remember the precise time when he became aware of his mother's homosexuality: "I was young, so I don't really remember an exact time that I realized it. I just sort of began to know." As with Chloe and Max, Josiah believed that he developed a strong sense of tolerance for differences in others.

———

All three teenagers were raised by openly lesbian mothers. All appeared to have close relationships with their mothers and did not feel that their mothers' sexual orientation created stress in their lives. In fact, when asked about their tolerance toward others, they all independently replied that their mothers' lifestyles enriched their lives by teaching them about tolerance for others who live "outside the norm." Like all other teenagers, these children of lesbian mothers played sports, worried about fitting in, liked to hang out with their friends, and talked on the phone for hours with members of the opposite sex. Their parents' homosexuality did not create a wedge between the mothers and children, change the teenagers' interactions with their peers, or affect the teenagers' identities and sexual orientations.

INDIVIDUAL EXPERIENCES
Characteristics Related to Visual Impairment

Tuttle and Tuttle (1996) wrote about the difficulty of establishing an identity and self-esteem, given the limitations that a visual impairment places on an individual. These limitations are evident in two ways: vulnerability to abuse and the subtleties of social interchanges that may be lost. Sobsey (1994) estimated as many as two out of every three women with disabilities may have been sexually assaulted, and Kapperman et al. (1993) reported that young adults with visual impairments are at a particular risk of sexual abuse or exploitation.

In the gay and lesbian community, individuals who have visible disabilities (such as physical impairments) are readily seen participating within the context of the community's social and political forums. Concerts, political rallies, and other large events routinely provide interpreters for homosexuals who are deaf or hard of hearing and ramp access for those who use wheelchairs. However, gays and lesbians who are visually impaired or blind are not as visible.

An interview with Miranda, the lesbian mother of a blind child, provides some insight into this phenomenon:

Having been a lesbian since her early teens, Miranda recalled the role that vision played in her ability to enter and actively participate in the lesbian community. She pointed out that despite great gains toward equality, being gay is still viewed as taboo in mainstream American society (see Leland, 2000). In Miranda's experience, most initial contacts among lesbians are dependent on visual cues. "There is a visual 'exchange' between two homosexual people that indicates, 'Yes, I am, too.' It would be very difficult for someone who was blind to pick up on these cues because they are very visually dependent." Miranda did not believe that there are no individuals who are blind and homosexual, only that it would be difficult to actualize one's sexuality if one could not see. "If one lost vision at a later age, sexuality would already be established and verbal cues would be easier to pick up on."

Among gays and lesbians, the ability to spot another person who is gay or lesbian is called "gaydar" (gay radar). It suggests that one can detect homosexuality by putting all the visual pieces together—dress, hairstyle, and other nonverbal cues, as well as the terms the person uses. Although this ability does not suggest that there are stereotypical gay or lesbian characteristics, it demonstrates the importance of reading a situation visually, formulating an appropriate response, and interpreting the result.

Individual Stories

The stories in this section of two lesbians and one gay man who are visually impaired are not intended to represent those of all gay men and lesbians with visual impairments. These individuals represent only themselves—people who have chosen to be out and who openly acknowledge their sexual orientation. They are not closeted, meaning that they do not hide their sexual orientation or allow others to assume they are straight (heterosexual). In today's society, discussing one's sexual choice in an interview exposes the person to the risk of ridicule and the fear of personal safety, so these stories should also be viewed as those of individuals who have chosen to be activists and are willing to stand up for others in a more public forum.

The recurring themes of fear, risk, anxiety, self-doubt, self-acceptance, judgment or prejudice, rejection, individuality, and the struggle between the sometimes competing forces of disability and sexuality that the following stories reveal are similar to the themes of the stories of other minorities presented elsewhere in this book.

Mary, a lesbian who lives in a southwestern state, has dealt with diabetes, a chronic health condition, for nearly 36 years. Initially, her health concerns were physical and affected her vision only minimally. Four years ago, the situation changed suddenly and took Mary by surprise. Mary was unable to continue working. "Because I'd worked in the field of disabilities," she said, "I kept thinking . . . this was like everything I studied about. I had to sort out what I really thought was important. I said to myself, 'It's time to practice what you know intellectually is important!'"

That was when Mary sought a support system. It was difficult for her to find others who understood her vision loss. When people would say, "Your eyes look OK to me," Mary would respond, "I don't care what they look like from the outside, it's the inside perspective I'm concerned about." Changes in all aspects of her lifestyle caused tension in her relationship with her parner, which was already rocky, and the relationship ended with her partner and her partner's son moving out.

Mary is an out lesbian. During the transition from having a minimal visual impairment to a more severe impairment, she contacted a heterosexual woman she knew who also had a visual impairment, so they could compare situations and emotionally support each other. It was hard to find someone who understood and could relate to her vision loss and the struggle she went through as she saw her independence slipping away and her dependence on others increasing. Some of her visual problems have resolved, but Mary feels more closeted about her visual impairment than she ever did about her sexual orientation before she came out, and she fears that her visual impairment jeopardizes her livelihood more than being a lesbian does. "If people can't deal with my sexual orientation, I don't really care. I have felt pretty 'closeted' about my visual impairment, in order to not be judged to do less than I can do, and wanting it to be *my* judgment call, since there is so much variation in my vision." Mary's doctoral dissertation was on lesbians with disabilities, and she is currently employed in a teaching position at a small college.

Nicholas, a single gay man who is studying for a master's degree in education in a southern state, has been visually impaired since birth, and is legally blind. He attended Catholic school when he was young and did not have role models when he was growing up who were either gay or visually impaired. Nicholas feels that being Italian American, gay, visually impaired, and an atheist are all parts of him and cannot be separated. His closest relationships are with others in the gay community because, as he said, "In the past, whenever I was involved with the V.I. [visually impaired] community, I ran into the same types of prejudice against gays that I run into elsewhere. Visually impaired individuals grow up in families, like everyone else, that are comprised of heterosexual parents that are maybe unfamiliar with gay people. They often are trained to hate 'gays' like anybody else. Whether they are visually impaired doesn't make a difference."

Nicholas, who has been openly gay since he was about 19 or 20, has been actively involved with the gay rights movement for many years. He has appeared on major television and radio talk shows to discuss the rights of gay people.

Jennifer, aged 43, lives in a northwestern state and has had diabetes since she was 5. By age 21, she had a severe visual impairment. Like Mary, Jennifer has been through many procedures to save her vision. She is now legally blind with a visual field of less than 10 degrees. She has a master's degree in social work and was employed as a social worker until a few years ago. Jennifer believed that the stress and demands of the job compromised her health and that her visual impairment got in the way of her work. She said: "There was lots of paperwork. I didn't use accommodations. I can read print, but at 50 words per minute, it makes reading hard and slow." In addition, she worked in an inner-city agency, and her visual impairment made her vulnerable to attack. She said, "I began meeting with clients in the office, and that changed the interactions we had."

Jennifer now resides in the country with her partner and is a potter. She stated that her visual impairment is an inconvenience to her, as did Mary and Nicholas. "You have to ask friends for rides and things like that. You have to plan more. You aren't as spontaneous. You have to pack a lunch just for a walk because of the diabetes!" she joked. Jennifer maintains a positive outlook on her visual impairment. Other than driving, there is really little that she does not do, although she is slow and sometimes does things her own way. For instance, when visiting the pyramids in Mexico, Jennifer had a hard time with depth perception, so she slid on her backside down the pyramids.

Jennifer believes that she is self-reliant and that if she tries to do something new, "all sorts of folks" will give her a hand. However, she acknowledged that she needs to do better asking for help when she needs it. Jennifer likes being around other lesbians with disabilities. As she put it, "I feel comfortable. It's nice not having to say what you need and being involved with creative problem solving. It's simple—there's no explaining needed. It's comfortable."

Acceptance

Where do individuals who are visually impaired and homosexual find acceptance? As the interviews with Mary, Nicholas, and Jennifer revealed, it depends on a person's needs at different times in his or her life. Mary sought members of the visually impaired community for support when her vision was changing. The intense relationships she developed with heterosexuals with visual impairments were transient, lasting only as long as the visual impairment and related issues had a high priority in her life. This commonality, the visual impairment, was not encompassing enough to sustain long-term relationships. Mary seemed to need enduring friendships that covered a greater gamut of interests.

Jennifer sought support from other lesbians, especially those who also had disabilities. Lesbians without disabilities did not always have the understanding and tolerance she needed. She did not always want or have the energy to educate others about visual impairment or to build relationships with people who had no idea of what it is like to be disabled. She stated it was just "more comfortable" to be with people with disabilities when she needed support for her visual impairment.

Nicholas reported some negative experiences with people who were visually impaired, although these experiences were no different from those he had with heterosexuals. His sexual orientation seemed to have a greater impact on his relationships than did his visual impairment. Nicholas was visually impaired from birth, whereas Mary and Jennifer dealt with changing vision throughout their lives. All three said that instead of being integrated, the blind community and the gay community were compartmentalized, so that they vacillated between participating in one or the other community to meet their needs at different times in their lives.

In the wake of the homicides of gay men in Colorado, Kentucky, and Texas, acceptance of people who are different seems to be a necessary goal. Ireland (1999, p. 8) pointed out that there is a great deal of homophobia among heterosexual adolescents, who use the term *faggot* as the "ultimate insult," to "designate those who are different or simply disliked, whether they are gay or not." As the president of the National Education Association (quoted in Ireland, 1999, p. 8) stated: "Schools cannot be neutral when we're dealing with human dignity and human rights—I'm not talking about tolerance, I'm talking about acceptance." Yet, "even acceptance . . . has come at the cost of self-censorship" (Leland, 2000, p. 49). For example, a homosexual who was interviewed for Leland's article said, "We make our inroads in society because we purposely make ourselves mainstream. Not that you deny your individuality or your sexuality. But you don't automatically say what you think" (p. 49).

Inconvenience

Mary, Nicholas, and Jennifer all reported that being visually impaired is "inconvenient" and sometimes interferes with their daily activities. Nicholas noted that he was sometimes excluded from sports and frequently had to ask someone to pick him up for social events he wished to attend, although most people in the gay community, he thought, were sensitive to his need for accommodations. Jennifer said that she often had to figure out her "own way of doing things." She admitted that she had to work on asking for help when she needed it, but that she did not like inconveniencing others and not being independent in some settings. She did her best to minimize her dependence on others by planning ahead for any accommodations she might need and figuring out a way that she could do something in return for those who help her out. For instance, because she knew she would be arriving at a campsite during the evening and would not be able to see well enough to set up her tent, she asked friends ahead of time to plan on helping her and her partner set up the tent. In return, she prepared the evening meal, an activity that was not dependent on her vision.

Perceptions of Services

Mary, Nicholas, and Jennifer let both heterosexual and homosexual friends know that they were visually impaired and what their needs were in relation to their impairment. However, they did not always disclose their sexual orientation when seeking services for their visual impairment because they do not always feel it is a safe thing to do and when they have occasionally disclosed it, they thought they received inferior service.

RECOMMENDATIONS FOR PROFESSIONALS

Professionals need to acknowledge and value a student or client who is visually impaired and homosexual for his or her individ-

uality, rather than allow their personal opinions to interfere with
the services they provide. In working with these students or
clients, it would be more productive to approach homosexuality
as a cultural difference that requires knowledge, understanding,
and ultimately adaptation. The following are some suggestions
for educational and rehabilitation professionals to enhance their
sensitivity and productivity in working with all clients, some of
whom are gay, lesbian, or bisexual:

- If a client or student tells you about his or her homosexuality, be cognizant of the risk he or she has taken and of the
  trust that the student or client places in you. Confidentiality is an ethical responsibility.
- Do not wonder about a client's or student's sexuality. It is
  not pertinent to the work that you do, and it creates an aura
  of suspicion and judgment that can eventually affect your
  relationship.
- Be cautious of assumptions that are not supported by the literature. In fact,
  1. Homosexuality is not a medical disorder and cannot be
     "cured" (American Academy of Pediatrics, 1993; Ameri-
     can Psychiatric Association, 1974; American Psychologi-
     cal Association, 1998).
  2. Gay men and lesbians do not sexually abuse children any
     more than heterosexuals do (American Psychological
     Association, 1998).
  3. The majority of child molesters are heterosexual men, not
     lesbian, gay, or bisexual people (Shepherd, 1998).
  4. "At this point in time, no single factor has emerged from
     the research as to what causes a homosexual orientation
     or any other sexual orientation" (Harrison, Thyer, &
     Wodarski (1996, p. 240).
  5. Gay men and lesbians do not have unstable relationships
     any more than the rest of society (Kurdeck, 1995).
  6. You cannot tell if someone is gay or lesbian by his or her
     appearance, mannerisms, or dress (Garnets & Kimmel,

1995), particularly when the person is visually impaired and may not know the implications of how he or she appears to others.

7. All gay men are not effeminate.
8. All lesbians are not butch.

Following these recommendations may begin to establish a culture of services "in which each diverse human gift will find a fitting place" (Mead, 1963, p. 322).

REFERENCES

American Academy of Pediatrics. (1993). Policy statement: Homosexuality and adolescence. *Pediatrics, 92,* 631–634.

American Psychiatric Association. (1974). Position statement on homosexuality and civil rights. *American Journal of Psychiatry, 131,* 497.

American Psychological Association. (1998, July). *Answers to your questions about sexual orientation and homosexuality.* Available at: www.apa.org/pubinfo/answers.html

American Psychological Association. (2000). Guidelines for psychotherapy with lesbian, gay, and bisexual clients. Available: http://www.apa.org/pi/lgbc/guidelines.html

American Psychological Association. (1998). Appropriate therapeutic responses to sexual orientation. Proceedings of the American Psychological Association, Inc., 1997. *American Psychologist, 53,* 882–939.

Blasch, B. B., Wiener, W. R., & Welsh, R. L. (Eds.). (1997). *Foundations of orientation and mobility* (2d ed.). New York: AFB Press.

Bledsoe, C. W. (1980). Originators of orientation and mobility training. In R. L. Welsh & B. B. Blasch (Eds.), *Foundations of orientation and mobility* (pp. 581–624). New York: American Foundation for the Blind.

Britzman, D. P. (1995). Is there a queer pedagogy? Or, stop reading straight. *Educational Theory, 45,* 151–165.

Capper, C. A. (1999). (Homo)sexualities, organizations, and administration: Possibilities for in(queer)y. *Educational Researcher, 28*(5), 4–10.

Centers for Disease Control. (2000). Commentary. *Surveillance Report, 11*(2). Available at: http://www.cdc.gov/hiv/stats/hasr 1102/commentary.htm

Cowen, T. (1988). *The lives of gay men and women who enriched the world.* New Canaan, CJ: William Mulvey.

Duberman, M. (1993). *Stonewall.* New York: E. P. Dutton.

Duberman, M. B., Vicinus, M., & Chauncey, F., Jr. (Eds.). (1989). *Hidden from history: Reclaiming the gay and lesbian past.* New York: New American Library.

Gallagher, W. F. (1988). Categorical services in the age of integration: Paradox or contradiction? *Journal of Visual Impairment & Blindness, 83,* 226–29.

Garnets, L. D., & Kimmel, D. C. (1995). *Psychological perspectives on lesbian and gay male experiences.* New York: Columbia University Press.

Griffin, P. (1996). *A research agenda on gay, lesbian, bisexual, transgender administrators: What can we learn from the research on women administrators, administrators of color, and homosexual teachers and youth?* (Cassette recording No. RA6–35.62). Paper presented at the annual meeting of the American Educational Research Association, New York, City.

Hammelman, T. (1993). Gay and lesbian youth contributing factors to serious attempts or considerations of suicide. *Journal of Gay and Lesbian Psychotherapy, 2,* 77–89.

Harrison, D. F., Thyer, B. A., & Wodarski, J. S. (1996). *Cultural diversity and social work practice* (2d ed.). Springfield, IL: Charles C Thomas.

Hetrick, E. S., & Martin, A. D. (1987). Developmental issues and their resolution for gay and lesbian adolescents. *Journal of Homosexuality, 14* (1–2), 25–43.

Honeychurch, K. G. (1996). Researching dissident subjectivities: Queering the grounds of theory and practice. *Harvard Educational Review, 66,* 339–355.

Hunter, J. (1992). *Health issues of gay and lesbian adolescents.* Unpublished manuscript, Columbia University, HIV Center for Clinical and Behavioral Studies.

Hyde, J. (1990). *Understanding human sexuality.* New York: McGraw Hill.

Ireland, D. (1999, June 14). Gay ed for kids. *The Nation, 268*(22), 8.

Kapperman, G., Matsuoka, J. C., & Pawelski, C. E. (1993). *HIV/AIDS prevention: A guide for working with people who are blind or visually impaired.* New York: AFB Press.

Kelly, G. (1990). *Sexuality today: The human perspective.* Guilford, NY: Duskin.

Kurdeck, L. (1995). Lesbian and gay couples. In A. D'Augelli & C. Patterson (Eds.), *Lesbian, gay, and bisexual lives over the lifespan* (pp. 243–261). New York: Oxford University Press.

Lang, S. (1998). *Men as women, women as men: Changing gender in Native American cultures* (J. L. Vantine, Trans.). Austin: University of Texas Press.

Lehman, M. (1993). *HIV/AIDS Surveillance Report, 5*(1). Atlanta, GA: Centers for Disease Control.

Leland, J. (2000, March 20). Shades of gay. *Newsweek,* pp. 46–49.

Lowenfeld, B. (1981). *Berthold Lowenfeld on blindness and blind people.* New York: American Foundation for the Blind.

Marcus, E. (1992). *Making history: The struggle for gay and lesbian equal rights, 1945–1990: An oral history.* New York: HarpersCollins.

Massachusetts Governor's Commission on Gay and Lesbian Youth. (1993). *Making schools safe for gay and lesbian youth: Report.* Boston: Author.

Mathison, C. (1998). The invisible minority: Preparing teachers to meet the needs of gay and lesbian youth. *Journal of Teacher Education, 49,* 151–155.

McNall, M., & Remafedi, G. (1999). Relationship of amphetamine and other substance use to unprotected intercourse among young men who have sex with men. *Archives of Pediatrics & Adolescent Medicine, 153,* 1130–35.

Mead, M. (1963). *Sex and temperament in three primitive societies.* New York: William Morrow.

National Gay and Lesbian Task Force. (1984). *National anti-gay/lesbian victimization report.* New York: Author.

Peyser, M., & Lorch, D. (2000, March 20). High school controversial. *Newsweek,* pp. 55–56.

Philadelphia Lesbian and Gay Task Force. (1992). *Discrimination and violence toward lesbian women and gay men in Philadelphia and the commonwealth of Pennsylvania.* Philadelphia: Author.

Radkowsky, M., & Siegel, L. J. (1997). The gay adolescent: Stressors, adaptations, and psychosocial interventions. *Clinical Psychology Review, 17,* 191–216.

Remafedi, G. (1987). Male homosexuality: The adolescent's perspective. *Pediatrics, 79,* 326–330.

Remafedi, G. (1999). Sexual orientation and youth suicide. *Journal of the American Medical Association, 282,* 1291–92.

Remafedi, G., French, S., Story, M., Resnick, M. D., & Blum, R. (1998). The relationship between suicide risk and sexual orientation: Results of a population-based study. *American Journal of Public Health, 88,* 57–60.

Sheperd, C. A. (1998, Sept. 23). *Quick facts about homosexuality.* Available: http://cqsa.virtualave.net/facts/html.

Sobsey, D. (1994). *Violence and abuse in the lives of people with disabilities: The end of silent acceptance?* Baltimore, MD: Paul H. Brookes.

Spungin, S. J., & Taylor, J. L. (1986). The teacher. In G. T. Scholl (Ed.), *Foundations of education for blind and visually handicapped children and youth* (pp. 255–264). New York: American Foundation for the Blind.

Tuttle, D. W., & Tuttle, N. R. (1996). *Self-esteem and adjusting with blindness: The process of responding to life's demands* (2d ed.). Springfield, IL: Charles C Thomas.

U.S. Bureau of the Census. (2000, February 14). Annual projections of the total resident population as of July 1: Middle, lowest, highest, and zero international migration series, 1999 to 2100 [On-line]. Available: http://www.census.gov/population/projections/natsum-T1.htm

U.S. Department of Health and Human Services. (1989). *Report of the secretary's task force on youth and suicide.* Washington, DC: U.S. Government Printing Office.

Wenger, B. L., Kaye, H. S., & LaPlante, M. P. (1996). *Disabilities statistics abstract No. 15: Disabilities among children.* Washington, DC: U.S. Department of Education, National Institute on Disability and Rehabilitation Research.

Wolfe, A. (1998, February 8). The homosexual exception. *New York Times Magazine,* pp. 46–47.

Youth Pride. (1997, April). *Creating safe schools for lesbian and gay students: A resource guide for school staff.* (Available from Office of Diversity Affairs, Council for Exceptional Children, 1920 Association Drive, Reston, VA 20191).

PART V

Professional Practices and Diversity

CHAPTER 12

Providing Professional Services to Individuals Who Speak English as a Second Language

**Madeline Milian
and Paula Conroy**

Language diversity has always existed in the United States, but only one language, English, has obtain the status of the dominant language. In the 1990s, laws designating English as the official language were passed in a number of states across this country. Supporters of this type of legislation maintain that these measures will speed the assimilation of those who are foreign born and their children (Lewelling, 1997). Proficiency in other languages does not receive the same status as proficiency in English, and adults who are unable to master the English language are often marginalized in low-paying jobs. Therefore, teaching English to individuals who speak languages other than English, whether they are visually impaired or sighted, is critical to helping them obtain educational and professional opportunities.

This chapter discusses issues that affect people who are blind or visually impaired and speak languages other than English. In essence, the same political and educational policies that apply to the general population of individuals who learn English as a second language also apply to those who are visually impaired. The chapter concentrates on strategies for identifying and assessing visually impaired students and clients who are learning English and methods for teaching them English. Two case studies are presented to illustrate the ideas discussed in this chapter and to offer suggestions to professionals who are providing services to individuals with visual impairments who are either foreign born or are members of non-English language groups.

LANGUAGE DIVERSITY IN THE UNITED STATES

Evidence of multilingualism can be traced to the Colonial period, when hundreds of languages were spoken by Native Americans, and Dutch, English, Spanish, and French were spoken by the European settlers (Dicker, 1996). In the 19th century, during the great waves of immigration, numerous other languages were spoken by newcomers, including Chinese, German, Yiddish, and various Slavic languages. According to the 1990 census (U.S. Bureau of the Census, 2000), almost 32 million, or 13.8 percent of people aged 5 and over who were living in the United States in 1990 spoke languages other than English at home. Spanish, French, German, Italian, and Chinese are the most common languages spoken in the United States, but a multitude of other languages are also spoken (Wiley, 1996). In addition, languages that were not previously represented in the United States are now being heard in communities across the country, and the use of low-incidence languages is increasing. For example, in New York City, the proportion of residents who spoke Hindi-related languages (Bengali, Gujarati, Malayalam, and Punjabi) increased from 0.2 percent to 0.5 percent from 1980 to 1990; the proportions who spoke Korean, Kru-Ibo-Yoruba, and Vietnamese tripled; and the proportions of those who spoke Hindi-Urdu, Chinese, Filipino, Arabic, and Persian doubled (Garcia, 1997).

The English proficiency of speakers of languages other than English range from those who speak English fluently to those who have limited or no knowledge of English. For example, in 1990 there were more than 6.3 million young people in the 5- to 17-year-old range, or 14 percent of the student population, who spoke languages other than English. In the same year, school districts reported that 2.2 million of these students, approximately 5 percent of the student population, were classified under the legal definition of limited English proficiency and needed either Bilingual Education or ESL services to learn English and to understand academic content. Since then, the number of students who have limited proficiency in English has increased, and in 1997 school districts reported that number to be 3.4 million students, or 7.4 percent of the student population (Macías, 1998; U.S. Bureau of the Census, 2000). Neither the total number of students with visual impairments who come from homes where languages other than English are spoken nor the level of English proficiency of those who speak other languages is known. However, efforts are being made to determine language diversity among people who are blind or visually impaired. For example, Milian and Ferrell (1998) reported that in a sample of 4,640 students with visual impairments in Arizona, California, Colorado, Florida, New Mexico, and New York, 1,267 (27.3 percent) students came from homes where languages other than English were spoken, and 382 (8.2 percent) of these students were identified by their teachers as having limited proficiency in English. Most important, these figures indicate that 30.1 percent of the students who came from homes where languages other than English were spoken were learning English.

Another study that gathered data on languages spoken by students with visual impairments was Project PRISM (Ferrell, 1998). This longitudinal study found that 87.5 percent of the parents of blind children who participated in the study spoke English at home, and the remaining 12.5 percent spoke either another language only or another language in addition to English.

There is no reason to believe that the population of individuals with visual impairments is not as linguistically diverse as the U.S. population as a whole or that their need to learn English is not the same. In fact, it can be argued that given the competitive nature of employment for people with visual impairments, becoming fluent in English and maintaining or developing literacy in their native languages will give individuals with visual impairments a tremendous advantage on the job market.

IDENTIFYING AND ASSESSING STUDENTS WHO SPEAK ENGLISH AS A SECOND LANGUAGE

Public school districts are required by federal civil right laws to provide assistance to all students who are learning English including those who are visually impaired, so the students can participate in educational programs. Before students can receive such assistance, however, they need to be identified and assessed.

Regulations for identifying students who are learning English are established by individual states, but most states have common basic requirements. First, the parents of all children who enter public schools must complete home language surveys or home language questionnaires at the time of enrollment. These surveys contain questions on the language or languages spoken to the children at home and the frequency with which these languages are used. The format and questions included in these surveys vary, depending on the state and sometimes on the school district or special school.

Second, for students whose family members stated that another language or additional languages other than English are spoken at home, schools follow up to confirm that the students have sufficient mastery of English to perform in English-only classrooms without modifications. Observations and language assessments begin at that point.

Teachers' questionnaires are frequently used to obtain informal ratings of students' English language proficiency. In addition, schools use formal language tests that have been approved by the state department of education and school district, including commercially available tests that are used nationwide. If a student is found to be functioning below the minimum English language level that a state sets for participating in an English-only classroom, modifications of the educational program need to be provided. In some cases, schools also test students' proficiency in their native language to determine if the students are performing at grade level in the native language.

When students score below the designated statewide level in a language proficiency test, other factors need to be considered. For example, if an evaluation has been recommended to determine academic or cognitive functioning, an evaluation conducted only in English is inappropriate because it does not indicate the student's actual academic or cognitive level. Assessment in the native language is an important and more appropriate procedure for students who do not speak English or have not mastered sufficient English skills.

Administrators of programs for students who are blind or visually impaired need to become familiar with the specific state regulations for students from non-English-speaking communities and provide needed services that target these students' language needs.

Language-Proficiency Tests

Typically, commercially available language tests are constructed with sighted students in mind in that they tend to have many items that require students to point to the correct item, identify the name of the object in a given picture, or create a story about a picture that is shown. Consequently, it is difficult to find standardized language proficiency tests that can be administered to blind or visually impaired students without modifications. In fact, teachers of students with visual impairments in Milian and Ferrell's (1998) study considered the assessment of ESL students to be extremely problematic because of the lack of valid assessment measures and qualified bilingual personnel to administer them.

Language-proficiency tests can be divided into two categories: those that measure only oral language and those that measure oral and written language. As with all commercially available tests, decisions need to be made on the basis of such factors as the use and quality of pictures, the reliance on pictures to answer information and comprehension questions, print size, and the visual requirements (such as depth perception) of individual items. Some of the most commonly used language-proficiency tests are reviewed next as a guide for professionals who are considering their use with blind and visually impaired students.

LANGUAGE ASSESSMENT SCALES

The Language Assessment Scales (LAS) is widely used to identify the language levels of students who are learning English. A Spanish version is also available to measure proficiency in Spanish. Although it is not difficult to administer the LAS, scoring the LAS can be tedious and requires training and practice.

Pre-LAS Oral. The Pre-LAS Oral is designed to measure young children's expressive and receptive abilities in morphology, syntax, and semantics. Of the six subscales—Simon Says, Choose a Picture, What's in the House? Say What You Hear, Finishing Stories, and Let's Tell Stories—some of the subscales require the use of a Cue Picture Book, so students can point to the correct answers. Pictures are typically free of complex details; however, the pictures used for the subscale What's in the House? include many details and fine lines. It may be possible to use this test with some modifications with students with low vision (those who can read large print) but it is not feasible to administer all the subscales to students who are blind because of the use of pictures.

LAS-Oral. The oral component of the LAS, for students in grades 1–12, measures vocabulary, comprehension, production, and aural discrimination and has a pronunciation component for students in grades 2–12. Oral language components include vocabulary, listening comprehension, and story retelling. The pronunciation component includes minimal sound pairs and phonemes. Cue pictures are required for some items.

Reading and Writing. According to the examiner's manual (Duncan & De Avila, 1988), the LAS Reading/Writing Scale measures skills in reading and writing English that are necessary for functioning in a mainstream academic environment. The test is used with ESL students in grades 2 to 9 or higher as a screening device for placement, and since it includes equivalent test forms that can be used to compare test/retest results, it can be used for reclassification. The test forms are printed in black and white, which allows for easy enlargement, and, for the most part, pictures are not complex, which makes it possible for students with low vision to use an enlarged version of the test. The seven subscales of the LAS Reading/Writing Scale are as follows:

Vocabulary. In grades 2–6 this subscale requires students to match pictures to words. Because of the reliance on pictures in the early grades, this subscale cannot be used with students in these grades who are blind. In grades 7–9 and up, however, students have to find synonyms or antonyms for the indicated words, and pictures are not used; thus, the subscale can be used with blind middle school and high school students.

Mechanics and Usage. This subscale measures knowledge of capitalization, punctuation, and grammar. Items are completed by filling in blanks, and no pictures are involved.

Fluency. This subscale measures overall language fluency and the ability to infer a missing word on the basis of knowledge of language usage and semantics. It uses fill-in-the-blank items, and pictures are not used.

Reading for Information. This subscale contains a story and multiple-choice questions that measure the ability to identify information in the story by reading; pictures are not used.

Finishing Sentences. In this subscale, students are given the first half of a sentence and are asked to finish the sentence. Pictures are not used.

What's Happening? This subscale contains pictures that are designed to elicit a sentence.

Let's Write! Pictures are used to elicit a writing sample in the form of a story.

In summary, it would be possible to use certain subscales of the LAS Reading and Writing test with blind students, but not the entire test. However, when modified as needed by enlarging the pictures, the test could be used with students with low vision. School personnel can also assess students in Spanish by administering the Spanish version of the LAS.

WOODCOCK-MUÑOZ LANGUAGE SURVEY

This instrument provides proficiency levels in oral language, reading, and writing in either English or Spanish. According to the test manual (Woodcock & Muñoz-Sandoval, 1993) the Spanish and English versions of the survey are specifically designed to determine cutoff points for five levels of proficiency in cognitive academic language in individuals aged 4 and over. The five levels are 5 (advanced), 4 (fluent), 3 (limited), 2 (very limited), and 1 (negligible). The scores assist school districts in determining if students need specialized language services.

The Woodcock-Muñoz survey uses an Easel Test Book that is arranged so the pictures or words face the student while the directions and answers face the examiner. There are five components of the test: picture vocabulary, verbal analogies, letter-word recognition, and dictation.

Picture Vocabulary. Since this part of the test measures the ability to name familiar and unfamiliar picture objects, it requires the ability to see pictures. A student is asked to place his or her finger on the picture that the examiner mentions (for example: "Put your finger on the flower") or to say the name of the picture when asked ("What is this?"). The pictures are in color and may be too small for some students with low vision to see. In addition, starting with item 9, there are two or more items or pictures per page, so examiners may want to show only the pictures that correspond with a specific item to avoid visual confusion.

Verbal Analogies. This part of the test requires a student to complete a logical word relationship verbally. Although written words are presented to students that emphasize the given analogies, these written words may not be necessary to answer the questions. Students can listen to the analogies and respond orally.

Letter-Word Recognition. The sample items and the first four items of this part require students to do some visual matching. Since the pictures presented are relatively small, they need to be enlarged for most students with low vision. Other items require students to name letters or read words. For students who read braille, it is necessary to braille the letters and words ahead of time. Some students who read large print may need to have the information enlarged for them.

Dictation. This part of the test measures skills that range from prewriting skills to word usage. Skills such as knowledge of letter forms, spelling, punctuation, and capitalization are included. Since students used a worksheet with small print to complete this part of the test, worksheets for students who read braille need to be brailled and those for students who read large print need to be enlarged. Adaptation of the worksheet would not require much time, since many of the items are given orally following a traditional dictation format.

The manual provides general test modifications for students with visual or physical impairments. Administration procedures are explained in the manual, and scoring and reporting disks are available from the testing company (see Woodcock & Muñoz-Sandoval, 1993) and provide age- and grade-equivalent scores.

BASIC INVENTORY OF NATURAL LANGUAGE

The Basic Inventory of Natural Language (BINL) assesses the oral language production of students in grades K–12 (Herbert, 1983). It can be administered in a number of languages provided that the examiner is fluent in them. The BINL is administered individually and uses large photographs to elicit an oral language sample, which is recorded on audiotape and then transcribed. It also includes a holistic scoring rubric for such areas as listening comprehension, fluency, vocabulary, pronunciation and grammar. This is a relatively simple tool to administer, and the transcribed oral sample can be sent to the publisher for scoring.

Because the photographs used for the BINL are large and colorful, many students with low vision will be able to see and talk about them without difficulty. When requested, the publisher will provide a set of questions for students who are blind that will also elicit an oral sample.

STUDENT ORAL LANGUAGE OBSERVATION MATRIX

The Student Oral Language Observation Matrix (SOLOM) (Los Angeles Unified School District, 1993) is an informal rating tool that can be used by teachers and other school personnel to assess students' oral language as used in school, on a five-point scale, in areas such as comprehension, fluency, vocabulary, pronunciation, and grammar. To ensure that the rating is meaningful, the person who completes the rating scale must be fluent in the target language and be familiar with the student.

This tool can be used with students with visual impairments without difficulty because it does not involve written language or pictures. Rather, the assessor uses his or her judgment to rate the student's oral language proficiency. The SOLOM is used widely in California and can be obtained from the California State Department of Education or the Los Angeles Unified School District.

OTHER FORMS OF ASSESSMENT

In addition to the assessment instruments just described, others are also frequently used by school personnel to facilitate their understanding of students' oral and written proficiency. Often, assessment tools are approved by a state's department of education for use in that state, and school district personnel select tools from the approved list of language tests.

Recognizing the limitations of standardized language assessments, programs for students with visual impairments may want to consider using what O'Malley and Valdez Pierce (1996, p. 14) called "authentic assessments," that is, "multiple forms of assessment that reflect student learning, achievement, motivation, and attitudes on instructionally-relevant classroom activities. Examples of authentic assessment include performance assessment, portfolios, and student self-assessment." Readers who want to use authentic assessment in their programs are encouraged to consult the books by O'Malley and Valdez Pierce (1996) and Fradd, Larrinaga McGee, and Wilen (1994). These two textbooks offer excellent examples of the activities that can be conducted with English language learners to follow their educational growth.

EDUCATIONAL PROGRAMS FOR LINGUISTICALLY DIVERSE STUDENTS WHO ARE VISUALLY IMPAIRED

It is important for educators to understand that program modifications are necessary to provide instruction to students who are learning English that will lead to both cognitive growth and language learning; without such modifications, these students may be at risk of academic failure. Programs for these students should, at a minimum, include ESL instruction. They may also include instruction in reading and language arts in the native language and English instruction in other subjects.

It is not clear if ESL students with visual impairments are participating in all available program options or only a few (for examples of program options see Milian, 2000). Milian and Ferrell (1998) found that 63.4 percent of the participating teachers reported that English-only instruction is frequently the only option available in their settings, and 73.9 percent reported that bilingual paraprofessionals are frequently used with ESL students who are visually impaired to facilitate understanding. Since this study was conducted in states with a large number of linguistically diverse students, the results may not be indicative of the situation in states with fewer ESL students.

Although all program options are not always available in every school district in the country, at least one option has to be offered in schools with students who are learning English. In general, program options tend to be either additive or subtractive (Cummins, 1989; Lambert & Tucker, 1972). Additive programs add the second language without replacing the native language of the student, while subtractive models only emphasize the second language leading to the replacement of the first language. Therefore, programs that only emphasize the teaching of English and do not encourage or make provisions for the development of literacy skills in first language are subtractive, while programs that focus on the development of literacy skills in the first language while also teaching English are additive.

To create appropriate educational programs for linguistically diverse students with visual impairments, teachers need to consider the attributes of a student that are critical to learning English and those that are crucial for participating in special education programs (Oxford-Carpenter, 1986). These essential attributes include the student's

- ◆ disability or disabilities
- ◆ current stage of second language acquisition
- ◆ strengths and weaknesses in listening, speaking, reading, and writing
- ◆ age, personality, and interests
- ◆ communication needs in the second language

- inclusion in the community of the target language
- language learning style

In general, the more factors addressed in planning instruction in English, the more successful the program will be for a linguistically diverse student with a disability.

The specific educational needs of students with visual impairments who are learning English determine the type of methods and strategies used for instruction. Some basic methods and strategies that could be used are total physical response, the natural approach, the language experience approach, and reading and writing workshops. These teaching approaches are based on theories of communicative competence, in which the main goal is to communicate meaning, not to use correct grammar (Canale & Swain, 1980). Although communicative approaches are popular, they have been criticized for promoting language fluency, rather than accuracy. Students in ESL classrooms where communicative approaches are used may be proficient in interacting socially with English speakers, but their academic language skills may be less well developed (Hammerly, 1991). Professionals who are interested in learning more about the methods mentioned here may want to examine the following texts: Crandall and Peyton (1993), Hagerty (1992), Larsen-Freeman (1986), and Ovando and Collier (1998).

Each teaching approach can be easily adapted or modified for use with individuals who are visually impaired, regardless of their age. It is important to note that these teaching approaches are not comprehensive literacy-instruction programs when used in isolation, but together with other programs, they can promote the development of skills in the four areas of literacy: listening, speaking, reading, and writing. Moreover, a number of other approaches used by ESL teachers have not been discussed. Professionals who want to learn about these other methods are encouraged to read one of the many textbooks on ESL methods, such as Celce-Murcia (1991), and Echerarvia and Vogt (2000).

Total Physical Response

Total physical response (TPR) is a teaching technique used by ESL teachers to instruct students who are in the beginning stages of learning English. A communicative approach, TPR incorporates the major premises of Krashen and Terrell's (1983) natural approach (discussed in the next section), which emphasizes communicating meaning, not learning grammatical structure. A "silent period" or a time when ESL learners are developing receptive skills and are not yet orally producing the new language typically takes place. When using TPR, this silent period is respected so that students can concentrate on understanding, rather than on producing, language.

TPR, developed by Asher (1966), is based on the theory that the way children learn a second language is similar to the way they learn their first language and that listening and comprehension are the bases for the later acquisition of speech. Asher found that language is more easily learned and retained when it is associated with simple body movements.

In TPR lessons, a teacher issues a series of directions using imperative statements, and students spend much of their time listening and physically responding to the teacher. As language learning progresses, the teacher adds more complete syntax, including interrogatives. As students grow more comfortable responding orally to commands and questions, they begin to give commands to the class, taking the role of teacher. The teacher is tolerant of students' errors; focuses on communication, not grammar; and allows students to begin to speaking when they are ready and does not force them to speak.

With the inclusion of some minor modifications, TPR is a viable way to begin ESL instruction with students who are visually impaired (Conroy, 1999). It is possible to begin using TPR by incorporating basic concepts needed to develop orientation and mobility (O&M) skills into language instruction. For example, for the command, "Put your cane to the right of the door," a student must use orientation skills to locate the door, directional/laterality concepts to put the cane to the right of the door, and mobility skills to travel to the door. At first, the teacher can accompany the student to the door as a way to model the behavior; then, the student can demonstrate the request by himself or herself. The following ideas should be taken into consideration when using TPR with ESL students who are visually impaired:

- Since the student cannot see the teacher well, the student must be put through the action or be allowed to feel the teacher demonstrating the desired response.
- Since there can be a certain degree of touching when illustrating concepts through TPR, teachers need to be aware of cultural norms related to touching. Are there parts of the body that are not appropriate to touch? Are there gender-based rules for touching?
- The use of pictures should be limited because students with low vision may not be able to identify and/or interpret the content of pictures, and those who are blind cannot see them at all. Only pictures that are large and simple enough to allow students with low vision to learn the required information should be used.
- At first, the pace of the lesson may have to be slower and the content may have to be less to allow the teacher to ensure that the student understands the concept thoroughly.
- The teacher must familiarize the student with the physical setup of the room and the location of objects that may frequently be moved.
- The student should learn and use protective techniques that ensure safety in the instructional environment.

TPR can provide a positive initial language-learning experience for ESL students with visual impairments. This method allows teachers to focus on teaching basic O&M skills and to use many commercially available books on the approach that detail specific lessons that teachers of students with visual impairments can easily modify.

The Natural Approach

The natural approach, described by Krashen and Terrell (1983), is one of the best-known communicative approaches for ESL instruction. In this approach, students participate in a variety of oral language activities in which they use the new language for meaningful communication, rather than for rote learning. The approach is appropriate when the major goal of language learning is develop interpersonal communicative skills, including the ability to engage in basic oral and written communication (Chamot & Stewner-Manzanares, 1985; Krashen & Terrell, 1983; Richards & Rogers, 1986).

According to the natural approach, all students progress through the same stages in language acquisition; the first stage is a silent period in which students develop language by listening to comprehensible input from English speakers (Krashen & Terrell, 1983; Savingnon, 1991). Teachers provide input in English at a level slightly beyond the students' current levels of proficiency and do not encourage students to speak before they are ready. When speech emerges, students typically use one or two words to respond to questions and communicate their ideas. Errors are not corrected; students gradually correct their own errors as they obtain more experience with the language. Reading and writing are taught as natural extensions of listening and speaking, and many different types of opportunities are provided for students to experience literacy.

Since teachers make lessons comprehensible by using visuals, real objects, gestures, role plays, and other context-enriching strategies, it is necessary to modify and adapt these strategies for use with students with visual impairments. The use of visuals should be based on a student's usable vision, gestures and role-plays need to be described and demonstrated to a student who cannot see the visual model, and a student may need to be put through the movements he or she is expected to imitate.

Language Experience Approach

In the language experience approach, students explore their own ideas through discussion and writing. To be able to build meaning from print, students must be able to predict the overall structure and some of the language of the reading material (Rigg, 1989). The more predictable the reading material, the easier it is for students to read. In the language experience approach, students generate ideas phrased in their own words, producing material that is, for them, highly predictable and therefore easy to read.

A lesson using the language experience approach starts with a clear purpose and a clear audience, which determine both the content and form. The teacher typically serves as a facilitator of the students' discussion and allows plenty of discussion time for students to plan what they will dictate. This discussion helps ensure that the dictated text is coherent, which is especially important in the early grades (Rigg, 1989). Each student dictates what he or she wants to say to the instructor, who writes it down exactly the way the student phrases it. After each sentence or phrase is written, the teacher reads it aloud to the student, running a finger under each word as it is read to call attention to the written word. Students who read braille should follow the reading with the instructor's guidance. Each sentence is read more than once, since repetition helps a student remember what he or she has expressed. It is important that the teacher does not change the student's phrasing, since doing so makes the material more difficult for the student to comprehend. If it is no longer written the way the student expressed it, the student may not be motivated to read because the writing may no longer feel like his or her language.

A primary principle of the language experience approach is

authenticity of task. Materials that are used (such as stories, letters, and poems) must be relevant to the students' home cultures and individual interests. Specific topics, determined by the students' interests, can range from cooking, family, pets, or what happened the previous day to what occurred on a field trip. Students must have their own reasons for dictating or wanting someone to write down their ideas. They must also have real people in mind to whom they want to read what they have dictated. Through the process of revision, students gain experience with the text and can easily remember the points they learned.

The language experience approach is ideal for use with students who are visually impaired because few modifications are needed and it can be used with an individual or a small group. Teachers write the stories dictated by students in either print or braille and then assist students when reading the stories. One benefit of this approach is that it combines experiential learning and oral and written language, areas that are of extreme importance for students with visual impairments.

Reading and Writing Workshops

Reading and writing workshops have been used in regular education classes for a number of years and have become popular for second language instruction (Samway, 1993). These workshops are considered a communicative approach because students write what is important to them, listen to one another, and make meaningful comments, rather than participate in make-believe dialogue centered on a grammar lesson (Au, 1993; Hudelson, 1989; Peitzman, 1992; Peyton, Jones, Vincent, & Greenblatt, 1994).

Although there is no set procedure for conducting reading and writing workshops, features common to all workshops include giving students opportunities to make their own choices and organizing lessons in a flexible manner to meet the unique needs of individual students. Gee (1996) reported that lessons usually consist of whole-group activities, small-group activities, and individual activities. Hagerty (1992) described the sequence of her reading workshops as follows:

1. a 5- to 10-minute minilesson
2. a 30- to 40-minute conferring activity in which students have the opportunity to work with the teacher and with each other on an activity directly related to reading
3. a 15- to 20-minute share session in which students share what they learned in a minilesson or a reading activity

Whole-group activities, such as shared reading or writing, are used to begin and end workshops. Students may not be able to read independently, but they can participate with the group. Short minilessons grow from the shared reading or writing activity or can focus on specific issues on which the teacher has determined that the students need to work and that have immediate value for the students (Strickland, 1992). Minilessons can be procedural, literary, or strategy/skills oriented (Hagerty, 1992).

A workshop starts with a brief planning period in which the teacher and students clarify how they will use their time, so that everyone knows what will happen and what is expected. As the students begin to see themselves as readers and writers, they gradually take over more of the planning (Reutzel & Cooter, 1991).

Individual activities are the core of workshops (Au, 1993). Although reading and writing are considered social activities, students need the opportunity to choose their own materials depending on their own interests and then explore and create meaning through writing (Peitzman, 1992). The teacher holds conferences with individual students to assess their development and determine their needs. Together, these whole-group, small-group, and individual activities can form the basis of a new literacy program or can enhance an existing one.

Teachers who use workshops with students who are visually impaired need to supply linguistic support and varied materials to enrich the context of reading and writing. Since language is made comprehensible by pictures, gestures, familiar formats and routines, and the use of the students' native languages when possible, teachers must be certain that students with visual impairments have access to clear information that will facilitate their comprehension and participation.

THE ADULT ESL LEARNER WITH VISUAL IMPAIRMENTS

Many of the teaching methods described in the preceding section are applicable to adult ESL students. However, the individual characteristics of adult learners, such as life experiences, motivation, immediate goals, and self-concept, make the teaching situation different from that of ESL students in elementary or high school (Graham & Walsh, 1996). For adults with visual impairments, the onset of the visual impairment and the reaction of the individual and the family to the situation needs to be considered. For example, an adult who has just experienced vision loss and does not speak English may benefit from rehabilitation services in his or her native language before the topic of learning English is introduced. Providing the skills that will facilitate adjustment is more important at first than introducing a new language.

Adults, unlike young children, may not be motivated to learn English unless they see a clear connection between doing so and their personal or professional goals. Furthermore, the teaching approach that an instructor uses may either motivate or discourage an adult from continuing to learn the language. An adult who has an immediate need to learn basic vocabulary to "get by" as an unskilled worker will be discouraged if an instructor emphasizes grammar and literacy skills. Conversely, an adult who has academic aspirations will benefit from such a program and will not be content with an approach that focuses on workplace vocabulary and drills.

Adults with low vision who want to learn English often attend adult ESL programs in their communities, whereas those who are braille users and want or need to learn the English braille code typically receive these services from a rehabilitation center. Communication and collaboration between these two settings will help ensure that an adult learns both English and the English braille code. Braille instructors need to modify their approach to teaching so that instruction is relevant to an individual adult's needs and to make adjustments according to the adult's level of fluency in English. Although braille instructors may not consider themselves to be language teachers, attention to language is essential when teaching the English braille code to ESL students.

TEACHING ENGLISH BRAILLE TO STUDENTS AND CLIENTS

One question that professionals often confront when working with ESL students and clients who use braille as a medium for written language is how to deal with braille contractions, or Grade 2 braille. This is indeed a difficult question to answer with certainty, given the lack of research in this area. In an effort to provide some ideas on how to deal with this issue, the authors offer the following suggestions that are based on their experiences teaching ESL students with visual impairments, the experiences of other teachers, and the experiences of blind students and clients who have either learned English as a second language or have studied foreign languages.

A number of characteristics appear to be relevant to deciding whether to introduce English Grade 2 braille to a particular student or client, including his or her age, proficiency level in the target language, literacy skills in the native language, and familiarity with the braille system.

As is true of all people who learn braille, other factors, such as additional disabilities and motivation, also need to be taken into account when considering the introduction of Grade 2 braille to ESL students or clients.

Age

Young students, particularly those who have entered school for the first time, need to develop the cognitive and literacy skills that will allow them to become readers and writers. The development of proficiency in oral English is a critical component of English literacy, for without it, students who speak a language other than English will not be able to succeed in written language activities. Young students who use braille and are still in the beginning stages of learning English benefit from using Grade 1 braille at first because it allows them to have more practice with individual sounds and spelling patterns. During the beginning stages of learning, the development of oral fluency and the connections between oral and written language should take priority. Later, as students become more proficient in oral and written English, contractions can be introduced as they appear in the texts that the students are learning to read. It is important to note that since English reading texts have been developed for English-speaking students, teachers have to spend more time explaining the meaning of words to ESL students because the students may not be familiar with many common words found in beginning reading and language arts textbooks.

Young adults who want to advance in their chosen profession, those who enjoy reading, and those who want to enter a vocational training program will need to learn Grade 2 braille. Some older adults may only wish to learn Grade 1 braille that will lead to functional skills, while others may want to learn Grade 2 braille so that they can continue to enjoy the pleasures of independent reading and writing.

Proficiency Level in the Target Language

Individuals who are learning English may be at different levels of proficiency, ranging from those who are working on the initial stages of receptive language to those who can make themselves understood orally (see Milian, 1997, for an explanation of the stages of acquiring a second language). During the first two stages, a greater emphasis is placed on learning the sounds, basic commands, and functional vocabulary of the new language. Professionals may want to wait to introduce Grade 2 braille until after students are able to ask and answer questions and express themselves. At this point, it may be possible to explain the use of contractions and their rules because the students have enough understanding of the language to understand the explanations and to ask questions when they do not understand what is being said.

Literacy Skills in the Native Language

The teaching of braille cannot be separated from the teaching of literacy skills, since braille is a medium for written language. This is a critical concept when professionals encounter individuals who need instruction in English braille but who may not have achieved sufficient levels of literacy in their native language. The ESL student who is not literate in his or her native language is confronted with the dual tasks of learning English and learning to read in English. A professional who speaks a student's or client's native language should consider introducing the braille code in this language to develop literacy skills. Once the person is familiar with the braille code in the native language, the transition to English Grade 1 braille will be easier because the person has a general understanding of the braille system and has acquired the necessary tactile perception skills. Grade 2 braille can be introduced when a student or client has gained greater fluency in English and his or her literacy skills have improved. Professionals who work with individuals who have low literacy skills and need to learn braille may want to refer to the adult literacy literature for ideas on how to introduce reading to these students or clients. The National Center for ESL Literacy Education (NCLE) has a number of publications that could be very helpful for instructors who work with adult ESL learners.

Familiarity with the Braille System

ESL students or clients may have different levels of familiarity with the braille system. Those who are congenitally blind may have grown up using braille, whereas those who recently lost their vision or never had the opportunity to learn braille may completely unfamiliar with it. Students or clients who have been using braille may understand the concept of contracted braille in their own languages, whereas those who recently became blind or never learned braille need to begin by developing tactile skills that will allow them to learn the braille code. As expected, those who know the braille system in their native language have a greater advantage and will be able to learn English Grade 2 braille much faster than those who are being introduced to the braille code for the first time.

USING INTERPRETERS AND TRANSLATORS

Ideally, individuals who conduct assessments, provide instruction, and establish and maintain communication with family members of non-English-speaking people who are blind or have low vision would be bilingual professionals with preparation in education or rehabilitation for individuals with visual impairments. Given the shortage of bilingual professionals, however, schools and rehabilitation centers often depend on interpreters and translators to assist with these important tasks.

The use of interpreters and translators can be a problem if measures are not taken to ensure that students' or client's needs are understood, appropriate instruction is provided, and effective communication is established with family members. The following suggestions, by the Council for Exceptional Children (1997) and Fradd and Wilen (1990), can be used as guidelines for professionals who provide services to ESL students with visual impairments and have to use interpreters and translators:

1. Avoid pulling nonprofessional bilingual persons from their regularly assigned duties to fulfill the role of interpreter/translator when they have not received appropriate training.
2. Use qualified bilingual professional personnel before seeking the assistance of interpreters or translators.
3. Determine the competencies of interpreters or translators before using their services. These competencies should include
   - knowledge of oral and written English
   - knowledge of the target language and the culture of the people who speak the language
   - knowledge of the U.S. culture and the culture of the institution providing services to the student or client
   - knowledge of typical professional terms used in the setting
4. Explain the importance of confidentiality when interpreting meetings or translating confidential documents.
5. Explain the importance of neutrality and impartiality in interpreting or translating. Omissions, alterations, additions, making personal statements, or offering opinions should be avoided.
6. Supervise interpreters and translators to ensure that they are not working in isolation. Their role is to assist professionals in completing assessment and instruction, not to conduct these activities themselves.

Professionals who use interpreters and translators need to know how to make appropriate use of these individuals' skills. A highly qualified person can serve as both the interpreter for a large meeting and the translator of an assessment report, whereas a less-qualified person may be able only to interpret at an informal meeting. Understanding the abilities of individual interpreters and translators is essential for determining assignments for them and creating successful situations.

FROM THEORY TO PRACTICE: CASE STUDIES OF ESL STUDENTS

Two case studies of ESL students with visual impairments are presented here to illustrate some of the ideas and suggestions introduced in this chapter. The information related to these two cases, while unique, may provide some guidelines for other professionals who work with linguistically diverse students who are blind or visually impaired.

Gao, a Kindergarten Student
BACKGROUND

Gao, a 5-year-old monolingual Hmong-speaking boy who is totally blind, moved to the United States with his parents from a refugee camp in Thailand. He lives in a medium-sized city with several aunts, uncles, and cousins who have been in the United States for several years. Gao lost his vision from an illness when he was 1 year old. His twin brother died from the illness, which the family thinks was caused by the father burying the wrong coin with the placenta when the boys were born, which brought bad luck to the boys.

The home situation is marked by acceptance and protectiveness of Gao. The entire extended family takes responsibility for Gao and provides assistance to ensure his safety. Gao plays with other children, but his mother does not allow him to participate in all types of activities, fearing for his safety.

An ophthalmologist examined Gao's eyes shortly after he arrived in the United States and recommended exploratory surgery, which the family refused because they were afraid that Gao would die as his brother did. Even after much counseling by Hmong-speaking medical professionals, the family refused the surgery, insisting that Gao would make the decision for himself when he is older.

IDENTIFICATION

The refugee agency that helped the family immigrate assisted them with immediate health and educational needs. It contacted the teacher of visually impaired students in the local school district, who began the special education process by alerting Gao's neighborhood elementary school and beginning to coordinate services. Next, the educational team, consisting of the ESL teacher, special education teacher, teacher of students with visual impairments, principal, kindergarten teacher, occupational therapist, speech therapist, and a special education administrator, was assembled. The team met to discuss what they thought were the necessary components of an appropriate educational program for Gao. The assignment from the school district of a native-language educational assistant was vital because there were no Hmong-speaking professionals in the school district.

The teacher of students with visual impairments sought resources in the following areas: the process of learning English, methods of teaching ESL, the Hmong culture, assessment procedures and adaptations, and strategies for merging English language instruction with all the typical components of an educational program for a student who is blind. Other types of resources made use of included university courses, consultation with university personnel, workshops, conferences, and literature on second-language learners with visual impairments. These resources gave the team ideas on how best to implement an educational program for a young ESL student who was blind.

COLLABORATION

When Gao arrived at the school, the team members sought advice from the teacher of students with visual impairments about how to work with him. The vision teacher used common sense, but knew that she was basing her actions on her experience, which did not include work with ESL students. The ESL teacher was frustrated because she would have to adapt her lessons for just one student and she did not have the time, resources, or knowledge to do so. She knew that Gao needed to receive special education services, but was reluctant to ask the special education program for advice.

The native-language educational assistant spent the day with Gao in kindergarten, helping him to understand what was happening in the class. The assistant also worked with the teacher of students with visual impairments, who spent time with Gao each day in his classroom, and translated what Gao was saying as closely as possible.

ASSESSMENT

Gao was assessed by each member of the educational team using alternative assessment strategies, including language samples, observation, interviews with the parents, and interviews with Gao. The essential attributes of Gao that were considered in creating his individualized educational program were his visual functioning; stage of learning English; strengths and weaknesses in listening, speaking, reading, and writing; age, personality, and interests; communication needs; preferred learning style (tactile or auditory); length of time in this country; and concepts already developed in his native language. The teacher of students with visual impairments assisted and gave advice to the other team members in adapting typical testing procedures and interpreting the information that was gathered.

The assessment, which was conducted after team members were sure that Gao was comfortable in his classroom and school, took a number of weeks. During the assessment, the team discovered that Gao had strong language skills and well-developed concepts in his native language, cognitive ability, no difficulty communicating in his native language, and strong fine and gross motor skills. His needs were in the areas of O&M, English braille literacy, nutrition, dental, and eye care.

PROGRAMMING

After all the assessment data were gathered, the team developed an educational program for Gao. The regular kindergarten curriculum was followed, with supplemental ESL and educational services from the teacher of students with visual impairments. The ESL teacher followed her regular curriculum, adapting lessons as suggested by the vision teacher. Collaboration between the ESL teacher and the vision teacher was key to the success of Gao's educational program.

The student was fully included in his regular education classroom, so the teacher of students with visual impairments integrated braille and O&M instruction into this curriculum. Basic concepts learned in ESL were enforced in lessons using TPR. Gao quickly learned the basic concepts and social language needed to function in the classroom.

After six months, Gao began to show interest in labeling objects in English braille. It should be noted that there is no braille code in his native language, Hmong, so literacy instruction began by teaching Gao basic concepts in English, exposing him to English braille in his environment, providing activities to develop discrimination skills, and teaching him to operate the braillewriter. If a braille code had been available in Hmong, it would have been the vehicle for instruction.

A major literacy breakthrough occurred when Gao realized that the braille dots stand for the names of objects. From then on, he worked hard to label as many objects around the classroom as possible. In time, Gao learned to associate the English letters with the sounds they made in words and could identify them tactilely. Initially, Grade 1 braille was used exclusively. When Gao learned the sounds of the English letters and blends, Grade 2 braille was introduced.

Julio, a Fourth-Grade Braille Reader

Julio is an adventitiously blind fourth-grade student who attended school in Mexico before he came to the United States. He had enrolled in the school a week before an informal assessment was conducted. The informal assessment was requested by the principal so the teachers would have some idea of how to work with Julio before the formal evaluation was completed by school district personnel. Since Julio had attended school in the United States only for one week, the assessment was conducted in Spanish. The teacher of students with visual impairments and the first author as a volunteer consultant, worked with Julio and met with his parents and teachers to gather information.

Information about Julio was gathered in the following areas:

1. educational history, obtained from his mother and father;
2. written language skills (spelling, punctuation, and spacing between words), based on a story that he summarized in Spanish braille after he heard an oral version;
3. reading skills (reading comprehension, rate, and grade level), based on Julio's reading of Spanish reading textbooks;
4. dictation skills, based on a passage from a third-grade science textbook in Spanish;
5. creative writing ability, based on the interview with the mother and father and a story Julio wrote on a theme of his choice; and
6. math skills, based on the interview with the mother and father and Julio's performance on computation worksheets with mixed operations.

EDUCATIONAL HISTORY

Julio was able to use his vision until he was in the first grade in a Montessori school in Mexico. When he lost his vision, he began receiving braille instruction from an itinerant teacher of students with visual impairments. Although Julio was able to complete his writing assignments in braille and his reading books were provided in braille, other content-area materials were not always available. Consequently, he used listening to learn content-area information. Julio enjoys listening to stories and participates by asking for clarification when he does not understand or by providing examples. It is evident that he has developed good listening comprehension skills.

His parents described him as highly independent and self-sufficient around the house and other familiar settings. Julio enjoys making friends and has never allowed his visual impairment to interfere with his social or physical activities. He is an active child who enjoys sports and has been able to participate in school and community-sponsored activities with some minor modifications.

Julio's parents said that in the small town in Mexico where they lived, most people knew each other and accepted Julio's disability, as did the school personnel. Since Julio was well known in the community, he was able to travel around the neighborhood without fear.

One goal that the parents mentioned is for Julio to be able to develop a social network and the same degree of independence at the new school and community as he did in Mexico. Academically, they would like Julio to be exposed to more written material in content areas, particularly math and science, so he can learn how to obtain new information from a written format and become less dependent on listening.

WRITING

The summary that Julio wrote in class of a story that was read to him was used to assess some aspects of his writing. The story was originally presented in English; then one of the bilingual students in the class translated the story for Julio, and Julio summarized the story in Spanish using braille. The assessment revealed that most of the errors he made were in spelling, punctuation, and the lack of spaces between words.

Spelling: Julio wrote *bruga* instead of *bruja, muiy* instead of *muy, bieja* instead of *vieja, bibia* instead of *vivia, ai* instead of *hay, boz* instead of *voz, lampara* instead of *lámpara, atras* instead of *atrás, pajaro* instead of *pájaro, bayas* instead of *vayas, entonses* instead of *entonces, i* instead of *y, quien* instead of *quién, mama* instead of *mamá, ba* instead of *va, boi* instead of *voy,* and *dises* instead of *dices.* As can be seen, his spelling difficulties consisted of the misuse of *g/j, i/y, v/b,* and *c/s;* the omission of h; and the failure to include accent marks in accented words—all of which are common spelling mistakes in Spanish. Julio also wrote the word *toco* as *tcco,* but this was more likely to be a braille mistake than a spelling mistake.

Punctuation: Julio used the capital sign at the beginning of the title, but rarely used it when writing proper nouns, including the name of the main character; and never used periods. He appropriately used a question mark at the beginning of a question, but then placed the closing question mark at the end of the answer, rather than at the end of the question. He also did not use quotation marks, or the *guión* (hyphen), also used in Spanish to indicate when someone in the story was speaking.

Spaces: Julio ran the following words together: *meboi; yosoy; itu; meba; mimama;* and *aiy.* When asked to read the story back, he was able to identify some of the mistakes he had made.

READING

When Julio was asked if he wanted to read from a number of Spanish stories written in braille, he eagerly answered that he did. He read a few pages from each story at different grade levels (grades 1 to 4). He then mentioned that he was familiar with some of the stories. His reading rate was slow, but his reading was accurate. His instructional reading level appeared to be at the third grade. When reading, Julio preferred to read with his right hand and often used his left hand only to locate braille lines.

DICTATION

When a selected passage from a third-grade science book was used for the dictation, Julio's errors were consistent with those in his previous writing—primarily spelling and punctuation mistakes and writing some words together. When he heard the word *algodón* (cotton), he asked if it had an accent. I did not answer, but when the assessor pronounced the word clearly enough so he would notice the emphasis on the accented vowel, he wrote the word correctly. When he used the braillewriter, Julio did not always use correct finger positioning; for example, he did not use his thumb to hit the space bar.

Spelling: Julio wrote *capsula*, not *cápsula*; *jeneralmente*, not *generalmente*; *cultiba*, not *cultiva*; *rojiso*, not *rojizo*; *comprenderas*, not *comprenderás*; and *espesies*, not *especies*. Again, his spelling errors were the failure to use accent marks with accented words and the misuse of *j/g*, *v/b*, *s/z*, and *s/c*.

Punctuation and Spaces: Again, Julio's punctuation errors were consistent with those he made in the writing component of the assessment. Julio did not use periods at the end of all sentences and treated each sentence as a new paragraph, rather than as part of the same paragraph, even though the reader said *"punto y seguido,"* which in Spanish indicates a period between sentences, not at the end of the paragraph. Julio also did not place a space between *a* and *las* and thus wrote the words as one word (*alas*).

CREATIVE WRITING

The assessors talked with Julio about writing a story and suggested some possible topics (such as his family, what he likes to do, his school, and his friends). Julio thought about it and then asked if he could write *"un cuento"* (a story) he knew. After he completed the story, the following spelling errors were observed: *bibia* for *vivia*, *pero* and *perrro* for *perro*, *entonses* for *entonces*, *carnisero* for *carnicero*, *codisioso* for *codicioso*, *corio* for *corrio*, *pedaso* for *pedazo*, *sirbio* for *sirvio*, and *lexcion* for *lección*.

Again, Julio was able either to recognize many of the errors as soon as he wrote them or to identify them when he reread what he had written.

BRAILLE CONTRACTIONS

When Julio was asked if he knew contractions (*estenografía*), he said he had just started learning the single letter contractions in

Spanish. He knew the following single letter contractions: b-*bien*, c-*con*, d-*de*, e-*el*, f-*fue*, g-*gran*, h-*haber*, j-*jamáz*, l-*le*, m-*me*, n-*no*, p-*por*, q-*que*, s-*se*, t-*te*, and v-*vez*.

MATH

Julio knew basic concepts of addition, subtraction, and multiplication, but had not been introduced to division. He identified numbers and was able to read addition, subtraction, and multiplication operations. The main concern was that he did not know how to solve written problems because instruction in math has been oral.

SUMMARY OF ASSESSMENT RESULTS

1. Julio needs to be more consistent in his use of punctuation.
2. His spelling errors are typical of those made by children his age. They consist of the failure to use accents and the use of b and *v; c, s,* or *z; g* or *j; i* or *y; h;* and *r* or *rr*.
3. Julio frequently writes words together, which could indicate a braille-writing difficulty. Further observation is required to determine the source of this problem.
4. Julio's reading rate is slow, and he appears to read at about the third-grade level.
5. When writing, Julio does not always use correct finger positioning, which could contribute to his tendency to write words together.
6. Julio has not been exposed to creative writing activities. He is able to summarize and retell stories in writing, but has limited experience composing his own stories.
7. Julio understands the concept of braille contractions and knows many of the single-letter contractions in Spanish.
8. Julio has limited experience with written mathematics.

THE TEAM'S RECOMMENDATIONS
FOR JULIO'S EDUCATIONAL PROGRAM

1. Julio will receive ESL instruction. The ESL instructor will give written work to the teacher of students with visual impairments for transcription.

2. Julio will continue to receive reading support in Spanish from the ESL teacher, who is bilingual in English and Spanish, until he achieves an intermediate level of English proficiency.
3. Julio will be encouraged to work with bilingual classmates, so they can assist with translations.
4. Julio will be encouraged to complete his work in either Spanish or English until he reaches an intermediate ESL level.
5. The teacher of students with visual impairments will provide direct instruction in math using the content covered in the classroom. She will also support the content covered by the ESL and classroom teachers.
6. Mobility instructor will concentrate on the route between the school and Julio's home.
7. All teachers will concentrate on helping Julio to make new friends at school.
8. English braille contractions will be introduced when Julio reaches the intermediate ESL level.
9. The teacher of students with visual impairments will work with Julio to improve his reading rate, use correct finger positioning on the braillewriter, and to use both hands when reading.

The cases of Gao and Julio offer different scenarios for educating ESL students with visual impairments. In Gao's case, using braille in the native language was not an option, but in Julio's case it became a vehicle for assessment as well as a means to transition into an English-only program. All situations are different, depending on each student's or client's characteristics, and on the resources and willingness of teachers and administrators to modify programs for ESL students. However, whatever basic modifications are provided to any ESL school-age student must meet state and federal requirements.

SUMMARY

Professionals who work with students and clients with visual impairments are likely to encounter those who come from linguistically diverse communities and are learning English as a second language. It is important for professionals to remember that gaining access to outside resources and information is crucial to the implementation of a program. Although the primary responsibility is to offer services that meet the vision needs of students or clients, it may not always be possible to do so without taking the students' or clients' language needs into consideration. By making use of resources and ideas from professionals who understand how languages are learned and taught, professionals in the field of visual impairment will create a better teaching environment for their ESL students or clients.

REFERENCES

Asher, J. (1966). The learning strategy of the total physical response: A review. *Modern Language Journal, 50*(2), 79–84.

Au, K. (1993). *Literacy instruction in multicultural settings.* Orlando, FL: Harcourt Brace Jovanovich.

Canale, M., & Swain, M. (1980). Theoretical bases of communicative approaches to second language teaching and testing. *Applied Linguistics,1*, 1–47.

Celce-Murcia, M. (Ed.). (1991). *Teaching English as a second or foreign language.* Boston, MA: Heinle & Heinle.

Chamot, A., & Stewner-Manzanares, G. (1985). *ESL instructional approaches and underlying language theories.* Washington, DC: National Clearinghouse for Bilingual Education.

Conroy, P. (1999). Total physical response: An instructional strategy for second-language learners who are visually impaired. *Journal of Visual Impairment & Blindness, 93*, 315–318.

Crandall, J. & Peyton, J. K. (Eds.). (1993). *Approaches to adult ESL literacy instruction.* McHenry, IL: Delta Systems.

Council for Exceptional Children. (1997). *CEC policies—Basic commitments and responsibilities to exceptional children* [On-line]. Available: http://www.cec. sped.org/pp/policies/cecpol.htm

Cummins, J. (1989). *Empowering minority students.* Sacramento: California Association for Bilingual Education.

Dicker S. J. (1996). *Languages in America: A pluralist view.* Philadelphia: PA: Multilingual Matters.

Duncan, S. E., & De Avila, E. A. (1988). *Language Assessment Scales.* Monterey, CA: CTB/McGraw-Hill.

Echevarria, J., Vogt, M. E., & Short, D. J. (2000). *Making content comprehensible for English language learners: The SIOP model.* Needham Heights, MA: Allyn and Bacon.

Ferrell, K. A. (1998). *Project PRISM: A longitudinal study of developmental patterns of children who are visually impaired (Final report).* (Field initiated research H023C101, U.S. Department of Education, Office of Special Education and Rehabilitative Services). [Available on-line from the Division of Special Education, University of Northern Colorado.]

Fradd, S. H. , & Wilen, D. K. (1990). *Using interpreters and translators to meet the needs of handicapped language minority students and their families* [On-line]. Available: http://www.ncbe.gwu.edu/ncbepubs/pigs/pig4.htm

Fradd, S. H., Larrinaga McGee, P., & Wilen, D. K. (1994). *Instructional assessment: An integrative approach to evaluating student performance.* Reading, MA: Addison-Wesley.

Freeman, D. E., & Freeman, Y. S. (1994). *Between worlds: Access to second language acquisition.* Portsmouth, NH: Heinemann.

Garcia, O. (1997). New York's multilingualism: World languages and their role in a U.S. city. In O. Garcia & J. A. Fishman (Eds), *The multilingual apple: Languages in New York City* (pp. 3–50). New York: Mouton de Gruyter.

Gee, R. (1996). Reading/writing workshops for the ESL classroom. *TESOL Journal, 5* 3, 4–9.

Graham, C. R., & Walsh, M. M. (1996). *Adult education ESL teachers guide* [On-line]. Available: http://humanities.byu.edu/elc/Teacher/Teacher/TeacherGuideMain

Hagerty, P. (1992). *Readers' workshop: Real reading.* New York: Scholastic.

Hammerly, H. (1991). *Fluency and accuracy: Toward balance in language teaching and learning.* Clevedon, England: Multilingual Matters.

Herbert, C. H. (1983). *Basic Inventory of Natural Language: Technical report.* San Bernardino, CA: CHECpoint Systems.

Hudelson, S. (1989). *Write on: Children writing in ESL.* Englewood Cliffs, NJ: Prentice Hall.

Krashen, S., & Terrell, T. (1983). *The natural approach: Language acquisition in the classroom.* Hayward, CA: Alemany Press.

Lambert, W. E., & Tucker, G. R. (1972). *Bilingual education of children: The St. Lambert experiment.* Rowley, MA: Newbury House.

Larsen-Freeman, D. (1986). *Techniques and principles in language teaching.* Oxford, England: Oxford University Press.

Lewelling, V. W. (1997, May). *Official English and English plus: An update* [On-line]. Available: http://www.cal.org/ericcll/digest/lewell01.html

Los Angeles Unified School District. (1993). *Sheltered instruction teacher handbook: Strategies for teaching LEP students in the elementary grades* Author. (Publication No. EC-617). Los Angeles: The Author.

Macía R. F. (1998). *Summary report of the survey of the state's limited English proficient students and available educational programs and services, 1996–97.* Washington, DC: National Clearinghouse for Bilingual Education.

Milian, M. (1997). Teaching braille reading and writing to students who are speakers of English as a second language. In D. Wormsley and F. Mary D'Andrea (Eds.), *Instructional strategies for braille literacy* (pp. 189–230). New York: American Foundation for the Blind.

Milian, M. (2000). Multicultural issues. In A. Keonig and C. Holbrook (Eds.), *Foundations of education: History and theory of teaching children and youths with visual impairments* (pp. 197–217). New York: AFB.

Milian, M., & Ferrell, K. A. (1998). *Preparing special educators to meet the needs of students who are learning English as a second language and are visually impaired: A Monograph.* ERIC Document No: ED426545.

O'Malley, J. M., & Valdez Pierce, L. (1996). *Authentic assessment for English language learners: Practical approaches for teachers.* Reading, MA: Addison-Wesley.

Ovando, C. J., & Collier, V. P. (1998). *Bilingual and ESL classrooms: Teaching in multicultural contexts.* New York: McGraw-Hill.

Oxford-Carpenter, R. (1986). *A new taxonomy of second language strategies.* Washington, DC : ERIC Clearinghouse on Languages and Linguistics, Center for Applied Linguistics.

Peitzman, F. (1992). Coaching the developing second language writer. In P. A. Richard-Amato & M. A. Snow (Eds.), *The multicultural classroom.* (pp. 198–209). White Plains, NY: Longman.

Peyton, J., Jones, C., Vincent, A., & Greenblatt, L. (1994). Implementing writing workshop with ESOL students: Visions and realities. *TESOL Quarterly, 28,* 469–487.

Reutzel, D., & Cooter, R. (1991). Organizing for effective instruction: The reading workshop. *Reading Teacher, 44,* 548–554.

Richards, J., & Rodgers, T. (1986). *Approaches and methods in language teaching.* New York: Cambridge University Press.

Rigg, P. (1989). Language experience approach: Reading naturally. In P. Rigg & V. Allen (Eds.), *When they don't all speak English: Integrating the ESL student into the regular classroom.* (pp. 65–76). Urbana, IL: National Council of Teachers of English.

Samway, K. (1993). "This is hard, isn't it?" Children evaluating writing. *TESOL Quarterly, 27,* 233–258.

Savingnon, S. (1991). Communicative language teaching: State of the art. *TESOL Quarterly, 25,* 261–278.

Strickland, D. (1992). Organizing a literature-based reading program. In B. E. Cullinan (Ed.), *Invitation to read: More children's literature in the reading program* (pp. 111–121). Newark, DE: International Reading Association.

U.S. Bureau of the Census. (2000). Table 2: Language use and English ability, persons 5 to 17 years, by state: 1990 census [On-line]. Available: www.census.gov/population/socdemo/language/talbe2.txt

U.S. Bureau of the Census. (2000, July). Table 4: Languages spoken at home by persons 5 years and over, by state: 1990 census [On-line]. Available: www.census.gov/population/socdemo/language/talbe4.txt

Wiley, T. G. (1996). *Literacy and language diversity in the United States.* McHenry, IL: Center for Applied Linguistics and Delta Systems.

Woodcock, R. W., & Muñoz-Sandoval, A. F. (1993). *Woodcock-Muñoz Language Survey: Comprehensive manual.* Chicago: Riverside.

Professionals
and Diversity

Jane N. Erin
and Madeline Milian

All professionals work with people whose characteristics are different from their own. The ability to understand, respect, and appreciate differences is an important factor in communicating successfully with others, including students, clients, and other professionals, as is the ability to establish a cooperative relationship with them. Planning and effort may be necessary for a professional to achieve a trusting relationship with a student or client, especially if there are wide variations in their backgrounds, values, and beliefs.

This chapter discusses issues related to self-awareness, communication, time and scheduling, customs and rituals, and socioeconomic status that are important to professionals in visual impairment who work with people with various characteristics. It also addresses the importance of training and recruiting a greater number of professionals of different races, religions, sexual orientations, and other sociocultural backgrounds to increase the diverse composition of the professional community.

Although not all individual variations relate to cultural characteristics, the literature in this area yields insights about constructive responses to human variations. The term *cross-cultural competence* describes "the ability to think, feel, and act in ways that acknowledge, respect, and build upon ethnic, cultural, and linguistic diversity" (Lynch & Hanson, 1993, p. 50). According to Lynch and Hanson (1998), the characteristics of a culturally competent professional include respect for people from other cultures, understanding of different perspectives, willingness to learn, and flexibility.

These characteristics can be applied to responses to religious variations, sexual orientation, and disabilities. Lynch (1998) identified four effective ways of learning about cultures that are different from one's own:

- reading, arts, and technology
- interacting with people who can act as mediators
- participating in typical life routines
- learning the language

The first three approaches can also be used to learn about individual characteristics other than culture. They enable professionals to appreciate human variations and to adapt their approaches to the characteristics of the individuals with whom they work. In the following example, a professional used all four methods to be effective in her new job.

Laura Harris accepted a position as an itinerant teacher on the Navajo Nation in northern Arizona. Laura was raised in New Jersey, and she knew that she would find a different lifestyle on the reservation. Before she moved there, she bought several books that were recommended by her new supervisor and attended a lecture on Native American arts at a university near her home. After she began her new job, she met with the principal of the high school that her students attended to ask about people in the community who could talk with her about local traditions and customs. When she went to visit the families of her students for the first time, she always asked a colleague who was Navajo to join her. At first, she was surprised that many family members were present for her visits, including grandparents, aunts, uncles, and cousins. When she was not sure whether to speak or behave in a particular way, she waited for her colleague to respond first. Her colleague told her that most families would offer food when she visited and that they would be pleased if she accepted their hospitality.

Although Laura often felt isolated and alone during her first month on the reservation, places and people soon began to seem familiar. After a few months, she was invited to community events. She came to look forward to the Friday "swap meets," and the family of one of her students invited her to a community festival in which there was traditional dancing and food. Laura became more comfortable with the quiet voices of the Navajo women and the pauses between sentences and no longer felt compelled to fill in silences with conversation. She became interested in the Navajo language and enrolled in a course in Navajo at the local community college. After four months, she felt comfortable living in the community, even though she knew that there were certain experiences she could not share because she was not a member of the Navajo culture.

SELF-AWARENESS

Professionals who are members of a majority group may assume, unconsciously or overtly, that certain behaviors or customs are "normal" and others are not. For example, formal altruism is expected in some cultural groups but not in others. Furthermore, in some cultures in which formal altruism is expected, such planned activities as volunteering at agencies, participating in fund-raising events, and establishing nonprofit organizations are unusual, and altruism is connected mainly with religious institutions. The motivations of "giving" and "caretaking," which often draw people to service professions, are "enculturated" characteristics—that is, their significance differs depending on the culture. Individuals who have not been raised in communities where people are paid for jobs in human services may view professional service providers as people who are establishing their own superiority or control, rather than as people who are motivated by consideration for others.

Webson and Vaughan (1996) identified some of these types of assumptions in their discussion of the establishment of rehabilitation agencies in other countries. They described the lack of established roles for rehabilitation workers, the mistrust of governmental agencies, and the culturally dictated roles of the agencies as obstacles to effective service delivery. Even though these challenges arose when attempting to apply a Western rehabilitation model in other countries, there may be similar obstacles to providing services using a traditional model with clients whose cultural backgrounds do not include experiences with human services delivered through established agencies.

Values such as the importance of promptness and scheduling, working toward a long-term goal or "dream," becoming independent from one's family, or acquiring newer and bigger material possessions are often viewed as typical characteristics in this society, but these values may not be shared by members of all cultural or social groups in the United States. Nevertheless, many professionals consider these values to be universal, failing to understand that individuals and families may vary in the importance they place on them.

Cultural self-awareness develops by first understanding one's own cultural background (Lynch, 1998). Talking with family members, researching genealogies, and exploring family records can encourage one to understand one's family heritage and changes across generations. Identifying beliefs and values that are associated with one's cultural background can enhance one's awareness of the family characteristics that are rooted in the culture. In particular, professionals will benefit from examining their own family values that may relate to their professional activities. For example, people who work with young children need to consider their own families' beliefs about encouraging independence and punishing inappropriate behavior in children, and those who work with adults need to examine their families' beliefs about male and female roles and attitudes toward money.

New professionals may experience initial discomfort or negative feelings based on their lack of experience with another person's characteristics. People vary in the ways in which they respond to that discomfort, and some of those variations are based on the attitudes they perceived or were taught in their own families. The ways in which one's parents responded to differences can provide a key to understanding one's own response. Did the family ignore unfamiliar behavior or characteristics? Talk about others? Approach others and ask questions in an effort to understand the differences? Make stereotypical generalizations? Laugh at the unfamiliar or become defensive? Recalling their own family's reactions can provide individuals with important clues to how they establish a level of comfort when they encounter the unfamiliar. If learned reactions to unfamiliarity are negative or inappropriate, professionals may have to work harder to respond naturally and constructively.

Professionals also need to be aware of any stereotypes or misconceptions they learned in their own families or communities. Homophobia is of particular concern because it is rarely addressed directly in the workplace, even though many work environments attempt to combat other types of discrimination based on culture or gender. Concerns about homosexuality are often expressed confidentially because homosexuality is not a visible characteristic, and many gay and lesbian people prefer not to discuss it in the workplace. Speculation and comments by others can have undesirable results, as in the following incident.

The supervisor of a program in a residential school was approached by the parents of a young child with multiple disabilities, who were concerned because another worker had told them that their son's caregiver was homosexual. They requested that their son's caregiver be changed. The supervisor explained that this was not a valid reason for making a change in staff and that the staff member was an excellent child care worker who was competent in his assigned role. The parents were unhappy with the supervisor's response and removed their son from the program at the end of the year.

Whether schools and agencies provide formal or informal mechanisms for staff to increase self-awareness, acknowledging the importance of this process will increase the effectiveness of services and communication among employees. Current resources on cultural competence can assist agencies or individuals in providing structured approaches to self-awareness as a foundation for developing professional competence in understanding diversity. Winzer and Mazurek (1998) recommend that employees need to be encouraged to do the following:

- write private biographies that ask people to compare and contrast themselves with others and to identify areas in which they feel superior and inferior,
- analyze their own affiliations with colleagues, including the reasons behind these affiliations; and
- write self-report inventories that describe their own attitudes toward multicultural variations

Even if formal methods are not encouraged in the workplace, individuals can develop their own responsiveness to differences by associating with people whose characteristics vary from theirs and by seeking information on the characteristics of their students or clients that may help them develop more relevant instructional or rehabilitative programs.

COMMUNICATION

How a professional communicates with others and adjusts his or her typical communication style can be a major influence on whether she or he can build a trusting relationship with students and clients. Factors to be considered in professional communication include conversational style, nonverbal characteristics, writing, and use of terminology.

Conversational Style

Individual styles of communication are influenced by one's family, community, education, culture, and gender identity. Because people adopt a communication style from those who are familiar to them, they perceive their own style as "normal." It requires a conscious effort to recognize that discomfort and inaccurate communication with certain individuals may be the result of differences in styles of communication, not just in the words that are said.

One aspect of communication style is how much talking is considered appropriate. A person who talks excessively may be viewed with mistrust, especially if he or she is not a member of the affiliated group or culture. Native American and Asian cultures are considered "high-context" groups in that their members speak less because communication is highly dependent on subtle expressions and gestures, as well as silences. Anglo-European cultures, known as "low-context" groups, depend on words for specific, direct meaning and may not be as sensitive to subtle gesture and cues, thereby missing valuable information that is being communicated. In addition, their use of many words may be viewed as an excess by people from a high-context culture (Lynch, 1998).

Interruptions and pauses in conversation also tend to vary widely among cultures, as well as between men and women. For instance, Tannen (1990) found that for some people, interruptions represent intensive involvement in conversation, whereas for others, they represent a lack of consideration. She presented cultural examples of this difference: When Midwesterners talked with New Yorkers, they thought that the New Yorkers were rude because they rarely paused, but when the Midwesterners talked with Athabaskan Indians, they became the interrupters because the Athabaskans expected longer pauses.

Acceptable topics of conversation vary, so people from some cultural groups may consider it inappropriate to discuss personal or negative topics, especially with strangers. As the following story illustrates, rapport must often be built before personal topics can be introduced.

An early childhood teacher was assigned to provide services to a Native American family in a small village in northern Alaska who had a young child with disabilities. On the teacher's first visit, she was served some food, and the parents sat down with her and talked about topics other than the family. Their daughter and her needs were never discussed or referred to, nor was the daughter brought into the room where the teacher and parents were sitting. On the second visit, the daughter was brought briefly into the room and introduced to the teacher, but interaction was not encouraged and the child's disability was not mentioned. On the third visit, the teacher was told that the child was disabled and was asked why she thought the disability had occurred. It took three visits for the family to feel comfortable enough to talk with this stranger about the child's disability. If the teacher had asked questions too early, the family might not have allowed her to return.

Questions can also carry powerful messages about control and dominance. Because a question structures another person's response and requests specific information, it can be perceived as an attempt to take control. Paradoxically, the questioner often perceives himself or herself to be in the less powerful position; for example, women tend to ask more questions than men during conversations, especially if they are talking with men (Coates, 1986; Fishman, 1983). In some cultures, questions may be seen as intrusive or prying, especially when the professional is new to the family. For example, some Native American groups obtain needed information by making indirect statements ("I will be selling these sheep soon"), rather than by asking directly ("Would you like to buy some sheep?").

This same indirect style is often evident in question responses by people from Asian cultures. Some people of Asian background may answer a question with a nod of the head and a spoken "yes." Even though they do not agree with the speaker's intent, this response avoids the appearance of displeasing the speaker or of not understanding the question (Chan, 1998). Similarly, Middle Eastern families may avoid a direct "no" answer out of consideration for the speaker's feelings, but they may not act on the professional's suggestions because they believe a recommended practice will not work for their family (Sharifzadeh, 1998).

As was already mentioned, the conversational styles of men and women also vary. Tannen (1990, 1994) described the extensive research on this topic, which verified that despite the changing views of gender roles, there are still clear differences between the ways in which most men and women communicate, and identified the following common differences:

- ◆ Men tend to impart information or create a "contest" in conversation, whereas women tend to try to establish or maintain connections.
- ◆ Because of their social priorities, women tend to use certain forms, such as questions and suggestions, rather than directives, more often than do men.
- ◆ Men are typically more comfortable with settings in which there is only a single speaker, such as formal presentations, while women often prefer interactive settings.
- ◆ Men generally interrupt more than do women, but women interrupt more than do men in situations in which there are multiple speakers.
- ◆ Women frequently address private or personal topics, whereas men frequently provide general information and are less interested in discussing personal issues.

Although not all men's and woman's communication styles reflect these generalizations, Tannen's research suggests that these differences are observable in most cultures. Variations in the conversational styles of men and women probably influence relationships between professionals and their clients or students. Female professionals need to be aware that supportive or sympathetic responses may be misinterpreted as agreement or even weakness by people whose conversational styles differ and that many men are not as comfortable as most women with sharing personal information, which is often encouraged in support groups. Male professionals need to be aware that many women alleviate anxiety by talking about their feelings. Thus, allowing time for conversation before or after a difficult mobility lesson or an unpleasant medical appointment may be more helpful for women than for men, whose anxiety may actually increase if they are asked to describe their feelings.

Professionals who have considered the influence of gender and culture on their conversational styles can deal better with imbalances or difficulties in communication in their professional practices. It may be helpful for new professionals to videotape themselves in informal conversations with others who are willing so that they can observe their own conversational habits.

Nonverbal Communication

Awareness of nonverbal communication is particularly important when interacting with visually impaired students or clients who may not be able to see the gestures of others or to monitor their own gestures to determine whether they are appropriate for a particular conversation. Professionals who work with people who are congenitally blind need to be aware of the uses of nonverbal communication in an individual's culture before they teach gestures as a supplement to conversation. Nonverbal communication may vary across cultures in its intensity, frequency, and significance.

Touching others can be interpreted differently according to the cultural context and ages and genders of the conversational partners. Varying interpretations of touch can have particular implications for orientation and mobility instruction, in which initial contact and use of the sighted guide technique may be viewed negatively by people from some cultural groups. In some cultures, there is a stigma associated with a man guiding a man or a woman guiding a man, based on gender stereotypes. Professionals should consider this possibility if a student or client is reluctant to use physical contact in real situations, especially with family members and others from their own culture. Discussing the advantages of the standard sighted guide technique and comparing this technique with less efficient alternatives will give the client or student information that will enable him or her to choose how to travel with others. It is also important, however, for the person who resists using the sighted guide technique to understand that interpretations of touch vary and that not all people view this technique as inappropriate.

Eye contact also has different meanings across cultures and between genders. Professionals in the field of visual impairment often emphasize the importance of establishing and maintaining eye contact during conversations and encourage students or clients to practice the appearance of eye contact. However, they should tell students or clients about variations in eye contact that may be useful, especially if the students or clients are congenitally blind.

Research on the communicative behaviors of men talking with men and women talking with women has consistently indicated that men tend to anchor their gazes on other objects when conversing with one another, whereas women tend to focus on one another's faces, with an occasional glance away (Tannen, 1990; 1994). Body orientation varies between the sexes as well, with women facing one another directly and men sitting or standing at an angle from one another. This information is important for visually impaired people who are working to include natural nonverbal communication in their interactions with others.

Similarly, some cultures have different expectations for eye contact, depending on the age and status of the conversants.

Some Native American or Asian American groups, for example, do not make eye contact with those who are viewed as having knowledge or authority (Chan, 1998; Joe & Malach, 1998; Orlansky & Trap, 1987); for this reason, children may not be encouraged to look an adult in the eyes. A professional who is not from an Asian or Native American culture may view the reluctance to make eye contact as rudeness or suspicion when it is actually a sign of respect.

Families who are African American or Hispanic often rely heavily on body language and personal delivery when communicating with others (Willis, 1998; Zuniga, 1998). Therefore, a professional who relies on lengthy explanation or written communication to convey information may not be trusted because familiar interpersonal features are absent. Written communication is especially open to misinterpretation by people who are not accustomed to communicating through print.

Written Language

Written letters and memos are a reliable form of communication among professionals because they are permanent and can be referred to in the future when confirmation of information is needed. For this reason, it is easy to overlook that written communication is not a trustworthy form of communication for some people, particularly if English is not their first language. Harry (1992) noted that Spanish-speaking families with children in special education regarded letters from the school district as a way for the schools to establish power and take control. Not only were the letters written in a language that was not their primary language, but they often contained complex professional jargon that was incomprehensible even when the parents spoke English. Parents often signed documents without fully understanding what they meant, only to discover later that their children had been placed in special education or tested without their knowledge.

These experiences support the importance of direct face-to-face communication between professionals and the individuals or families with whom they are working. When a change is to be made in the education or rehabilitation program, a meeting is usually more effective than a written notice, particularly if the individual or family does not speak English well. The presence of an interpreter who is not a friend or relative of the family can ensure that accurate information is conveyed and can help to establish two-way communication. When a document must be signed, the professional should clarify the understanding of the material before he or she asks the person to sign it by saying, for instance, "Please tell me about what this paper means to you." It may not be sufficient to ask "Do you understand what the paper says?" since many people will say yes because they do not want to offend the professional or be thought of as ignorant. This is especially true for such cultural groups as Asian Americans, who place a high priority on respecting authority.

Use of Terminology

It is sometimes difficult to know how to talk about differences when a speaker must refer to an individual characteristic. Terms that were considered appropriate in one generation may become negative or even pejorative in the next; examples include the shift from *colored* to *black* or *African American,* or the increasing stigma attached to *idiot* and *imbecile,* which were once clinical descriptors of intellectual variations.

Accepted terminology may also vary across social and socioeconomic groups. The term *chick* to refer to a woman may be acceptable and even positive in some social groups, but it is considered demeaning among many educated or feminist women. Even when people share a characteristic, they may not agree on what term they prefer to use in talking about it, just as people with disabilities vary in whether they prefer to describe themselves as "disabled" or "handicapped," "legally blind," or having "low vision."

In talking with clients or students, professionals should choose terms that are neutral, standard, and clear. The use of slang can be misinterpreted or viewed as an effort to become too familiar, even if the client, student, or family uses it. Some people use negative terms in their own groups that would be offensive if used by others who do not share their experience. It is risky for a professional to participate in this kind of joking because members of a group or family may interpret it as a false attempt to establish membership in or intimacy with the group.

Conversely, terminology that is formal or represents professional jargon can also interfere with clear communication and be viewed as the professional's attempt to appear superior or better educated. Technical terms should be briefly described and related to the student's or client's experiences, especially with people who speak English as a second language.

The following questions can help professionals decide what terms are appropriate when referring to individual characteristics:

- Is it necessary to refer to a characteristic at all?
- Can the characteristic be described, rather than labeled? (for example, "Does your family come from Mexico?" instead of "Are you Hispanic?")
- What terms do the individual and family use when they describe the characteristic to non-family members?
- Can you comfortably ask about the preferred terminology? (for instance, "This application form asks about ethnic background. What do you want me to write there?")

Spoken and written communication must convey a clear message and should transmit respect for the experiences of the receiver. To do so, the professional may have to follow the student's or client's lead with respect to communication style and structure, which also may help to develop the trust necessary for learning to take place.

TIME AND SCHEDULING

People from different cultures often vary in how they view time. Asamoah (1996) described cultures as being past, present, or future oriented. Those that focus on the past emphasize the importance of history in learning. Many Asian American cultures are past oriented, honoring ancestors and celebrating death dates. Cultures that value the present, including Native American and African American groups, tend not to emphasize detailed planning for the future. Euro-Americans are often future oriented, sacrificing present experiences to ensure the future.

Family and cultural background can influence how an individual approaches scheduling. This can be a difficult issue for professionals, who must usually plan a specific time to provide services and must make their plans well in advance of the contact date. The following suggestions may be helpful in working with people who are not accustomed to the clock-driven schedule that is common in professional environments in the United States:

- Establish a consistent schedule and telephone the person before the appointment to remind him or her of the meeting.
- Provide clear information about time constraints, but do not be judgmental. For example, "I am available to you between 2:00 and 3:00 in the afternoon on Thursdays. It is important that we have this time to meet so that I can find out what kind of education your son will need. If we cannot meet this week, I can make another appointment to meet next Thursday at the same time."
- If a client or student fails to keep the appointment, determine whether the issue is a different interpretation of time or a reluctance to participate in services. If it is time, explain it as a mutual frustration: "I wish I could spend more time, but other people also need to talk with me. There is a woman across town who has just become blind, and I must

take the bus to see her, so I can only be here between 2:00 and 3:00 in the afternoon."

For some people, it may be necessary to adhere to unfamiliar time arrangements to benefit from scheduled events and services. To an individual from another country, the professional can provide a source of information about how time is perceived and measured in the United States, which will ultimately enable the person to adapt to mainstream behaviors.

CUSTOMS AND BELIEFS

Professionals occasionally meet individuals or families who have negative attitudes toward blindness, why it occurs, and what blind people can do. The following examples illustrate such beliefs:

- ◆ A well-known anthropologist, John Gwaltney, lived among the Chinantec villagers in Mexico while doing research for the National Institutes of Health. Gwaltney, who is blind, used a metal cane that was unfamiliar to the villagers. One woman believed that the cane was a magic stick that could be used to turn the villagers into pigs (Kent & Quinlan, 1996).
- ◆ A man who was blind was brought up to believe that he should not touch or be touched by anyone because touching could cause blindness to be passed on to others (Wagner-Lampl & Oliver, 1994).
- ◆ Many folktales and stories describe water as a "cure" for blindness. In Hungary, the dew on the night of the new moon was thought to restore sight, and in Mississippi, water from the first snowfall was recommended as a way of regaining vision (Wagner-Lampl & Oliver, 1994).
- ◆ Some religious communities think that blindness is retribution for sin, a belief that a blind person who is raised with this religious belief can also have (Wagner-Lampl & Oliver, 1994).

When a family or an individual has a strong belief that is inaccurate, direct opposition is rarely effective in changing it. A well-meaning professional who attempts to explain why the belief is inaccurate is likely to alienate himself or herself from the family or the individual. A more successful approach may be to talk with the family or individual about the belief in an effort to learn more about it. Often it will become apparent that the belief is a family story or that it is repeated because an older family member believes it to be true. Younger family members may be aware of the inaccuracies but may not acknowledge them out of respect for the older member.

If a negative perception is pervasive and seems to affect a family's willingness to encourage learning, it may be useful to involve a respected member of the community, such as a religious leader, an adult who is blind, or a member of a family who has positive beliefs about blindness. Professionals should keep in mind that stereotypical explanations of blindness are especially common right after a student or client is newly diagnosed and that these explanations may represent a sincere attempt to explain an unexpected and unwanted occurrence. If the diagnosis is recent, a clear explanation of the origin of the impairment may be helpful.

If a negative belief about blindness is repeated in front of a child who is blind or visually impaired, it may be helpful to talk with the parents about how this belief may affect a child's feelings or sense of self-worth. Without disagreeing with the belief, the professional can talk about how important it is for children to be encouraged to try to do things for themselves and that they may not do so if they come to believe that blindness is a punishment or is going to be "cured" before they grow up. In rare situations, the professional may need to tell the child that people believe different things about why blindness occurs, but that it has nothing to do with what kind of person the child is or decides to become.

Sometimes the strength of a family's religious convictions seems to create barriers to the child learning important skills.

Professionals have occasionally described families who have not accepted braille instruction because they believe their children's blindness will be "healed" or who have regularly taken children out of school to visit faith healers. It may be helpful to talk with these families about their children's short-term need for a skill or to explain that this skill is important so the children can teach others even if they regain their sight. It is usually unwise to disagree with a family's beliefs because family members may lose trust in the professional as an instructor. Families who hope for miraculous changes in their children's vision often gradually come to understand that their children are valuable individuals, blind or sighted. They may continue to connect their natural hope to their religious beliefs; however, if a trusting relationship with a professional is developed, many families will reinterpret the need for new learning in the context of their beliefs.

POVERTY

Unlike other characteristics described in this book, poverty is not permanent or cultural. Nevertheless, it is discussed here because it is an individual variation that can be affected by social attitudes. Poverty is experienced by individuals in all the groups who have been described here. In 1999, 11.8 percent of the U.S. population (or 32.2 million people) were living in poverty, which reflected the third consecutive year of decreases in the poverty rate and the first year in which the poverty rates of all racial and ethnic groups dropped. The poverty rates also dropped for people aged 25–44, elderly people, and children, although the poverty rate for children—16.9 percent—was higher than for any other age group (U.S. Bureau of the Census, 2000). The national definition of poverty varies according to the number of individuals in a family, with an income of $13,290 considered to be the poverty line for a family of three and an income of $17,029 considered to be the poverty line for a family of four in 1999 (U.S. Bureau of the Census, 2000).

The proportion of people with visual impairments whose incomes are below the poverty line is significantly higher than that of the general population. According to Halfmann and Schmeidler (1998), for example, more than a third of the people who were homeless in Los Angeles County were visually impaired, although this number may have included individuals whose visual impairment was correctable. For people with visual impairments, reduced income can restrict access to services and equipment, which are sometimes the very items that can allow them to develop the skills to move out of poverty.

The large number of people with visual impairments who are poor also reflects the general characteristics of people in poverty in the United States. The most notable change in the demographics of people living in poverty from 1950 to 1984 was the greater number of female-headed households with dependent children (Rodgers, 1986; Skog, 1987). According to Rodgers, people living in households headed by single women represented the largest percentage of poor people in every ethnic group, reflecting an increase of 168 percent in the number of poor households headed by single women between 1959 and 1984. However, according to the U.S. Bureau of the Census (2000), the poverty rate for female-headed families dropped markedly in 1999—to 27.5 percent, the lowest rate in 20 years. Nevertheless, it should be noted that the poverty rate for children under age 6 in female-headed families was 50.3 percent, compared to 9.0 percent for their age-mates in married-couple families.

A number of stereotypes persist about people who live in poverty that are often unconsciously perpetuated by professionals. The most common belief is that individuals in poverty have no motivation to work and could change their situation if they desired. Another stereotype is that specific racial or ethnic groups have higher rates of poverty. Although African American and Hispanic people are overrepresented among the poor, their numbers are decreasing in proportion, and people in poverty represent only small percentages of these groups (23.6 percent of African Americans and 22.8 percent of Hispanics in 1999; see U.S. Bureau of the Census, 2000). Recent studies have reported that people have more in common with others of a similar socioeconomic level than they do with people who have the same ethnic background but different socioeconomic levels. Nevertheless, many people continue to make assumptions about economic levels based on race or ethnicity.

Professionals should consider the specific circumstances of a student's or client's economic need and try to assist the student or client to take appropriate steps to ease the effects of poverty and eventually to become self-sufficient. In the case of a school-aged student, professionals should have access to social workers or others in the area who can provide information about financial assistance for families in need. In addition, information regarding Supplemental Security Income and Social Security Disability Income should be available, and individuals who qualify for benefits should be informed of how to obtain this assistance as well as opportunities for developing work skills and earning some income while receiving assistance.

SUPPORTING PROFESSIONAL DIVERSITY

People who are blind or visually impaired represent all cultures, religions, and gender orientations. The community of professionals who provide services, however, does not reflect the same diversity.

Diversity among Vision Professionals

Women constitute the majority of professionals who work with blind and visually impaired individuals, especially in education. According to a survey by Head (1987), teachers of visually impaired students who entered the profession from 1962 to 1983 were predominantly female (83 percent) and white (92 percent). Although orientation and mobility began as a predominantly male profession, by 1985 that professional group also included mainly young white women (Uslan, Hill, & Peck, 1989). It is not surprising that there are no data on the number of gay and lesbian professionals in the field of visual impairment. Because homosexuality is not a visible characteristic, awareness of a given professional's sexual preference depends essentially on whether the person chooses to inform colleagues about it.

People from ethnic minorities are significantly underrepresented in professional work with visually impaired individuals. The rate of visual impairments in the United States is the highest among African Americans (20 percent versus 12 percent of the total population) and Hispanic people have a similar rate of visual impairments as do white people (Schmeidler & Halfmann, 1998). It is important that the professional community reflect the diversity that provides role models and those who have similar cultural experiences to assist clients in dealing with their own cultural views of visual impairments. Nevertheless, the profession of work with people who are visually impared does not include racial and ethnic diversity that reflects the general population. According to Head (1987), the percentages of minority participants in teacher preparation programs in visual impairment between 1966 and 1983 ranged from no minority participants in 1972 to 9.9 in 1982. During these years, 91.6% of teachers were white, and 83% were female. In a survey of 361 teachers and orientation and mobility instructors of students with visual impairments from seven states, Milian and Ferrell (1998) reported a similar underrepresentation of professionals from minority groups. In this study, 1.4 percent of the respondents were African Americans, 0.9 percent were Asian Americans, 84.2 percent were European Americans, 5.5 percent were Hispanic Americans, 2.9 percent were Native Americans, 2.9 percent were of mixed racial backgrounds, and 2.3 percent listed themselves as "other."[1]

---

[1] As Milian and Ferrell (1998) explained, the respondents seem to have confused the terms Native American and European American, which may have resulted in an overrepresentation of those who classified themselves as Native Americans. Since the total proportion of Native American teachers in the United States is only 0.7 percent (American Association of Colleges for Teacher Education, 1994), it is unlikely that 2.9 percent of vision and mobility professionals are Native Americans.

This underrepresentation may magnify the role of individuals from minority groups who do enter the profession. A professional who is a member of a minority group can be a key contact for people from ethnic minorities who are receiving services, but may also find himself or herself cast in the role of a representative of his or her own ethnic group, regardless of how he or she feels about it, as shown in the following example:

Eve, a rehabilitation teacher, works for a private agency for the blind in a major city where 60 percent of the clients are African Americans. As an African American woman, she has become a resource for the two other rehabilitation teachers in the agency who are not African American. These teachers ask her for advice about their clients' family situations, and when an African American client seems resistant to learning new skills, Eve is often asked to talk with the client and his or her family. Although she likes to be seen as essential to the organization, she sometimes feels the pressure of her role. "Everyone figures I know all the answers and I understand the black people" she says. "Sometimes I don't have any better ideas on what to do than the others, but I feel like I have to act like I do. And when someone who is black comes in for classes the first time, I know they feel better when they see me."

Professionals who are the only member of a minority group at an agency may experience stress because of their role as a liaison with students or clientele and may need administrative support to maintain a balance in work responsibilities. Ultimately, the solution to this issue is the inclusion of a more diverse professional staff.

Perhaps the most important step to ensuring that diversity is valued in the profession of visual impairment is the active recruitment of professionals from diverse backgrounds. With increased diversity, the profession can provide models for all students and clients and can more effectively communicate the message that vision is just one of many characteristics that varies among individuals. People from all backgrounds can develop the skills to live comfortably with visual impairments, and they should have the opportunity to learn these skills in partnership with professionals who represent a breadth of experiences.

Promoting Diversity in Preparation Programs

The literature supports the usefulness of multicultural course work and experiences in the preservice professional curriculum. Pohan's (1996) study reported that there was a strong positive relationship between multicultural course work and cultural responsiveness in 492 teachers from four universities. It also found a strong relationship between cross-cultural experiences, such as time spent in another country or tutoring ethnically diverse students, and cultural sensitivity. These findings support the importance of preservice preparation that includes information about cultural variations and encourages contact with people from different cultural backgrounds to prepare future professionals to work with people from diverse backgrounds.

Preparation programs in the field of visual impairments may choose from a number of approaches to facilitate competencies that address diversity concerns. One approach may be to ask trainees to take courses that address general topics of diversity, which are typically taught in every university to meet the licensure requirements of individual states and tend to have such titles as Pluralism in Education, Diversity in Our Schools, or Multicultural Education. However, these courses typically do not directly address the intersection of culture, gender, race, class, religious beliefs, sexual orientation, and disability, leaving students to connect the pieces of the puzzle and figure out how the information taught applies to individuals with visual impairments. Another approach is to offer a course in the special education or rehabilitation department that deals with diversity in the special education or rehabilitation context, in addition to the general diversity course. These courses generally have such titles as Bilingual Special Education, Teaching Linguistically Diverse Learners with Disabilities, Diversity and Special Education, or Health Issues in Multicultural Communities. Although it is difficult to generalize, these courses tend to address the multiple dimensions found in individuals with disabilities more directly than general diversity courses do. A third approach is to require trainees to take both the general diversity course and a course dealing specifically with diversity among people with disabilities and then address diversity concerns in a number of other courses as appropriate. This approach infuses concerns about diversity throughout the curriculum in a natural sequence. It provides ample opportunities for trainees to become competent in issues related to diversity, provided, of course, that the issues are covered accurately and in depth.

Milian and Ferrell (1998) presented a list of suggested competencies related to cultural diversity and language in the population of individuals with visual impairments that will be useful for programs that are planning to infuse this content into their courses or to develop specific courses dealing with these areas. These competencies, which are listed in Sidebar 13.1, are divided into two sections: cultural diversity and language diversity.

These competencies are offered as a guide for developing activities that address a number of culture and language concerns for students and clients with visual impairments and their family members who come from multicultural communities. Individual programs may incorporate all or some of these competencies into their programs, depending on local and state needs. Professionals may want to collaborate with colleagues in other disciplines to infuse diversity competencies into their existing programs. In addition, they may also want to attend conferences and lectures offered at the national and state level to improve their knowledge of issues related to diversity.

There is no doubt that promoting diversity in preparation programs for individuals with visual impairments represents an additional challenge to programs that are typically already saturated

≋ Sidebar 13.1.
Competencies Related to Cultural Diversity and Language

The following are suggested competencies for programs to consider in incorporating content related to cultural diversity and language among people with visual impairments into other courses or to develop courses that focus specifically on these topics. Programs and instructors can select appropriate competencies for particular courses and use them as a basis for creating suitable activities.

Cultural Diversity

1. Explore personal attitudes toward culturally and linguistically diverse individuals.
2. Understand the concept of diversity in its broadest sense.
3. Understand differences in the view of various cultures regarding the acquisition of independent living skills.
4. Understand how social and recreational skills may differ in content and importance among various cultures.
5. Understand the need to be sensitive to cultural concerns.
6. Understand families' views of independence that are related to their cultural and child-rearing beliefs.
7. Identify cultural variables that may have an impact on the delivery of orientation and mobility services.
8. Understand how family structure, roles, and responsibilities may differ according to families' cultures.
9. Explore how discipline may be perceived by different cultural groups.
10. Explore cultural, religious, and spiritual beliefs as coping resources.
11. Understand issues of transition from school to work and how culturally diverse families may view the process.
12. Understand how families' beliefs, stigmas of visual disabilities, and treatment of children with visual impairments influence their views of school programs.

(continued on next page)

13. Understand the medical, educational, and economic needs of families of students with visual impairments who come from linguistically diverse communities.
14. Understand how blindness affects the family dynamics of various cultures.

Language Diversity
Instruction
1. Discuss issues related to the use of both native language and English versus English only with students with visual impairments and those with multiple disabilities.
2. Discuss ways to incorporate a student's native language into the educational program.
3. Identify program modifications necessary when providing orientation and mobility services to students with limited knowledge of English.
4. Identify how the roles of itinerant, resource room, and residential school teachers can change when providing services to students who are visually impaired and are learning English as a new language.
5. Identify the instructional needs of students with visual disabilities who are learning English.
6. Identify approaches to teaching languages and examine their use with students with visual disabilities who are learning English.
7. Examine reading methods and their use with students with visual impairments who are learning English.
8. Examine effective teaching strategies to improve the education of students with visual impairments who are learning English.

Assessment
1. Demonstrate familiarity with assessment instruments that are available in languages other than English.

(continued on next page)

2. Adapt commercially available assessments and develop strategies for assessing visually impared students who are learning English as a new language.
3. Review bilingual assessments and evaluate their use with students who have visual impairments.
4. Understand informal and authentic assessment strategies and their use with bilingual students who are visually impaired.

Communication

1. Transcribe written materials in Spanish using the Spanish braille code.
2. Understand the advantages and disadvantages of using interpreters when communicating with non-English-speaking clients and families.
3. Discuss strategies for communicating with non-English-speaking clients and families.
4. Develop an understanding of communication techniques to use with parents of students with visual impairments from various cultural backgrounds.
5. Demonstrate familiarity with teaming strategies for teaching and assessment.
6. Demonstrate familiarity with listening and communication techniques to facilitate culturally sensitive, nonjudgmental home visits.

Technology

1. Identify available software to facilitate the teaching of English.
2. Identify available software to support the teaching of languages other than English.
3. Identify keyboard functions needed to write in a language other than English.
4. Identify hardware with access to languages other than English.

(continued on next page)

> **Sidebar 13.1.** *(continued from previous page)*
>
> *Instructional Materials*
> 1. Demonstrate familiarity with obtaining materials for students who speak and read languages other than English.
> 2. Become familiar with language arts materials in languages other than English and their availability for students with visual impairments.
> 3. Review and evaluate English as a second language materials and those written in languages other than English and determine their use with second language students and clients with visual impairments.

with state and national requirements. Given the nature of the population of students and clients that trainees will work with, however, it would be a disservice to the professionals in training and to the students and clients they will work with not to do so.

CONCLUSION

Professionals who recognize the value of diversity can more easily become a force in creating positive change. For some people, this recognition is a natural element of their own background; for others, sensitivity toward others will require recognition of their own needs and a plan for expanding their perspectives. Human diversity adds texture to the experience of interacting with others. The professional who appreciates the richness of individual variations will be not only more effective in working with others, but constantly renewed by the opportunity to discover new facets of human experience.

REFERENCES

American Association of Colleges for Teacher Education. (1994). *Teacher education pipeline III: Schools, colleges, and Department of Education enrollments by race, ethnicity, and gender.* Washington, DC: Author.

Asamoah, Y. (1996). *Innovations in delivering culturally sensitive social work services: Challenges for practice and education.* New York: Haworth Press.

Chan, S. (1998). Families with Asian roots. In E. Lynch and M. Hanson (Eds.), *Developing cross-cultural competence* (pp. 251–344). Baltimore: Paul H. Brookes Publishing Company.

Coates, J. (1986). *Women, men, and language.* New York: Longman.

Fishman, P. (1983). Interaction: The work women do. In B. Thorne, C. Kramarae, & N. Henley (Eds.), *Language, gender, and society.* (pp. 89–101). Rowley, MA: Newbury House.

Halfmann, D., & Schmeidler, E. (1998). Visual impairment among homeless people. *Journal of Visual Impairment & Blindness, 92,* 90–91.

Harry, B. (1992). *Cultural diversity, families, and the special education system.* New York: Teachers College Press.

Head, D. (1987). Minority participation in teaching programs. *Journal of Visual Impairment & Blindness, 81,* 269–164.

Joe, J., & Malach, S. (1998). Families with Native American roots. In E. Lynch & M. Hanson (Eds.), *Developing cross-cultural competence* (pp. 127–158). Baltimore, MD: Paul H. Brookes.

Kent, D., & Quintan, K. (1996). *Extraordinary people with disabilities.* New York: Children's Press.

Lynch, E. (1998). Developing cross-cultural competence. In E. Lynch & M. Hanson (Eds.), *Developing cross-cultural competence* (pp.). Baltimore, MD: Paul H. Brookes.

Lynch, E. W., & Hanson, M. J. (1998). Steps in the right direction. In E. Lynch and M. Hanson (Eds.), *Developing cross-cultural competence* (pp. 491–512). Baltimore: Paul H. Brookes Publishing Company.

Lynch, E. W., & Hanson, M. J. (1993). Changing demographics: Implications for training in early intervention. *Infants and Young Children, 6,* 50–55.

Milian, M., & Ferrell, K. (1998). *Preparing special educators to meet the needs of students who are learning English as a second language and are visually impaired: A monograph.* ERIC Document No. ED426545.

Orlansky, M., & Trap, J. (1987). Working with Native American persons: Issues in facilitating communication and providing culturally relevant services. *Journal of Visual Impairment & Blindness, 81,* 151–155.

Pohan, C. (1996). Preservice teachers' beliefs about diversity: Uncovering factors leading to multicultural responsiveness. *Equity & Excellence in Education, 29,* 62–69.

Rodgers, H. (1986). *Poor women, poor families: The economic plight of America's female-headed households.* Armonk, NY: M. E. Sharpe.

Schmeidler, E., & Halfmann, D. (1998). Race and ethnicity of persons with visual impairments. *Journal of Visual Impairment & Blindness, 92,* 539–540.

Sharoifzedah, V. (1998). Families with Middle Eastern roots. In E. Lynch and M. Hanson (Eds.), *Developing cross-cultural competence* (pp. 441–478). Baltimore: Paul H. Brookes Publishing Company.

Skog, S. (1987). Reaganomics, women, and poverty. In F. Jimenez (Ed.), *Poverty and social justice: Critical perspectives*. Tempe, AZ: Bilingual Press, Inc.

Tannen, D. (1990). *You just don't understand: Women and men in conversation.* New York: Balantine Books.

Tannen, D. (1994). *Gender and discourse.* New York: Oxford University Press.

U.S. Bureau of the Census. (2000, September 26). Poverty rate lowest in 20 years, household income at record high, census bureau reports [On-line]. Available: http://www.census.gov/pub/Press-Release/www/2000/cb00-158.html

Uslan, M., Hill, E., & Peck, A. (1989). *The profession of orientation and mobility in the 1980s: The AFB competency study.* New York: American Foundation for the Blind.

Wagner-Lampl, A., & Oliver, G. (1994). Folklore of blindness. *Journal of Visual Impairment & Blindness, 88,* 267–276.

Webson, W., & Vaughan, C. (1996). Social correlates of successful rehabilitation programs in diverse cultural settings. *Journal of Visual Impairment & Blindness, 90,* 536–540.

Willis, W. (1998). Families with African American roots. In E. Lynch and M. Hanson (Eds.), *Developing cross-cultural competence* (pp. 165–202). Baltimore: Paul H. Brookes Publishing Company.

Winzer, M. A., & Mazurek, K. (1998). *Special education in multicultural contexts.* Upper Saddle River, NJ: Merrill.

Zuniga, M. (1998). Families with Latino roots. In E. Lynch and M. Hanson (Eds.), *Developing cross-cultural competence* (pp. 209–245). Baltimore: Paul H. Brookes Publishing Company.

Resources Related to
Disability and Diversity

A wealth of resources exist to assist practitioners who work with people from diverse backgrounds. Presented here is a representative selection of these resources for both professionals and consumers that relate to the topics discussed in this book. Among the listings are organizations and other sources of information and referral in the areas of visual impairment, disability, and diversity, as well as resources for services, such as the transcription of materials into braille, large print, or other alternate media. More extensive listings, including additional sources for the production of alternate media, can be found in the *AFB Directory of Services for Blind and Visually Impaired Persons in the United States and Canada*, published by the American Foundation for the Blind.

Readers are cautioned that postings on the Internet change rapidly. Although the information listed here was accurate at the time of publication, website addresses are subject to change, and any information derived from these sites ought to be verified.

BLINDNESS AND VISUAL IMPAIRMENT

NATIONAL BLINDNESS ORGANIZATIONS

American Council of the Blind
1155 15th Street, NW, Suite 720
Washington, DC 20005
Phone: (212) 467-5081 or (800) 424-8666
fax: (202) 467-5085
E-mail: ncrabb@access.digex.net
Website: http://www.acb.org

This organization promotes the effective participation of blind people in all aspects of society. It provides information and referral and assistance with legal issues, scholarships, advocacy, consultation, and program development and publishes the *Braille Forum*.

American Foundation for the Blind
11 Penn Plaza, Suite 300
New York, NY 10001
Phone: (212) 502-7600 or (800) 232-5463
TDD: (212) 502-7662
fax: (212) 502-7777
E-mail: afbinfo@afb.net
Website: http://www.afb.org

AFB is a national information, consultative, and advocacy resource for people who are visually impaired and their families, the public, professionals, schools, organizations, and corporations and operates a toll-free information hotline. AFB conducts research and mounts program initiatives to promote the inclusion of visually impaired persons, especially in the areas of literacy, technology, aging, and employment; advocates for services and legislation; and maintains the M. C. Migel Memorial Library and the Helen Keller Archives. It also produces videos and publishes books, pamphlets, *the Directory of Services for Blind and Visually*

Impaired Persons in the United States and Canada, the Journal of Visual Impairment & Blindness, and *AccessWorld: Technology and People with Visual Impairments.* AFB maintains the CareerConnect web site (www.afb.org/CareerConnect), a free resource for people who want to learn about the range and diversity of jobs performed by adults who are blind or visually impaired throughout the United States and Canada; a National Literacy Center in Atlanta; a National Center on Vision Loss in Dallas; AFB TECH, which focuses on assistive and mainstream technology, in Huntington, West Virginia; a National Employment Center in San Francisco; and a Public Policy Center in Washington, DC.

American Printing House for the Blind
1839 Frankfort Avenue
Louisville, KY 40206-0085
Phone: (502) 985-2405 or (800) 223-1839
fax: (502) 899-2274
E-mail: info@aph.org
Website: http://www.aph.org

APH's mission is to promote the independence of blind and visually impaired individuals by providing special materials and tools needed for education and life. Under the 1879 Act to Promote the Education of the Blind, APH is the official supplier of educational materials for visually impaired students below the college level in the United States and its territories. It also produces materials for visually impaired young children, adults, and senior citizens who are not in the K–12 population mandated by the act.

Association for Education and Rehabilitation of the Blind
    and Visually Impaired
4600 Duke Street, Suite 430
Alexandria, VA 22304
Phone: (703) 823-9690
fax: (703) 823-9695
E-mail: aernet@aerbvi.org
Website: http://aerbvi.org

AER is a professional organization that promotes all phases of education and work for people of all ages who are blind and visually impaired. In addition to disseminating information, AER sponsors an international conference every other year and publishes *RE:view* and the *AER Report.*

> Council for Exceptional Children
> Division on Visual Impairments
> 1110 North Glebe Road, Suite 300
> Arlington, VA 22201-5704
> Phone: (703) 620-3660 or (888) CEC-SPED
> TDD: (703) 264-9446
> fax: (703) 264-9494
> E-mail: service@cec.sped.org
> Website: http://cec.sped.org
> Division on Visual Impairment website:
>   http://www.u.arizona.edu/~rosenblu/penny/dvi.htm

CEC's mission is to support special education professionals and others who work on behalf of individuals with exceptionalities. It advocates for newly and historically underserved individuals with exceptionalities and for appropriate governmental policies, sets professional standards, provides continuing professional development, and helps professionals achieve the conditions and resources necessary for effective professional practice. CEC also has resources on cross-cultural issues for educators and publishes numerous related materials, journals, and newsletters.

> National Federation of the Blind
> 1800 Johnson Street
> Baltimore, MD 21230
> Phone: (410) 659-9314
> fax: (410) 685-5653
> Website: http://www.nfb.org

NFB strives to improve the social and economic conditions of blind persons. It provides public education about blindness,

Newsline and Jobline, information and referral services, scholarships, publications on blindness, adaptive equipment for blind people through its International Braille and Technology Center, advocacy services, and services to protect civil rights. NFB has affiliates in all 50 states plus Washington, DC, and Puerto Rico, and 700 local chapters. Its publications include the *Braille Monitor*, *Reflections*, and *Voice of the Diabetic*.

National Library Service for the Blind and Physically
　Handicapped
Library of Congress
1291 Taylor Street, NW
Washington, DC 20542
Phone: (202) 707-5100 or (800) 424-8567
fax: (202) 707-0712
Website: http://www.loc.gov/nls

NLS conducts a free national library program of braille and recorded materials for individuals who are blind or have physical disabilities. It selects and produces full-length books and magazines in braille and on recorded disks and cassettes and distributes the materials to regional and local libraries, where they are circulated to eligible borrowers.

Specific Visual Conditions

The Achromatopsia Network
P.O. Box 214
Berkeley, CA 94701-0214
Phone: (510) 540-4700
E-mail: futterman@achromat.org
Website: http://www.achromat.org

The Achromatopsia Network provides information and support for individuals with this rare inherited vision disorder and their families.

Foundation Fighting Blindness
Executive Plaza 1, Suite 800
11350 McCormick Road
Hunt Valley, MD 21031
Phone: (410) 785-1414 or (888) 394-3937
TDD: (800) 683-5551; local TDD: (410) 785-9687
fax: (410) 771-9470
Website: http://www.blindness.org

The foundation funds research on the causes of and treatments, preventive methods, and cures for retinitis pigmentosa, macular degeneration, Usher syndrome, and other retinal degenerative diseases at over 50 U.S. and foreign institutions. It provides public education, information and referral, and workshops and publishes *Fighting Blindness News*. It has offices in California, Florida, Georgia, New York, and North Carolina, and the Western Region and lists contact persons on its website.

Glaucoma Research Foundation
200 Pine Street, Suite 200
San Francisco, CA 94104
Phone: (415) 986-3162 or (800) 826-6693
E-mail: info@glaucoma.org
Website: http://glaucoma.org

GRF is a national organization dedicated to protecting sight. It publishes fact sheets and booklets on glaucoma, publishes a free newsletter, provides funding for research, and conducts a number of other services aimed at preventing glaucoma.

National Organization for Albinism and Hypopigmentation
P.O. Box 959
East Hampstead, NH 03826-0959
Phone: (800) 473-2310
fax and phone: (603) 887-2310
Website: http://www.albinism.org

NOAH is a volunteer educational organization for persons with albinism and their families. It sponsors workshops and conferences on albinism; publishes a newsletter, *NOAH News,* and information bulletins on living with albinism; has a network of local chapters; and promotes networks of support groups.

Online Blindness Resources

New York Institute for Special Education
999 Pelham Parkway
Bronx, NY 10469
Phone: (718) 519-7000, ext. 315
fax: (718) 231-9314
E-mail: ilumin@earthlink.net
Website: http://www.nyise.org/index.html

The New York Institute for Special Education (originally founded as the New York Institution for the Blind) provides educational programs for children who are blind or visually disabled, emotionally or learning disabled, and developmentally delayed. The Blindness Resource Center section of its website contains a wide range of information. Individuals with visual impairments, teachers, administrators, and the general public can find information on blindness, braille history and literacy, deaf-blindness, eye conditions, other disabilities, low vision resources, research, organizations, university programs, and vendors. Its website also includes resources on diversity for educators.

GENERAL DISABILITY RESOURCES

Berkeley Policy Associates
440 Grand Avenue, Suite 500
Oakland, CA 94610-5085
Phone: (510) 465-7884
fax: (510) 465-7885
TDD: (510) 465-4493
E-mail: info@bpacal.com
Website: http://www.bpacal.com/

Berkeley Policy Associates provides research and consulting services related to education and child/youth development, employment and training, welfare policy, disability policy research, the Americans with Disabilities Act, and small business and economic development. Its aim is to increase social and economic opportunities for those with disabilities. Its website has an excellent bibliography on women with disabilities.

Disability Organizations

Center on Human Policy
Syracuse University
805 South Crouse Avenue
Syracuse, NY 13344-2280
Phone: (315) 443-3851
fax: (315) 443-4338
TTY: (315) 443-4355
E-mail: thechp@sued.syr.edu
Website: http://soeweb.syr.edu/thechp

This center is involved in policy, research, and advocacy to ensure the rights of people with disabilities and has been involved in the study and promotion of inclusive communities for people with disabilities. Its website contains a report on women with disabilities.

Center for Research on Women with Disabilities
Department of Physical Medicine and Rehabilitation
Baylor College of Medicine
3440 Richmond Avenue, Suite B
Houston, TX 77046
Phone: (713) 970-0505 or (800) 44-CROWD
fax: (713) 961-3555
E-mail: crowd@bcm.tmc.edu
Website: http://www.bcm.tmc.edu/crowd

CROWD focuses on issues related to health, aging, civil rights, abuse, and independent living. Its purpose is to promote, develop, and disseminate information that will expand the life choices of women with disabilities. Its researchers develop and evaluate intervention models that specifically address problems affecting women with disabilities.

Consortium for Citizens with Disabilities
1730 K Street, NW, Suite 1212
Washington, DC 20006
Phone: (202) 785-3388
fax: (202) 467-4179
E-mail: info@c-c-d.org
Website: http://www.c-c-d.org

This consortium is a coalition of approximately 100 national disability organizations that work together to advocate for national public policy that will ensure the self-determination, independence, employment, integration, and inclusion of children and adults with disabilities in all aspects of society.

Disability Advocates of Minority Organization
P.O. Box 31024
Oakland, CA 94604
Phone: (415) 841-5953 or (510) 234-5278

This organization was established to represent and promote the welfare and equal opportunities of members of ethnic minorities with disabilities by encouraging and developing education, self-advocacy training, networking, and consulting.

> Disability Social History Project
> 255 3rd Street, Suite 202
> Oakland, CA 94607
> E-mail: sdias@disabilityhistory.org
>   pchad@disabilityhistory.org
> Website: http://www.disabilityhistory.org

The purpose of this project is to document the rich history of individuals with disabilities. Some topics that are included are biographies of disabled activists and philosophers; the history of the disability rights movement; the history of institutions, including schools for the deaf and blind and state institutions for people with developmental and psychiatric disabilities; and the history and culture of "freak shows" in the 19th century.

> National Clearinghouse on Women and Girls with Disabilities
> 114 East 32nd Street
> New York, NY 10016
> Phone: (212) 725-1803
> fax: (212) 725-0947
> E-mail: 75507.1306@compuserve.com

This clearinghouse aims to increase public awareness of specific issues faced by women and girls with disabilities. It conducts national advocacy efforts, publishes manuals and directories specifically for women and girls with disabilities, and provides referrals to local resources.

Online Disability Resources

Family Village
Waisman Center
University of Wisconsin-Madison
1500 Highland Avenue
Madison, WI 53705-2280
E-mail: familyvillage@waisman.wisc.edu
Website: http://www.familyvillage.wisc.edu

Family Village describes itself as a global community of disability-related resources. It integrates information, resources, and communication opportunities on the Internet for persons with cognitive and other disabilities and their families and providers of services and support. Some topics included on the website are information on specific diagnoses, communication connections, adaptive products and technology, adaptive recreational activities, education, worship, health issues, and disability-related media and literature.

National Women's Health Information Center
Women with Disabilities
Phone (800) 994-WOMAN
TDD: (888) 220-5446
E-mail: 4women@soza.com
Website: http://www.4women.gov/wwd/index.htm

NWHIC is a service of the Office on Women's Health, U.S. Department of Health and Human Services. Its website addresses numerous issues of particular interest to women with disabilities, such as abuse, parenting, and sexuality. The center also provides general resources about critical health issues for a variety of disabilities, including visual impairments.

DIVERSITY RESOURCES

Diversity Organizations

Early Childhood Research Institute: Culturally and
    Linguistically Appropriate Services
University of Illinois at Urbana-Champaign
Children's Research Center
51 Gerty Drive
Champaign, IL 61820-7649
Phone: (800) 583-4135 (V/TTY)
fax: (217) 333-3767
E-mail: clas@uiuc.edu
Website: http://ericps.ed.uiuc.edu/clas

This federally funded collaborative effort to improve services to young children with disabilities and their families acquires and evaluates materials and assesses practices developed for early intervention and preschool services with children and families from culturally and linguistically diverse backgrounds and for the professionals who work with them. Its aim is to create a resource bank and catalog of validated, culturally and linguistically appropriate materials and effective strategies that are sensitive and respectful to children and families from culturally and linguistically diverse backgrounds.

Research and Training Center on Rural Rehabilitation
    Services
Montana University Affiliated Rural Institute on Disabilities
University of Montana
32 Campus Drive, Suite 7056
Missoula, MT 59812-7056
Phone: (888) 268-2743 or (406) 243-2448
E-mail: fowler@selway.umt.edu
Website:
    http://ruralinstitute.umt.edu/rtcrural/Indian/AmI.htm

The center's American Indians with Disabilities project develops and evaluates culturally acceptable methods that tribal members with disabilities can use to initiate long-range planning and development discussions on their reservations, with an emphasis on disability issues and accommodating people with disabilities. It offers a number of research reports, monographs, fact sheets, and resources specific to this population and of particular interest to those who work in rural areas.

Online Diversity Resources

Internet and Web Resources on American Studies,
    Multiculturalism, and Diversity
University of Wisconsin-Milwaukee
Professor Gregory Jay
e-mail: gjay@uwm.edu
Website:
    http://www.uwm.edu/~gjay/InternetResources.htm

This website includes information on 16 areas related to diversity, including specific ethnic and racial groups, women, gay and lesbian concerns, disability, and Holocaust studies.

WWW Virtual Library—American Indians
Index of Native American Resources on the Internet
Website: http://hanksville.org/NAresources/

This virtual library includes a number of topics that will be of interest to professionals who work with Native American students and clients. Some of the topics covered are culture, language, history, education, organizations, books, and nations.

ENGLISH AS A SECOND LANGUAGE AND BILINGUAL RESOURCES

ESL Professional Organizations

Teachers of English to Speakers of Other Languages
700 South Washington Street, Suite 200
Alexandria, Virginia 22314
Phone: (703) 836-0774
fax: (703) 836-7864
E-mail: info@tesol.org
Website: http://www.tesol.org

TESOL is a professional organization for ESL teachers. Its website has links to state, local, and international affiliates; information on advocacy and membership; publications; and information on other services it provides.

National Association for Bilingual Education
1220 L Street, NW, Suite 605
Washington, DC 20005-1829
Phone: (202) 8898-1829
fax: (202) 789-2866
E-mail: NABE@nabe.org
http://www.nabe.org

This professional organization for bilingual educators has state chapters, holds state and national conferences, and issues publications.

Online ESL Resources for Professionals

Adult Education ESL Teachers Guide. By C. Ray Graham and Mark M. Walsh. Adult Education Center, Texas A&I University, Kingsville, TX. Available at http://humanities.byu.edu /elc/Teacher/ TeacherGuideMain

Online manual for those with little or no experience teaching ESL includes information on adult ESL learners, language teaching, ESL placement, and program organization. It also presents lessons for teaching beginning, intermediate, and preliterate learners.

Center for Applied Linguistics
4646 40th Street, NW
Washington, DC 20016-1859
Phone: (202) 362-0700
fax: (202) 362-3740
E-mail: info@cal.org
Website: http://www.cal.org

This website has links to publications and searchable directories on foreign and second language education, ESL, dialects, bilingual education, and education of refugees.

Center for Canadian Language Benchmarks
200 Elgin Street, Suite 803
Ottawa, Ontario, K2P 1L5 Canada
Phone: (613) 230-7729
fax: (613) 230-9305
E-mail: info@language.ca
Website: http://www.language.ca

This French and English site supports the development of national performance standards for adult ESL instruction. It has links to other related sites and publications containing ESL-related materials.

ESL Start-Up Kit
Website: http://cls/coe.utk.edu/lpm/esltoolkit/

This website includes theoretical and background knowledge on the acquisition of languages, English language instruction, and

teaching adult learners and a collection of teaching tips and suggestions for activities.

LINCS Adult ESL Special Collection
National Institute for Literacy
1775 I Street, NW, Suite 730
Washington, DC 20006-2401
Phone: 202/233-2025
fax: 202/233-2025
Website: http://www.literacynet.org/esl

LINCS—the Literacy Information and Communication System—a cooperative electronic network of the National Institute
for Literacy, encompasses dozens of literacy-related databases
and websites, more than 50 discussion lists, and instructional
materials on a variety of topics. The LINCS Adult ESL Special
collection includes materials and web resources about teaching
ESL to adults.

National Clearinghouse for Bilingual Education
George Washington University
Center for the Study of Language and Education
2011 I Street NW, Suite 200
Washington, DC 20006
Phone: (202) 467-4283 (within the DC area)
E-mail: askncbe@ncbe.gwu.edu
Website: http://www.ncbe.gwu.edu

This national clearinghouse, operated by George Washington
University's Graduate School of Education and Human Development, Institute for Education Policy Studies, is funded by the
U.S. Department of Education's Office of Bilingual Education
and Minority Languages Affairs to collect, analyze, and disseminate information related to the effective education of linguistically and culturally diverse learners. It provides information

through its website, produces a biweekly news bulletin, and manages a topical online discussion group. It has a searchable bibliographic database and a library of hundreds of full-text online documents, reports, and resources in Spanish for parents and educators.

National Clearinghouse for ESL Literacy Education
4646 40th Street, NW
Washington, DC 20016-1859
Phone: (202) 362-0700, ext. 200
fax: (202) 363-7204
E-mail: ncle@cal.org
Website: http://www.cal.org/ncle

This website features ERIC digests on the topic, a newsletter, and other publications; has links to other adult literacy and ESL sites; and presents answers to frequently asked questions about teaching ESL to adults.

Recursos en Español (Resources for Spanish Speakers)
U.S. Department of Education
Office of Intergovernmental and Interagency Affairs
400 Maryland Avenue, SW
Washington, DC 20202-0498
Phone: 1-800-USA-LEARN
Website:
    http://www.ed.gov/offices/OIIA/spanishresources

This website, sponsored by the U.S. Department of Education, has a number of documents in Spanish that are useful to teachers and administrators who work in school districts or programs with Spanish-speaking children.

GAY AND LESBIAN RESOURCES

Gay, Lesbian, and Bisexual Veterans of America
Membership Services
P.O. Box 29317
Chicago, IL 60629
E-mail: membership@glbva.org
Website: http://www.glbva.org

This chapter-based membership association of active, reserve, and veteran members of the U.S. armed forces is dedicated to full and equal rights and equitable treatment for all present and former servicemen and servicewomen. The website provides addresses for the state chapters.

GLSEN (Gay, Lesbian, and Straight Educational Network)
National Office
121 West 27th Street, Suite 804
New York, NY 10001
Phone: (212) 727-0135
fax: (212) 727-0254
E-mail: glsen@glsen.org
Website: http://www.glsen.org

GLSEN's mission is to ensure that each member of every school community is valued and respected, regardless of his or her sexual orientation. With chapters across the country, it provides technical support to schools; creates and distributes teacher training materials and curricular resources to elementary and secondary schools; and advocates at the federal, state, and local levels to protect lesbian, gay, and bisexual youths in schools.

ONE Institute: International Gay and Lesbian Archives
909 West Adams Boulevard
Los Angeles, CA 90007
Phone: (213) 741-0094 or (310) 854-0271
E-mail: oneigla@usc.edu
Website: http://www.usc.edu/isd/archives/onegla

ONE is an independent California educational institution that houses the world's largest research library on gay, lesbian, bisexual, and transgender heritage and concerns.

PFLAG: Parents and Friends of Lesbians and Gays
P.O. Box 82762
San Diego, CA 92138
Phone: (619) 579-7640
Website: http://www.pflag.com

PFLAG promotes the health and well-being of gay, lesbian, bisexual, and transgender persons and their families and friends through support, education, and advocacy.

RELIGIOUS RESOURCES

National Religious Organizations

Association of Jewish Special Educators
Special Education Center
Board of Jewish Education
426 West 58th Street
New York, NY 10019
Phone: (212) 245-8200, ext. 385

Christian Council for Persons with Disabilities
7120 West Dove Court
Milwaukee, WI 53223
Phone: (414) 357-6672

Christian Reformed Church
Division of Disability Concerns
2850 Kalamazoo Avenue, SE
Grand Rapids, MI 49560
Phone: (616) 246-0837

Evangelical Lutheran Church in America
Disability Ministries, Division for Church in Society
8765 West Higgins Road
Chicago, IL 60631-4187
Phone: (800) 638-3522, ext. 2692

National Catholic Office for Persons with Disabilities
P O. Box 29113
Washington, DC 20017
Phone: (202) 529-2933

National Church Conference of the Blind
P.O. Box 163
Denver, CO 80201
Phone: (303) 789-7441
The Electronic Church (echurch)
Forum for Blind Christians
E-mail: echurch-l@netcom.com

National Organization on Disability
Religion and Disability Program
910 16th Street, NW
Washington, DC 20006
Phone: (202) 293-5960

United Synagogue of Conservative Judaism
Committee on Accessibility
155 Fifth Avenue
New York, NY 10010-6802
Phone: (212) 533-7800, ext. 2614

PRODUCERS OF RELIGIOUS MATERIALS IN ALTERNATE MEDIA

(An asterisk indicates that materials are available in languages other than English.)

Abingdon Press
201 8th Avenue South
Nashville, TN 37203
Phone: (800) 251-3320

*Access USA
P.O. Box 160, 242 James Street
Clayton, NY 13624
Phone: (800) 263-2750

Bibles for the Blind and Visually Handicapped
3228 East Rosehill Avenue
Terre Haute, IN 47805
Phone: (812) 466-4899

Braille Bible Foundation
PO. Box 948307
Maitland, FL 32794-8307
Phone: (407) 834-3628 or (800) 766-9080

*Braille Circulating Library
2700 Stuart Avenue
Richmond, VA 23220
Phone: (804) 359-3743

Catholic Guild for the Blind
180 North Michigan Avenue, Suite 1700
Chicago, IL 60601-7463
Phone: (312) 236-8569

Christian Education for the Blind
P.O. Box 6399
Fort Worth, TX 76115
Phone: (817) 923-0603

Christian Services for the Blind International
P.O. Box 26
South Pasadena, CA 91031-0026
Phone: (818) 799-3935

Evangelical Lutheran Church in America
Braille and Tape Service
Augsburg Fortress Publishers
426 South Fifth Street, Box 1209
Minneapolis, MN 55440-1209
Phone: (612) 330-3300
(800) FORTRESS

Gospel Light Foundation for the Blind
485 Tewsbury Lane, NE
Palm Bay, FL 32907
Phone: (407) 724-9036

*Hosanna
2421 Aztec Road, NE
Albuquerque, NM 87107-4200
Phone: (800) 545-6552

*International Bible Society
1820 Jet Stream Drive
Colorado Springs, CO 80921-3696
Phone: (719) 488-9200

*Jewish Braille Institute of America
110 East 30th Street
New York, NY 10016
Phone: (212) 889-2525

*Lutheran Braille Workers
P.O. Box 5000
Yucaipa, CA 92399
Phone: (909) 795-8977

*Lutheran Large Print Workers
495 Ninth Avenue
San Francisco, CA 94118
Phone: (415) 751-6184

Lutheran Library for the Blind
Lutheran Church
1333 South Kirkwood Road
St. Louis, MO 63122-7295
Phone: (314) 965-9000 or (800) 433-3954

Moravian Church in America
1021 Center Street, P.O. Box
Bethlehem, PA 18016-1245
Phone: (610) 867-0593

Morehouse Publishing Group (Episcopal)
P.O. Box 132
Harrisburg, PA 17105
Phone: (800) 877-0012

Narrow Way Ministries
6948 Highway 212, North
Coveting, GA 30209
Phone: (404) 786-6649

National Braille Association
3 Townline Circle
Rochester, NY 14623
Phone (716) 427-8260

Thomas Nelson Publishing House
P.O. Box 141000
Nashville, TN 37214-1000
Phone: (800) 251-4000

Reorganized Church of Jesus Christ of Latter-Day Saints
Services to the Blind
P.O. Box 1059
1001 West Walnut
Independence, MO 64051
Phone: (816) 833-1000, ext. 1460

Sunday School Board of the Southern Baptist Convention
127 Ninth Avenue North
Nashville, TN 37234
Phone: (800) 458-2772

Taped Ministries of the Northwest
122 SW 150th Street
Burien, WA 98166-1956
Phone: (206) 243-7377

Xavier Society for the Blind
154 East 23rd Street
New York, NY 10010
Phone: (212) 473-7800

Index